Global Health for All

Global Health for All

Global Health for All

Knowledge, Politics, and Practices

EDITED BY
JEAN-PAUL GAUDILLIÈRE
ANDREW McDOWELL
CLAUDIA LANG
CLAIRE BEAUDEVIN

RUTGERS UNIVERSITY PRESS
NEW BRUNSWICK, CAMDEN, AND NEWARK,
NEW JERSEY, AND LONDON

Library of Congress Cataloging-in-Publication Data
Names: Gaudillière, Jean-Paul, 1957 editor. | McDowell, Andrew, editor. |
  Lang, Claudia, editor. | Beaudevin, Claire, editor.
Title: Global health for all: knowledge, politics, and practices / edited by Jean-Paul
  Gaudillière, Andrew McDowell, Claudia Lang, and Claire Beaudevin.
Description: New Brunswick, NJ: Rutgers University Press, 2022. |
  Includes bibliographical references and index.
Identifiers: LCCN 2021029927 | ISBN 9781978827400 (paperback) |
  ISBN 9781978827417 (hardcover) | ISBN 9781978827424 (epub) |
  ISBN 9781978827431 (mobi) | ISBN 9781978827448 (pdf)
Subjects: LCSH: World health—20th century. | World health—21st century. |
  Public health—International cooperation. | Globalization—Health aspects. |
  Health policy. | Ethnology.
Classification: LCC RA441 .H439 2022 | DDC 362.1—dc23
LC record available at https://lccn.loc.gov/2021029927

A British Cataloging-in-Publication record for this book is available from the British Library.

References to internet websites (URLs) were accurate at the time of writing. Neither the author
nor Rutgers University Press is responsible for URLs that may have expired or changed since
the manuscript was prepared.

♾ The paper used in this publication meets the requirements of the American National Standard for Information Sciences—Permanence of Paper for Printed Library Materials, ANSI
Z39.48-1992.

www.rutgersuniversitypress.org

Manufactured in the United States of America

Contents

Global Health for All

Prologue

A STORY WITH SIXTEEN TELLERS

Andrew McDowell, Claire Beaudevin,
Claudia Lang, and Jean-Paul Gaudillière

This volume has at least two beginnings. One occurred just south of Paris, in a conference room in what was once the morgue of a hospital but is now an academic building. There we discussed the outcome of our now five-year-long research program and debated about how to stitch together our disparate pieces of data. As medical anthropologists, historians, and sociologists, we had amassed hundreds, if not thousands, of hours of interview and participant-observation data and collated thousands of texts from archives on four continents. We each knew our own research project and its topical or disciplinary intervention, but in the morgue, we began wondering if telling these stories together might have something to contribute to the scholarship on global health. Resolved to write this larger story together, we struggled to collectively make sense of how to combine our disciplinary concerns, our individual interpretations, and our diverse research foci.

This discussion had not been our first meeting at the Parisian morgue. We often met there to build and refine a data collection and interpretation strategy that would help us understand health at a global scale. From the very beginning, we had organized our team into four groups. Each was in charge of examining actors, targets, tools, and practices associated with a specific domain of global health: tuberculosis (TB), global mental health, Asian medicines, and medical genetics. Together, we reflected on each domain and what it might teach us about the phenomena that, in those days, we called international and global health.

Our four-member TB team examined the intersection of social life, institutions, and the tuberculosis mycobacterium in order to analyze standardization and prioritization in global health. Historian Christoph Gradmann visited institutional archives in Europe and Tanzania to observe changing regimes of care. Sociologist Fanny Chabrol joined him in Tanzania to document stories about past and present-day practices at the national TB hospital. Anthropologist Andrew McDowell spent time talking with TB research scientists in India to learn about what it meant to be a TB expert there in the 1990s. Vegard Sture spent many hours in a Tanzanian clinical laboratory observing the performance of rapid molecular TB tests. Together, the TB team aimed to understand the globalization of a specific treatment program—namely, the directly observed treatment short-course (DOTS) strategy.

Our mental health team was comprised of four anthropologists focusing on depression and schizophrenia. Anne Lovell and Papa Diagne in Senegal focused their efforts on the local trajectory of psychiatry, the changing forms of expertise, and the emergence of global mental health as an international movement. Claudia Lang interviewed clinicians, health workers, and family members of people diagnosed with depression in Kerala, India. Ursula Read researched the ways that human rights language affects formal and ad hoc mental healthcare in Ghana. Together, they investigated the contemporary regime of global health and its hotly debated but growing interest in noncommunicable illness. Theirs was a vibrant conversation about global mental health's contested classification categories and the changes that transformed an initial interest by the World Health Organization (WHO) in international psychiatric epidemiology into mental illnesses' near universality.

Another team collaborated to study the globalization of traditional medicine. This group focused on Asian traditional herbal therapeutic preparations, their industrialization, and their market development. Anthropologist Laurent Pordié and historian Jean-Paul Gaudillière interviewed officials and examined archives at institutions and firms working to systematize and sell Ayurveda in India. Anthropologist Caroline Meier zu Biesen talked with Ayurvedic pharmacists and pharmaceutical producers about the circulations of Ayurveda between India and East Africa. Sociologist Simeng Wang contributed data from her work, which traced Chinese international aid and traditional medicine to and from Europe. Sociologist Jessica Pourraz also introduced material and analysis from her own comparative ethnographic study of pharmaceutical industries in Benin and Ghana. Together, the team traced the dynamic, shifting role and meaning of traditional medicines from the late 1970s, when states like China and India, the WHO, and firms and practitioners of Asian medicine took herbal preparations global.

Our fourth group focused on medical genetics and genomics. The team examined the processes that struggle to put genetics on the international public health and global health agenda. Sociologist Lucile Ruault explored the recent history of medical genetics on a global scale by visiting the WHO archives and interviewing retired WHO experts working to develop community genetics. Anthropologist Mandy Geise conducted participant-observation studies in a nascent institute for genomics and field genetic studies in Mexico, and anthropologist Claire Beaudevin shadowed and interviewed medical geneticists and nurses working in Oman's healthcare system. Political scientist Sameea Ahmed Hassim researched medical genetics and screening programs in the Cuban healthcare system. By focusing on community genetics, sequencing technologies, screening programs, and the epigenetics of noncommunicable disorders, the team explored a medical specialty that has been slow to enter global health.

Jean-Paul Gaudillière roved across and knit together each group. His interests in metrics, markets, TB, and traditional medicines took him to numerous sites in search of documents concerning the economization of health and primary health care's trajectory as a marker of the transition toward global health. His early findings inspired the creation of a fifth group, which attended to primary health care as both a strategy and system of practice. Historian Olivia Fiorilli worked with him to examine the archives and texts produced by the WHO, the World Bank, and several governments during the heyday of the primary health care movement, and Claudia Lang conducted participant-observation in a primary health clinic in South India.

Working concurrently but in these thematic groups, we were able to examine various parallels in configurations of health and disease for continuity and change over time. We were all challenged by the questions that juxtaposing memories and archives posed for our own disciplines. We worked through them together, each individual finding one's own way to treat these materials. In so doing, groups and disciplines kept bumping into each other and nourishing each other's thinking. Historians and anthropologists visited Tanzania and India together. We found ourselves exchanging notes on food options at the World Bank's Washington, D.C., cafeteria, and on several occasions we filled the WHO Geneva archive to capacity.

The book's second beginning was in September 2017, in a tiny village in the northern French Alps. In an attempt to synthesize what we had collected in the previous years and initially discussed in the morgue, our group converged on the Alps from Paris, Germany, the United Kingdom, and Norway. This retreat was meant to assess strategies for developing a composite voice that could combine our parts without needing to chase its product to the ends of the earth. Each contributor wrote a short reflection on a theme encountered in the field or archive. As we convened at a large table looking out over the alpine forest's changing colors, we discussed each theme and how it resonated with the others. After two days of debates and walks that refined, renamed, recentered, or even rejected particular themes, we agreed on the chapters of this volume and distributed the responsibilities of their writing among us. Each group of writers happened to be of radically different composition than the research teams, yet by the end of the three days in the Alps, we had plotted a course for the chapters you will soon read.

Over the next two years, we met again and again in small groups and as a collective to discuss each chapter. During this process, every chapter has been enriched by the collective's insights and interventions. As such, the story told here is as much about separate inquiries, which examined archives at sites as diverse as Dar-es-Salaam and Stockholm and engaged people from Kolkata to Muscat and Mexico City, as it is about the polyvocal, shifting strategy necessary to research and write about health at global scale. This broader strategy and story first came together there, in the Alps.

As a result of this integrated collaborative research and writing strategy, we follow specific trajectories of localization, circulation, generalization, and routinization in the histories in this volume. We examine the increasing discursive visibility of mental health over the last two decades; the ubiquity of the DOTS TB program in the 2000s; and the growing then fading presence of medical genetics at the WHO from 1980 to 2010. In so doing, we rely on archival documents created before 1970; on archives and personal interviews from the 1970s to the 1990s; and on a combination of comprehensive ethnography, personal interviews and archival materials for the most recent period. We chose to trace these changes, historically and ethnographically, in particular sites of intervention and policymaking across the globe. They included Tanzania, the birthplace of DOTS; Geneva, site of the WHO archives and innumerable expert meetings; Mexico, where a massive diabetes epidemic has triggered genomic research; Washington, DC, where major steps of the transition we trace took place at the World Bank; India, where mental health has gained importance, especially in Kerala, where community mental health focuses on depression; Oman, where comprehensive primary health care is integrating genetic medicine; and Kenya, where the market of Ayurvedic medicines is unfolding.

Despite lacunae, there are many things a polyvocal story has to say. Primarily, this book is not an edited academic volume; it is a collectively written book. This distinction is important: our sixteen-member group working together in Paris from 2014 to 2019 and our repeated writing sessions are the main ingredients that flavor this book. Together, the variety of our writing styles, the large scope of our fieldwork sites, the range of our research objects, and the spectrum of our theoretical inquiries shape and ground our claims about global health and its main features, foundations, weaknesses, and promises. Our goal has never been comprehensiveness. Instead, we have struggled to tell a story about health from many perspectives in hopes of creating what Michael Jackson (1989) has called radical empiricism. It is just that—an attempt. Our story of many perspectives remains fragmented even as it works to represent something of the world from our viewpoint. Though many voices are joined here, other voices and perspectives remain just over the mountain from our alpine table. We encourage readers to consider the ways that their own voices and perspectives may or may not be part of the story we tell.

Regardless of where it began, this book has arrived in your hands after a collective labor of intense conversation and an attempt to craft a story with sixteen tellers.

Introduction

HEALTH UNIVERSALISM AND
THE HEALTH OF OTHERS

Jean-Paul Gaudillière, Andrew McDowell,
Claire Beaudevin, and Claudia Lang

A compact building sits in a walled compound a few meters off a north-south artery that connects Mumbai's crowded western suburbs. This unassuming municipal tuberculosis (TB) clinic has been a buoy on the shifting seas of twentieth- and twenty-first-century health interventions. Though dusty, the clinic has been a locus of change and continuity in the entanglement of health, knowledge, and governance over the past one hundred years. A brief float with it on the currents of time introduces the central questions of this book.

In the early 1960s, just over a decade after India's independence, Mumbai's municipal government constructed this five-room building to be one of the city's six TB clinics. It was an example of the many infrastructural projects built and staffed as part of the decolonization process. Yet, since its inception, the clinic has been a site of care within global flows of medical ideas, materials, and people. Its construction as an outpost of care and governance within a rapidly expanding suburban space highlights health's centrality to postcolonial projects of internationalism, bilateral cooperation for development, and the new world order of global politics.

Starting at its founding and until the 1990s, the clinic served Mumbai's northwestern region and oversaw the treatment of some of the millions of Indians affected by TB. It housed a doctor, nurses, and technicians, as well as drugs, microscopes, and an x-ray machine. Physicians and nurses from across the city's hospitals and dispensaries referred patients they worried might be afflicted by TB to this particular clinic. Once a patient arrived, the clinician made a diagnosis and provided a month's course of medicine from the clinic's stocks. Health workers sent patients letters at home reminding them to take their medicine and attend monthly appointments. Coordinating treatment, distributing medicines, and caring for people who were spread across one-sixth of the growing city was a challenge, but one faced by many similar clinics across the country.

The TB care available here and throughout India followed a paradigm designed by an interdisciplinary group of Indian, UNESCO, and World Health Organization (WHO) experts at India's National Tuberculosis Institute. This group of experts based their protocol for in-home treatment of TB on a British Medical Research Council trial in Chennai—a city in southern India. This trial, in turn, had scaled up methods designed at a TB clinic in Delhi. The Delhi clinic's work was inspired by care given at a facility in Edinburgh. Already we can see the way flows of global and local knowledge intersected in the creation of the national treatment regime. Ultimately, the group hoped that the treatment program would be a temporary solution until a postcolonial India eradicated the disease through development.

In the early 1990s, however, global health experts began to question the program's efficacy. Epidemiologists worried that India's efforts had produced no documented epidemiological effect after thirty years. As these concerns reached the WHO and other institutions like the World Bank, actors there began to encourage India's minister of health to align the country's TB care with an emerging, standardized, WHO-supported intervention model. The clinic in northwest Mumbai was selected as a site to test the model, and quickly changes began to occur. Mumbai's municipal health authority, which had staffed, managed, and stocked the clinic since its opening, relocated the clinic's physician to make room for a clinician from the municipal TB department.

Funded by the bilateral agreement with Sweden that had earlier paid for TB drugs, and supervised by India's Ministry of Health and the WHO, the project carved out a small part of the clinic's catchment area to test a similar global health program within the Indian health system. For five years the clinic simultaneously ran two TB programs, the Indian program and the emerging global one. While India's existing system relied on patients' perceived needs, flexible diagnostic criteria, and monthly distribution of medicine, the new global health paradigm was characterized by urgency, intensified documentation, surveillance of patients as they took their medicine every other day at a health center, house-to-house patient follow-up, statistical measures of efficiency, and standardized drugs and diagnostic regimens. Eventually, the World Bank funded an expansion of this new program, and the clinic's remaining seven TB wards were decentralized. From 1997 onward, any municipal health center could provide TB treatment and any clinician was authorized to diagnose TB using a standard diagnostic protocol. Patients no longer needed to visit a specialized clinic; instead, they could get TB care from health workers in their neighborhoods. By 2000, the Mumbai clinic's paint had chipped and its gardens were overgrown. The region's supply of drugs and data flowed through the clinic, but patients rarely visited.

Unsurprisingly, the clinic languished, and in 2010 a local legislator proposed expanding the building and turning it into a TB hospital (Gurav 2011). The city government, however, denied the request, saying that TB was on the decline and there was no need for such a hospital (Banerjee 2012). Just two years later, Mumbai was launched back into the global health spotlight, this time because the city became a hotspot when a nearby private hospital reported several cases of extremely drug-resistant TB bacteria (Udwadia, Amale et al. 2012). Quickly, the Mumbai clinic was transformed into an administrative center housing the area's district TB officer—a technocrat in charge of the management of TB services. By 2019, the clinic had a new coat of paint but the district TB officer has moved. Today, it serves as a laboratory identifying about ten new drug-resistant TB patients each month and provides TB treatment to about a hundred patients. Those with drug-resistant forms of the disease receive a week's worth of medicine. Others receive a month-long course of medicine, as they had thirty years before. But all of them now also get a mobile phone–based treatment adherence system. Today's patients also receive a nutritional supplement or conditional cash transfer and access to a counselor who has a master's degree in social work to help with this multidrug resistant tuberculosis. In addition, each patient is tested for HIV and diabetes before beginning TB treatment. What was once a vertical, disease-specific approach to TB intervention seems to have grown branches. The clinic is once again a node in a larger health apparatus linked to priority diseases, psychosocial support, and new forms of governance through incentives. Each step of the way, the clinic, though a constant site of health intervention, has been deeply changed by global transformations.

This clinic is an example of what we call *health universalism*. Health universalism is a constellation that includes ideas about health's universal possibility, practices of making health universally recognizable and measurable, and discourses on universal human rights. The relations between each of these components has shifted through time. These shifts allow health universalism to encompass our three, often separately studied, domains of research: international health, global health, and health globalization processes. Throughout this book we engage health universalism as an often failed aspiration for human commensurability and ubiquitous development that grounds and authorizes important ways of knowing and intervening in health at a global scale. Though we take a critical lens on health and other forms of universalism, health universalism is an essential if not unquestionable social fact for the actors we observe, read about, and exchange with.

For historians, this particular clinic's place in health universalism raises a question of periodization. It simultaneously confirms and troubles narratives of a transition from a regime of international health, characterized by national boundaries and bilateral aid, and a model of global health, crowded by nonstate actors who determine priorities and fund health interventions across borders. The clinic shows something else. It suggests that though the 1990s brought significant change, important aspects of previous health interventions continue. This book works through this paradox of continuity and rupture to consider the practices that make global health simultaneously new and deeply marked by a history of infrastructures, markets, and circulations of objects and ideas.

This problem of change and stability strikes anthropologists, too. In more anthropological language, the question of global health and this specific Mumbai clinic is one of event and continuity (Sahlins 1981; Das 1996; Caton 2005). Does a shift in meaning and practice always make an event? Does the pilot project that shifted the way TB care was practiced here, and in India more broadly, constitute an event across other scales? Or does attention to the long process of change in the postcolonial world better situate practice and meaning? *Global Health for All* works through these issues of history and social life as continuity or rupture by carefully tracing the emergence of a global health regime from within a model of international health. Even though we use the term "global health" to describe the current discourse, the book shows that these two paradigms are not entirely separate entities but rather parallel ways of thinking about health.

We define "global health" as an umbrella term created by European and North American organizations working self-consciously to advance health and development on a global scale. Global health is neither a discipline nor a discrete set of practices that scholars can easily delineate. Instead, the term encompasses thirty years of multifaceted and diverse interventions on the health of others, particularly people considered vulnerable and living in "low- and middle-income" countries. Global health is a grand narrative, but one that, in practice, rarely lives up to proclamations about what it is, does, or will do. Like its constituent parts—medicine, science, governance, globalization, and markets—it operates on multiple levels. Each instantiation of global health—the actors involved, the forms of knowledge produced and mobilized, the targets selected, the tools tested and implemented—is therefore context-specific, locally situated, and bound to time.

Simultaneously, global health, as a powerful field of interventions and practices, is a social, historical, and political construct of the late twentieth century. Its existence has deep roots in the neoliberal project, its agenda, and its constellation of tools. These tools affect the government of lives based on a number of factors: economic discourses of performance and cost-effectiveness; the reinvention of public institutions and state bodies as regulators for markets; and the promotion of individual responsibility and rational investments (i.e., governmentality in health). In other words, we contend that global health is not a mere reflection of epidemiological data or pressing (basic) needs: it is a biopolitics of disease and development.

We make the following arguments. First, understanding global health across time and space requires mapping the entanglements of the field of global health—which is a set of institutions, forms of knowledge and instruments mobilized in programs, and actors who understand themselves as practitioners of global health—and less formal and more varied arenas of health globalization such as circulations of health personnel, patients, or drugs. Second, global health moves across multiple scales. In order to understand how its knowledge, interventions, and practices crosscut levels from the local to the global, it is indispensable to attend to their entanglements and look at the ways in which these scales become contextually relevant and mobilized. Third, global health's practices of knowing and doing are forms of neoliberal rationality and economization that disguise the political processes of technocratic governing and apportioning of collective resources in vocabularies of evidence-based intervention, efficiency, inclusion, and operability. In many but not all of our contexts, the state's role as provider and organizer of healthcare has been transformed by neoliberal reason and its advocates to render it an implementer of health programs rather than a space for debate about them.

Thus, we suggest that local interventions facilitate the spread and standardization of projects, politics, and subjectivities authorized by neoclassical economic concepts of efficiency, competition, and human capital instead of rights, politics, and public debate. We contextualize the stakes of these arguments by introducing the themes of periodization, scale, standardization, and neoliberalism.

Periodization

Defining historical periods is an important part of a historian's work, and the historiography of international health has produced its own delineation of the path to the regime of global health. The idea that post-1945 international health initiatives belong to three very different moments may not be uncontested, but it has acquired definite currency (Brown, Cueto et al. 2006; Birn 2009; Packard 2016). Scholars thus argue that the emergence of global health signals the end of an exceptional moment, the decades from 1965 to 1985, that had in turn supplanted an earlier moment of postcolonial and postwar reorganization of powers and infrastructures in the 1945–1965 period.

Historians suggest that during the 1960s and 1970s, self-defined Third World countries led and benefited from widespread critiques of colonial legacies and the hegemony of industrialized countries, pushed for alternatives to the international economic order and classical development strategies, and allied with international health experts. Together, they created what became known as the Primary Health Care Strategy, an original form of social medicine for the Global South. Then, the neoliberal reforms of the 1980s and 1990s brought that moment to an end and enabled the rise of global health. Although often viewed as a third period in this tripartite narrative, global health shares many features with the early days of international health. Continuities include a strong endorsement of biomedicine, the priority given to vertical programs targeting infectious disorders, and the decisive role of bilateral aid (from the United States or Scandinavian countries).

Our aim is not to offer an alternative narrative, perhaps stressing, for instance, the novelty of the global health decades with their unprecedented conjunction of actors, targets, tools, and modalities of intervention. Rather than defining a new regime, the book tries to change the granularity of the time line, looking at the juxtaposition between heterogeneous temporalities and between various combinations of change and continuity. We show, for instance, that depending on programs, countries, or collectives observed, what happens within and around the WHO blurs the classical tripartition of the period between 1945 and 2010, revealing decisive continuities through the 1960s and 1970s and the 1990s and 2000s.

Diversifying the lens on change and continuity through time also challenges the narrative of the WHO as a dominant, international, and social-medicine-oriented organization. Even during the 1970s, the years of its most visible influence, the WHO remained a weak institution. By mandate and intention, it did not operate on its own. It relied on a web of collaborations with powerful players like the World Bank or the United States Agency for International Development (USAID), and it was often disconnected from the dynamics of health planning in individual countries. The economization of health issues, a pattern emblematic of the WHO's adaptation to the new international order (Chorev 2012), will thus appear as a new form of prioritization. It is characterized by new tools for evaluating cost and effectiveness, but we show it is also rooted in previous and more political forms of triage that is applied when prioritizing health issues.

Attentiveness to space as well as time does not imply that our chapters avoid any kind of periodization—that is, any attempt at identifying patterns of action and assessing their coalescence in time. Four chronological premises, whose meaning will unfold through the entire book, are essential. First, a major reorganization of international health took place in the 1990s in concert with the neoliberal redefinition of the international economic and political order. This reorganization affected actors, targets, and the tools of intervention. Second, many priorities for integrating health, development, and economic growth that emerged in the 1990s have never become targets of global health investment or intervention. As a consequence, global health shares many characteristics with international health as it existed in the immediate postwar period. Third, the "Third World" has vanished in a world deeply affected by the end of the Cold War and industrial delocalization. As a result, the Global South lost its political and economic influence. Rapidly increasing inequalities within countries and new international hierarchies have emerged—for instance between new global players like China and those who have benefited less from globalization, like most countries in sub-Saharan Africa. Fourth, the 2010s were years of mounting challenges to global health as a domain of action built on the fundamental premise that resources and expertise reside in the Global North while most pressing health problems affect populations in the Global South. The 2009 economic crisis and its cortege of austerity policies, first of all in Europe, have indeed made visible the shared and mounting importance of scarcity and economic triage beyond the usual divide between our health and the health of others. Ten years later, the COVID-19 pandemic has revealed other—even less expected—layers of circulation and convergence with material resources, as well as social and technical means of intervention imported on a grand scale from Asia into Euro-America as well as Africa.

In other words, rather than offering one single alternative periodization, *Global Health for All* suggests that different time frames are needed to render the multiple ways in which the past of international health is shaping the present of global health.

A FIELD AND WHAT ELSE?

What is global health as an object of study? Is it a material thing? An obscure creation of the imagination? An empty signifier? If we start from the term itself, we see a fairly recent departure from earlier vocabularies of international health governance. Before the late 1980s, medical and public health literature barely used the term "global health" (Gaudillière 2014a; Weisz, Cambrosio et al. 2017). During the

1990s, however, the term began to spread through articles, editorials, statements, and annual reports as a neologism used by new health actors to describe their work and their goals. It was particularly common in documents emanating from a seemingly new set of actors and institutions, such as the Bill and Melinda Gates Foundation, the Harvard Initiative for Global Health, The Lancet, the Global Fund, the TB Alliance, and the Global Alliance for Vaccines and Immunization (known as Gavi, the Vaccine Alliance), among others.

Global health's claims for novelty, however, go beyond its name and those organizations described by it. Global health also includes targets and tools designed to consciously differ from what had come before. These new targets were novel diseases, such as HIV/AIDS or multidrug-resistant tuberculosis (MDR-TB), but also an unprecedented rise of noncommunicable diseases including mental health issues. Medical and public health literature endorsing the global health label stresses an unprecedented epidemiological situation in which a burden of chronic disorders is now shared between industrialized countries and large segments of the population in middle- and low-income countries. Proposals and pleas for action also place global health at arm's length from early developments in international health, particularly programs and strategies now perceived to be failed or obsolete, such as primary health care or centralized, state-run interventions. Champions of global health stress the need for participation and individual empowerment. They argue for a new ethic of efficiency and for the reliance on tools such as policy-making trials, audits, and cost-benefit analysis. All of these ideas are folded into the new term.

These particularities suggest that global health is not simply a domain or a specialty within the vast world of health. It is a field with its own rules and practices. As Pierre Bourdieu argued, the notion of "field" is useful in thinking about a certain genre of social spaces that are not only sites of interactions but abstract territories that gather together a limited set of actors, assembled in a closed space, to engage in a competitive game governed by formal as well as many informal rules (Bourdieu 1976, 1984). Following Bourdieu, the social sciences have theorized the field as a set of relationships and rules between actors animated by the same values, pursuing the accumulation of varied but shared forms of capital (Martin 2003). When in a shared field, actors "feel" the same kind of constraints, have tacit agreements about how to perform certain actions, and understand their rights and responsibilities. They are equipped with acquired dispositions and learned habitus indispensable to playing the game. The concept of field thus resonates with ideas of norms, boundaries, coherence, and homogeneity.

Approaching global health as a field is therefore a convenient way to think about its institutional, political, and economic dimensions. It allows us to look at the ways in which entities claiming to foster and practice global health implement similar resources and (mostly tacit) rules for their researchers and experts, their financing mechanisms, their measurements and evaluation procedures, their priority targets and programs, their own implementing bodies, and their local partners. Such a perspective echoes attempts to understand globalization as the making of specific fields beyond the boundaries of the nation-state, from geopolitics to humanitarianism (Go and Krause 2016).

For a decade, historians have been the most effective promoters of an understanding of global health as a field. They suggest that the field is made of new institutional and political arrangements for intervening in the health of others. They have accordingly argued that global health is regulated or dominated by institutions, like those we listed earlier, which define and implement disease-oriented, technology-driven, and highly selective programs that funnel funding and attention to the big three communicable disorders (HIV, TB, and malaria), as well as maternal and child health. Historical work identifies structures and instructions that define, act in, and police the global health field. *Global Health for All* follows this work in the sense that we argue that global health has emerged as a field following transformations that started in the 1980s, lasted for a quarter of a century, and remain active but contested.

Leaving things at that would, however, be deeply insufficient because global health is not merely a field. Anthropologists most often consider local iterations and particular projects in which global health actors figure as distant donors. From their perspective, the very people who act on behalf of global health seem to figure in the scene from offstage. While historians have looked at global health as a field, the anthropological approach addresses the shortcomings of the field model by exploring multiple and not necessarily overlapping circulations of concepts, techniques, people, and goods. They aim to synthesize global health as a field *and* the circulations that enter, transect, or encircle it, by arguing that the existence of global health as a field depends on the much broader processes of health globalization that take place both within and outside it. We call these processes of health *globalization arenas*.

A comparison of how globalization operates in domains as diverse as tuberculosis or Asian traditional medicines illustrates why distinguishing between global health as a field and health globalization as a series of arenas is useful. Global tuberculosis management is a paradigmatic example of the vertical logic that historians of global health have singled out. Tuberculosis intervention follows the rules of the global health field and defines its boundaries, while existing studies show a web of actors—such as the Global Fund, the World Bank, the WHO, more than a hundred nation-states, and an even more diverse palette of nongovernmental organizations (NGOs) in the field of global health's TB interventions (Koch 2013; McMillen 2015; Brimnes 2016). These actors engage and stabilize the field by following the rules of standardized, single-disease, low-cost, high-effect programs. Together, this network promotes the DOTS (directly observed treatment short-course) strategy, a standardized and focused package of medical knowledge, accounting, and pharmaceuticals. DOTS and its implementers have so effectively followed the rules of the field that it has retained a central place in global health for nearly thirty years. Metrics depict DOTS as one of the most cost-effective interventions in global health, and treatment strategies that diverge from it are quickly escorted off the field, portrayed as naïve alternatives or costly utopianism.

Conversely, we can view the growth of markets for traditional medicines as operating outside the logic of global health while adjacent to its networks. Therapeutic preparations found in the Chinese and Indian medical traditions have become major health products. They circulate all over Asia as well as East Africa, well beyond their initial territorial base. This circulation has, however, taken place outside the global health field, circumventing its players and rules and only occasionally breaching its borders. Unsurprisingly, historians and anthropologists have not accounted for this circulation when considering contemporary health universalism. In spite of the WHO's proclaimed push for the integration of "traditional medicines," these medicines circulate without the endorsement of any significant global health institution or actor, not even the WHO. Asian herbal formulations are therapeutic goods made global through processes of industrialization and trade whose circulation and use are invisible in the global health field.

In other words, the DOTS strategy against tuberculosis is integral to global health as a field while the circulation of traditional medicines has little obvious connection to it. However, this circulation reveals a global collection of actors, tools, and targets related to the most recent wave of economic globalization. When viewed from the perspective of these traditional medicines, the globalization of health is made possible by processes ranging from the direct transfer of industrial goods manufactured in Asia to the generalization (and contestation) of intellectual property rules. Large foundations and their intervention programs are nowhere to be found, but this is a form of health globalization nonetheless. Such goods and services emerge around the field as an effect of processes and patterns of action unconnected with the game. These ensembles of ideas, practices, objects, and actors are the arenas where the globalization of health takes shape.

Building on both historical and anthropological studies of globalization, this book thus proposes to supplement the notion of the field with the idea of arenas. Arenas are the less homogeneous and more dynamic social worlds where the processes of health globalization operate (Bonneuil, Joly et al. 2008). Health globalization as discursive and material engagement that makes health-related entities movable, and perhaps general, is thus not reducible to the global health field described by a set of dedicated programs and institutional actors. It also involves the worlds of finance, commerce, industry, development, education, international law, as well as traditional and social media. Looking into arenas of health globalization brings to the fore other dynamics and tensions than those at stake in the big programs and their focus on drug access, and helps escape a strictly North American and European understanding of what global health is, or should be, about. Such a perspective allows this book to move beyond the silo logic that has characterized much social science scholarship on global health and health universalism, viewing it only from the inner circle of global health actors.

It takes a bit of work to think through the intersection of the circulation of arenas and the structure of a field. Critics suggest that "circulation" as an analytical category tacitly endorses the idea that the world is a flat and empty space where entities move freely escaping power structures. As the historian Frederick Cooper once pointed out, stressing circulations and their role in globalization often goes with a certain fascination with flows, hubs, connectivity, and openness without much attention granted to the question of how the very same circulations are predicated on—and reinforce—strong hierarchies (Cooper 2005). Two examples of arenas emerging around and intersecting with the field of global health—the investment gap in noncommunicable diseases with its links to the circulation of biomedical pharmaceuticals, and biosecurity—may help elucidate their relationship.

The relationship between the global health field and its contiguous arenas of health globalization is not always smooth, and the question of power often results in tensions and unmet aspirations. One such tension exists in the difference between the importance attributed to noncommunicable diseases (such as cardiovascular diseases, diabetes, and mental health disorders) by global health actors and the actual funding allocated to treatment of these types of health challenges, what some have called "the investment gap." This discrepancy between stated priorities and funding may be interpreted in two different, though not incompatible, ways. A field approach focuses on the global health field and its actors; the other attends to health globalization arenas. A field interpretation focuses on the actors, structures, and deeply seated imaginaries that participated in the emergence of global health and characterize its current operations. This interpretation reveals the power of a historical focus on infectious disease and highlights an overwhelming continuity between international health and global health. It suggests that the investment gap is the predictable result of a field in which noncommunicable diseases, by virtue of their chronic status and their absence of cure, cannot play by the rules. An arena or health globalization interpretation in contrast reveals the massive circulation and consumption of pharmaceuticals for noncommunicable diseases.

Looking at the pharmaceuticals that enter the field of global health or circulate in the arenas of health globalization working in and across investment gaps reveals hierarchies and power relationships that we call arenas. The contemporary flows of pharmaceutical goods, whether formal or informal, go hand in hand with the preserved influence of North American and European pharmaceutical corporations and the growth of a new international trading order starting in the early 1980s. The new ways that goods are produced and travel, value is created, wealth is appropriated, and markets are constructed have radically altered North-South as well as South-South circulations and power gradients. In short, an analysis of global health as only a field fails to register innumerable forms of health at a global scale and the multiple arenas like these pharmaceutical flows.

Biosecurity is also an arena of health globalization. Biosecurity's concern is a globally universal risk of infectious disease, which is a form of health universalism, but its practices of preserving rather than producing health cannot reconcile with the rules of practice in the global health field. Scholars have shown that biosecurity concerns the planning, preparedness, and buildup of systems to stabilize existing health infrastructure and physical as well as economic well-being in emergencies (Collier, Lakoff et al. 2004; Lakoff and Collier 2008; Lakoff 2010a, 2010b; Caduff 2015;

Lakoff 2017). These concerns are quite different from global health's usual interventions on the health of others through patching broken systems, treating endemic infectious disease, and assessing the need and efficacy of treatments to bring about health. Biosecurity was surprisingly absent from our sites and archives of practice. Biosecurity's absence in these spaces suggests that although it affects the operation of global health, it is peripheral to the everyday practices of imagining and implementing global health interventions, revealing an autonomous arena.

An understanding of global health across time and space requires understanding the entanglements of the field of global health—as a set of institutions, forms of knowledge and instruments mobilized in programs, and actors who understand themselves as representatives of global health—and the less formal and more varied arenas of health globalization—such as circulations of health personnel, patients, or drugs. To do so, we suggest that scholars must also attend to scales and take a roving perspective.

The Game of Scales

Global health moves across multiple scales. Its knowledge, interventions, and practices crosscut the globe, region, community, and nation. Inspired by French historians who argued for the methodological importance of scale (Revel 1996), we follow moves between scales, attending to their entanglements and looking at the ways that scales become contextually relevant and practically mobilized.

We take scaling in global health as our object of investigation. The problem of generalization and localization and of scalable and nonscalable knowledge and action lies at the heart of the very pretense and the actual practice of understanding the health of others and intervening in it. A primary health care depression program in Kerala, India, crosses scales by linking local development priorities and the government of health with global agendas of moving mental health from the margins to the center of development programs. A GeneXpert machine in a hospital in Tanzania or India tells us as about tuberculosis as a priority of global actors and about local policies and health systems, genomic technology markets, global health infrastructures, and "off the grid" technological fixes. It tells as much about failures as creativity. These grids and the question of what is included in them relate to scale and scalability as well as issues of coverage, penetration, and implementation that reveal globalization's motors and global health's values.

Focusing on configurations of knowledge and action while considering the multiple social worlds of global health, we create a historiography and ethnography of shifting health configurations—international public health and global health—deployed at multiple scales. By working at the sites and in the archives of global-health-oriented knowledge production and practical intervention, we reveal actors, processes, and forms of action that transcend the distinctions between the global, the national, and the local. Combining scales allows us to consider specific diseases, care practices, technologies, and medical specialties, not only in relation to transnational health management and larger social and economic patterns but also within their local and concrete historical settings. We cross and combine scales by exploring globalization processes, looking at the making of knowledge, the production and commercialization of health goods, the implementation of public health programs, and routine medical work.

Using the case studies drawn from our own mobile and roving fieldwork as well as iterative, comparative conversations about findings in other sites and other times, we aim to understand how categories, standardized diseases and treatment regimens, industrial products, management tools, and specialties have become elements in the global government of health. We look at the production of the World Bank's pathbreaking "World Health Reports" in New York, as well as the negotiations around antimalarial medicines at the WHO in Geneva. We follow the circulation of international experts seeking to implement programs in national contexts and observe care in research, treatment, and management sites. We explore the reconfigurations of health regimes and the peculiar assemblages of science, medicine, economy, and politics associated with global health by telling big stories alongside and sometimes through small ones. What we face are, for example, global health actors in Washington producing documents that are supposed to organize Ghana, India, or Senegal, or, on the other hand, policymakers in Kerala trying to redefine development on the basis of their own terms while avoiding most but not all of global health's infrastructure.

Following global health actors, targets, and tools, as well as processes of health globalization, across scales resembles multisited ethnography. In the last decades, multisited ethnography has emerged as a methodology for exploring a field dispersed across space and scale by following people, technologies, and techniques in various locations (Marcus 1995). Crosscutting dichotomies such as the global and the local, multisited research allows an ethnographic engagement with large-scale entities even while focusing on everyday life and small-scale events and processes. Anthropologists have most fruitfully used this method to explore political, economic, environmental, or scientific global assemblages (Ong and Collier 2005). In the process, they have created opportunities to understand a convergence of new historiographic registers and structures while remaining attentive to local processes.

By ethnographically and historically following global health across sites and scales, *Global Health for All* engages the global and the local as sites as well as processes of siting or localizing at the same time. We follow global health across scales even while we take scaling processes and their frictions in global health as our object of investigation. What emerges is more than a multisited ethnography and history of global health. It is an assemblage of inquiries showing that scalability or the ability to expand is both difficult and central to global health, made possible by manifold, intense standardizations.

STANDARDIZATION

Anthropologists and historians have developed a great number of anxieties while studying global health's practices of standardization. For those whose interest and livelihood is the local and particular, global health's foundational assumptions, discourses, and practices are alarming in their dismissal and erasure of local particularities and complexities in favor of efforts to scale up and compare However, when we take steps to understand how standardization works among those hoping to achieve it and those at whom it is aimed, we find new insights about global health's inner-workings.

Comparability is both a necessary condition and an effect of technology, metrics, and medicine itself. Making bodies, communications, diseases, pharmaceuticals, and molecules comparable if not standard is central to knowing and intervening in global health. It also makes aspirations of universal health possible. With the transition from international public health to global health, a global scale of comparability that was once unnecessary and impossible moved to center stage because global health requires comparability of intervention, data collection, and the linking of cause and effect across locations and contexts.

Standardization, like comparability, is a double object. It is both a process and a product. We engage it in both forms. As process, standardization abides in practices that define and police an acceptable range of diversity as a basis for comparison and scaling up. For example, continuous and iterative standardization operates in practices that identify the acceptable range of variation in a pharmaceutical's active ingredient content or those that develop ranges of safe and unsafe blood pressure. Based on expert opinions of normal and abnormal, standardization moves processually from deciding on acceptable ranges of variation to describing appropriate actions based on these identified variables. The results of these practices bring us to a second kind of standardization. Standardization as product is the state of being standard or fitting into these ranges of acceptable variation.

Standardization tools pervade and animate the work of the WHO, the Gates Foundation, and the Institute for Health Metrics and Evaluation (IHME). The WHO constructs standards of care, like DOTS for TB or mental health interventions. Markets and regulators develop guides for technical specifications of drugs and technologies. Unified tools like disability-adjusted life years (DALYs) aspire to build standardized measures of cause and effect. Nonetheless, even in the center of the global health field, where these processes, constructions, and developments are put into practice, their effects remain slippery. They rarely bring about stable standardization as a product. Standardization as similarity is partial and as much a motor of diversity as uniformity. Noelle Sullivan provides an example of the tension between standardization as process and product in her study of the ways that global health funders' financial accounting and transparency techniques produce standardized reports of supported activities despite incredible diversity (Sullivan 2017). She shows that although Tanzanian grantees returned financial report worksheets to funders in the necessary standardized format, the very process that these reports represented relied on divergent ways of knowing and representing the world. Similarly, Wenzel Geissler argues that standardization processes that do not necessarily lead to standardized practice are part of global health's "unknown knowns" (Geissler 2013a). Replete with failed standardization and "unknown knowns," our work shows that more than standardization occurs when standardized metrics, technologies, pharmaceuticals, and ways of knowing are put to work.

Our inquiries reveal four points of comparability that guide practices of standardization within global health. They coalesce to enable the field's tentative imagination of a globally similar humanity and the interventions designed for its health. They include standardization of pharmaceuticals, biological commensurability of bodies, metrics, and universalist knowledge.

First, the standardization of pharmaceuticals means that the production of health requires globally shared processes of comparability in biomedicine and its pharmacopoeia, but also processes and protocols that are standard enough to move across production contexts and locations. The tightly coupled activities of drug companies, physicians, pharmacists, the public, and judicial actors, in addition to administrative and state actors, regulate and standardize the development, marketing, and use of pharmaceuticals (Gaudillière and Hess 2013). Because global health relies on drugs and their markets, many of these pharmaceutical standardization practices occur through the international regulation of drug development, circulation, and use. Regulations are negotiated in diverse places, such as WHO expert committees, Lancet commissions, international medical societies, OECD (Organization for Economic Cooperation and Development) commissions, and all these organizations produce systematic reviews outlining best practices.

Randomized control trials (RCTs) became the standard protocol for pharmaceutical innovation and drug development in the 1960s and have expanded into complex experiments in the era of global health (Marks 1997; Gaudillière 2008; Gaudillière and Hess 2013). Aiming to demonstrate safety and efficacy, these trials are grounded in supposedly universal biological bodies and ignore the social contexts in which pharmaceuticals and other interventions operate (Biehl and Petryna 2013; Brives, Le Marcis et al. 2016; Hardon and Pool 2016; Hardon and Sanabria 2017). Commercial interests and the power of the industry shape these standardized practices of evidence-making (Petryna 2009; Sunder Rajan 2017), and clinical trials shape pharmaceuticals' action in bodies. Pharmaceutical standardization through RCT experiments—often outsourced to research areas such as India, Poland, or Gambia—reconfigure patients and their value by assuming that all nonpathological bodies are generally interchangeable. Similarly, global "harmonization"—a process linking places through commensurable standards—brings national laws in line with global regulatory frameworks and thus facilitates clinical trials' offshoring (Petryna 2009; Sunder Rajan 2017). We add to this discussion showing that pharmaceutical standardization is also shaped by the production and circulation of drugs in markets. While bioequivalence and prequalification standards regulate the market by creating equivalences between global health drugs and their effects, networks and practices of illicit political economies subvert these very standards of drug markets and their transactions.

Standardization regimes also govern the development and circulation of traditional medicines such as Ayurveda or Chinese medicine that, although not part of global health as a field, have become important factors in larger processes of health globalization. Standardization in industrialized Ayurvedic drugs not only produces uniform combinations of plants, good production practices, and laboratory-based quality control but also neotraditional drugs that address standardized, and presumably universal, diseases and biological bodies (Pordié and Gaudillière 2014a, 2014b). Combined, these two dimensions of standardization have major effects on the construction of markets and the global circulation of these products.

These forms of pharmaceutical or industrial standardization result in a second form of global health comparability that Lock and Nguyen (2018) have called "biological commensurability" to describe changes in the body and ways of thinking about the body made possible by biomedicine. Biological commensurability "allows people to be sorted into standardized groups and populations because their biology is assumed to be the same" (Lock and Nguyen 2018, 176). Biomedicine uses biology to compare bodies and lives globally by measuring them as deviations from norm. Biology's standardized bodies are both the basis and the effect of global health's universalizing practices of knowing and intervening in the health of others. Universalized biomedical diseases in commensurable bodies are enabled and reinforced by standardized global health policies, research, and interventions. Biologically commensurable bodies are the basis for an understanding of globally shared risk (of being exposed to pathogens) and universalism or "biological humanism" in global health (Rees 2014). Anthropologists have challenged the idea of universal bodies, and the tendency to disentangle bodies from social relations, by emphasizing variation and situatedness of knowing and experiencing not only health and disease but also, and more importantly, biologies and vitalities themselves.

The third process of comparability in global health occurs through metrics. Metrics in global health hold the promise of an economic calculus that allows experts to know, count, and intervene in bodies in a value-neutral, politically unbiased way. We carefully document the centrality of the Global Burden of Disease studies and its DALY metrics in global health and follow its production and use over time and space. The DALY metrics as the epitome of the "economization of life" (Murphy 2017) in global health provides a technoscientific imaginary of comparison, linking disability, morbidity, risk, and productivity.

Finally, global health also knows and intervenes on bodies through universalist knowledge produced in research collaborations between NGOs, philanthropic foundations, hospitals, and universities. Research sites with highly standardized protocols turn vitalities and suffering into countable statistical units, measurable outcomes, and fiscal value; produce well-resourced islands or enclaves of global health science, care, and data (Geissler 2013a; Adams 2016a, 2016b; Sullivan 2017; Mahajan 2018); and aspire to shape policies, guidelines, and standards. Critics have contested the preference for hegemonic forms of knowledge production over slow qualitative research by asking what counts as knowledge and whose knowledge counts in global health (Reid-Henry 2010; Adams and Biehl 2016). Processes that simultaneously create standards, foster global equivalence, and bracket context represent a troubling set of changes in global conditions of possibility and imagination. They allow global health to appear as rational and natural despite the unsuccessful imposition of standardization, which actually opens spaces of unpredictability, chance, and diversity. While we agree with critics who point to the seductiveness and danger of standardizing processes for knowing and intervening in global health, we contend that although processes of knowing the world may be harmonized, ways of being and taking action in the world are rarely as uniform as they might seem. In short, life overflows and subverts standardizing biopolitics.

Tracing standardization as these four processes and products, our inquiries reveal little of the standardized fiscalization of lives—the turning of lives and vitalities into fiscally meaningful forms—that Adams (2016a) and other critics of globalization warn of. Social life is far too audacious to be completely controlled and stabilized. Even those physicians and healthcare workers intensely enmeshed in global health's standardizing impetus seem to muddle attempts to engage processes of standardization and to bring about prescribed forms of bodily existence. Nonetheless, comparability makes up one of the key tenets of global health and its entanglement with accounting brought about by neoliberalism.

What Is Neoliberal about Global Health?

Neoliberalism—a theory of economics that rejected Keynesian planning in favor of unplanned markets and streamlined bureaucracies—is folded into the tools and systems that guide global health. Throughout this book, we will explore some of the ways that neoliberalism entered global health and its effects on health interventions at a global scale. Attention to global health's neoliberal proclivities is not new. Global health scholars—historians as well as anthropologists—suggest that neoliberalism entered global health during the meteoric decline of state services ushered in by the structural adjustment programs of the 1980s and 1990s (Escobar 1995; Kim 2000; Comaroff 2007; Fassin 2007; Pfeiffer and Chapman 2010; Packard 2016; Erikson 2019). They argue that structural adjustment programs promoted a form of neoliberalism—called anarchic-neoliberalism—in which the market is deemed the sole organizing force in social and political life. These programs orchestrated the decline of state-run health infrastructures like clinics and hospitals, while the NGOs, philanthropies, and market strategies that funded care in the state's absence reinforced neoliberal ideology's power in global health. These same scholars suggest that by the dawn of the twenty-first century, neoliberalism had taken over global health and eroded the state's role in healthcare. They point to examples like the Bamako Initiative's misguided revolving drug fund, increases in the private provision of care and diminishing state services, and the supranational priority-setting role of organizations like the Gates Foundation, the President's Emergency Plan for AIDS Relief (PEPFAR), and the Global Fund (Pfeiffer 2013;

Keshavjee 2014; McGoey 2015; Adams 2016b). Nonetheless, analyses of what makes these projects neoliberal and market-based, or what role the state might now be playing, are limited. Even fewer have examined the individual recipients of health interventions or the social effects of neoliberalism in health.

Many who reveal strong links between global health and the spread of markets organized by neoliberalism have focused on post-Soviet or Soviet satellite states during the turbulent period created by the fall of the Soviet Union and World Bank intervention in the former Soviet bloc (Farmer 2005; Petryna 2009; Collier 2011; Koch 2013; Keshavjee 2014). These are illuminating but extreme examples of the state retreating from its role as caregiver. Developing our understanding of a global phenomenon based solely on these cases overlooks the processes of evaluation and triage used by technocrats and global health experts in order to make collective decisions about which public services should be shed and which strengthened. In most cases of global health restructuring, particularly in those contexts less affected by the fall of the Soviet Union, the state's role in attending to its citizens' health was deeply transformed, but not necessarily reduced, through subtle processes of optimization, partnership, and evidence-based policy.

Although neoliberalism cuts across public, private, and global health spheres, the state remains part of global health conversations and data-making. It is a bearer of expertise, policy, and institutional power; a configuration of jurisdictional and regulatory space; and a provider of pastoral care for populations. Despite its persistence, the state is inflected by neoliberalism precisely through the tools and value systems that state actors—politicians, technocrats, and physicians—use to interpret action and make decisions about health. In this way, the state and national bureaucracies remain stakeholders in global health while their roles, processes of legitimation, and logics of social organization have changed. How can the shared role of state and nonstate global health actors be understood and critically analyzed in light of the relationship between global health and neoliberalism?

To address this question, we find new strategies for interpreting neoliberal theory and its impacts on the state. Accounts of global health by anthropologists often interpret the field's ways of knowing and intervening as politics and antipolitics (Ferguson 1990; Harper and Parker 2014; Parker and Allen 2014; Taylor and Harper 2014). In other words, they attend to the ways that some forms of global health action are debated while others are seemingly uncontestable. They are concerned about the ways many global health actions seem uncontestably practical, to the extent of foreclosing politics, debate, and alternative action. We extend these critiques by focusing on the ways that global health's practices of knowing and doing are forms of neoliberal reason and economization, which disguise the political action of governing and apportioning collective resources in vocabularies of evidence-based intervention, efficiency, inclusion, and operability. In many but not all of our contexts, the state's role in healthcare has been transformed by neoliberal reason and its advocates from a space for debate about health priorities to a simple implementer of health programs. We suggest that interventions facilitate the spread and standardization of projects, politics, and subjectivities authorized by neoclassical economics' concepts of efficiency, competition, and human capital instead of rights, politics, and public debate.

David Reubi has identified what he calls "audit epidemiology" as one effect of the efficiency, performance, and management discourse in global health (Reubi 2018). Drawing from scholarship on neoliberal audit practices that govern and incentivize efficiency in business and the public sector (Power 1997; Strathern 2000), Reubi argues that just because large global health foundations and institutions lack public accountability and democratic processes in their decision making, it does not mean that no accountability exists. Rather, accountability, like the state, persists but is transformed. He shows that neoliberalism shifts accountability away from elected political actors, who voters could potentially hold responsible, to sites of policy-making, in which experts make decisions about which programs to attempt or continue on the basis of performance, efficient use of funds, and promise of epidemiologically verifiable effects (Nguyen 2009). Indeed, neoliberal thinkers like Ludwig von Mises (1944) argue that this method is more equitable than decisions based on political gain or bureaucratic inertia. In its own eyes, neoliberal reason enters healthcare through discourses and practices of efficiency, performance, optimization, and measurement linked to fairness and equity. This entry gives economic logic and epidemiological audit central roles as forms of moral conduct devoid of political machination. They also hinge on a positive evaluation of competition and human capital as catalysts for health and development. However, as we show, neoliberal prioritizations are political decisions framed as practical ones.

In reality, growth-related priorities and neoliberal vocabularies replace other logics of healthcare provision, like human needs or citizenship, with its own. Wendy Brown writes of neoliberalism's tendency to reconfigure values by suggesting that "neoliberalism is a distinctive mode of reason, of production of subjects, a 'conduct of conduct,' and a scheme of valuation. It names a historically specific economic and political reaction against Keynesianism and democratic socialism, as well as a more generalized practice of 'economizing' spheres and activities heretofore governed by other tables of value" (Brown 2015, 21). Brown's omnibus mode of thinking about neoliberalism, as the economization of spheres—in our case health—and systems of value—in our case democratic decision making and state services as part of the social contract—, is essential to our understanding of neoliberalism throughout this text. We present narratives that outline how "neoliberal political rationality does not merely marketize in the sense of monetizing all social conduct and social relations, but, more radically, casts them in an exclusively economic frame, one that has both epistemological and ontological dimensions" (Brown 2015, 62). For our purposes, we examine transitions in the "conduct of conduct" and the "tables of value" that state and other actors use to assess health-related activity to consider neoliberalism and global health's ways of imagining what is possible and practical. We find it an imagination in which both the possible and the practical are understood in selective economic terms. This monetization and transformation of social conduct and imaginary is the economization of health or even life.

Economization, or what Brown calls neoliberalism's conduct of conduct, does not supplant the state but enters it, "as Foucault puts it, to 'regulate society by the market'" (Brown 2015, 62). Michelle Murphy's work suggests that the economization of life "names the practices that differently value and govern life in terms of their ability to foster the macro-economy of the nation-state, such as life's ability to contribute to the gross domestic product of the nation" (Murphy 2017, 6). We define the economization of health as the evaluation of processes designed to transform illness into health based on their effects on well-being as part of national and international economies. More precisely, these economic effects include the production of goods and services as well as the capacity of those transformed lives and health to consume, innovate, and maximize market potentialities. From this perspective, economization situates neoliberalism as just one of multiple and competing political economies jockeying to negotiate and interpret the relationship between populations, governance, and economics. It is one among several possible conducts of conduct that state and nonstate actors might use to attend to health.

Examining neoliberal reason first highlights its ability to move institutions away from existing values by reconfiguring reflexive systems of evaluation and interpretation. Second, it foregrounds neoliberalism's variability across space and time, allowing us to consider the ways that neoliberal reason shifts across contexts. In realms of health, neoliberal reason is always changing as it adapts to the kinds of political, economic, and health systems it meets. *Global Health for All* engages neoliberalism, then, as a variable process of economizing health that works through the use of tools to know, assess, and make decisions based on the zero-sum games of money and action. When viewed through the lens of neoliberalism, interventions based on other sets of values inevitably look like failures. Moreover, these tools make new projects seem like major breaks regardless of their similarity to earlier interventions. This is one part of global health's ambiguous origins.

We examine several examples of tools and discourses for a conduct of conduct aimed at maximizing a health investment's effects by optimizing its performance. They include metrics and the famous DALYs; the shifting role of expertise from clinicians to epidemiologists and economists; and new forms of prioritizing or triaging diseases based on effect on human capital and feasibility of intervention. We trace each to show how these forms of program evaluation at the birth of global health were part of the processes that proclaimed international health a failure. Similarly, we show how they continue to paint most interventions in the health of others as lacking efficiency, hampered by scarce resources, replete with gaps in capacity, and mired in local context, while insisting on the promises of effectively verified and documented cost-effective activities.

From the World Bank's 1993 report on investing in health to contemporary discourses of universal health coverage, competition and human capital have become central organizing tropes in global health's "conduct of conduct." Competition between public and private sectors to manage disease, as well as managing each other, is a way to compete for attention and funding through the introduction of neoliberal reason in health. However, competition between the state and market are not the only forms of competition at work. We also find technologies competing for WHO and funder endorsement, competition between maladies for visibility, competition between hospitals and clinics, even competition between experts throughout the field. Each must prove its superiority through a series of inscription techniques and evaluative technologies that promise to maximize health with lower investments of money, capacity, and time (Akrich 1992). This is based on the presumption that quality of care in each sector increases when markets, states, and donors compete to provide the best care at the lowest cost. Decisions about an intervention's competitive advantage are made with built-in assumptions about who will pay, who can pay, and whose values count. It is crucial to remember that these assumptions guide the work of bureaucrats as well as global health funders, both of whom have bought in to neoliberal strategies of maximizing growth potential by identifying low-cost, high-margin products and interventions. The assumptions that structure the field do not overtly suggest that patients themselves compete for global health resources but that diseases, treatments, and forms of care are in competition to access scare resources. In most cases, these competitions are adjudicated based on what Reubi calls audit epidemiology: a combination of their modeled potential effects on a population and their cost. We engage competition throughout the text by considering development, metrics, triage, and markets.

We also trace neoliberalism in global health by attending to human capital. Ideas about human capital economize health and make it a tool for speculative, neoliberal projects that encourage market participation, maximize the effects of minimal expenditure, and foment economic productivity. Despite its centrality, the idea of intervening in health in order to enhance human capital is rather new. For much of the twentieth century, economists considered health a positive side effect of state-led development. In a landmark reversal, however, in 1993 the World Bank health economists who authored the *World Development Report: Investing in Health* publicly argued that improving health would catalyze economic development, rather than result from it, primarily through an improvement in human capital. These economists and their entourage use "human capital" to refer to a whole theory of production that understands people as "ability-machines" with a combination of innate and learned capabilities necessary to produce goods and services (Foucault, Senellart et al. 2008, 226). Health interventions, they posited, would enhance these capabilities and thus individuals' participation in national cycles of production and consumption. They imagined that once set in motion, increased human capital's potential effects on gross national product and global economies would be exponential, almost utopian. Indeed, in the human capital imaginary, the pastoral state acts to render itself obsolete. It must organize healthcare to start the cycle and then recede. At the same time, recipients of state care are no longer bearers of rights or citizens or even infectious risks to national populations. Instead, the state must triage individuals to funnel resources to people it identifies as potential producers, inventors, market innovators, and consumers. It hopes these individuals will, in turn, improve their health, grow their human capital, and participate in development. Global health's logic of human capital neoliberalizes and economizes health and human flourishing as sources of economic value and human capital rather than valuable in and of themselves. We trace the effects of this neoliberal economization across the field of global health.

Neoliberalization and its rationality has certain central tenets when it comes to health: namely, competition, efficiency, auditing, human capital, and triage. However, we have been careful to recognize that neoliberal logic results in specific assemblages that occasionally coalesce in shared values like efficiency, competition, and human capital. By doing so, we do not avoid the cold truths that healthcare infrastructures—often considered the state's purview—are generally in wretched states in contexts where global health is powerful. Rather, we understand this state of affairs to be both a condition of possibility for localized forms of neoliberal healthcare interventions and an effect of them. Neoliberalism in global health, though context-specific and situated, is alarming in its scope, its ability to expose health and life to the market, and its use of logics of economic gain to justify and critique national social safety nets. That it has entered the state's provision of care policies is even more concerning than the state's retreat from healthcare wholesale. We encourage readers to keep in mind that neoliberalism is inflecting the conduct of conduct, the players, and the game itself throughout this text. Our chapters considering triage, metrics, and markets reveal this influence directly, while other chapters highlight moments of contestation, elaboration, and infiltration.

Multi-Scalar Methodologies

The fifty-year-old TB clinic where we began is one of the many places that we take our readers on this anthropological and historical journey. Like any journey with two guides, the path is not always direct. At times, it veers off to consider objects that appear more interesting to one guide or the other, but the richness of the conversation, we hope, makes the journey worth its deviations and pauses. This is the nature of our collective exploration and conversation. Our five-year project traverses four continents, thirteen countries, and sometimes peculiar parts of the Internet. It draws the authors into conversation about four topics that illustrate the range of different domains touched by global health today (tuberculosis, mental health, Asian medicines, and medical genetics). We approach health universalism by anchoring it in the past and present experiences of many of its protagonists—nurses, physicians, policymakers, staff of the WHO or the World Bank, and entrepreneurs.

In our work, we privilege no single site of truth or validity and pursue the epistemic goal of understanding health universalism on the basis of, first, the addition of unexpected sites for observing interventions; second, a complementary focus on several knowledge- and evidence-producing locations; third, our decision to not favor one particular type of data over another. We look at the "local" beyond its role as a space for the application of norms or programs and contend that it is a multiplex space that produces and is produced by health universalism. This approach explains our focus on the conventional core of global health (e.g., diseases like TB and malaria and organizations such as the WHO and the World Bank), as well as some of its less explored margins (e.g., issues such as mental health, genetics, and traditional medicine and regions like the Middle East). Dealing simultaneously with these different streams and scales allows us to better differentiate the field of global health and its contiguous arenas of health globalization. By exploring these spaces, we tell a story complementary to mainstream international and global health narratives. We explore the global health beyond the headlines, which often focus on innovation, the Gates Foundation, and other global-scale actors, HIV and Ebola, and an "ailing" African continent. Our exploration spans the second half of the twentieth century through the beginning of the twenty-first, with a specific focus on the transition from international health to global health during the mid-1990s. Dealing with this period allows us to combine interviews, ethnographic observation, and access to archives up to the late 1990s in "global" (the WHO, the World Bank, the Swedish International Development Agency) as well as "local" (the Kerala Health Secretariat, the Kibong'oto hospital, researchers' personal libraries) sites of memory and history. Our dual approach combines the interest of historians of health for what people say and do at a particular moment in time and medical anthropologists' focus on what these very people mean to be saying or doing.

Admittedly, people in the field grant anthropologists and historians a certain— and shifting—place on the power ladder, defining what studying up or down means and where it might lead (Conti and O'Neil 2007). Moreover, in a multi-scale, multisited, and multidisciplinary endeavor like ours, the variation of positionality is significant. Our way through these shifting sands was regular, collective, and comparative discussions of the main arguments of this volume, which reached an apex in the collaborative writing of the book itself. This difficult separation of the researcher's own positionality and the webs of significance and sociality that ensnare a researcher is more obvious in a collaborative project like ours. Research collectives often shape perceptions, and as our conversations turned into collective writing, our ethnographic gazes, whether informed by training in anthropology or history, tended to settle on similar objects (Latour and Woolgar 1979). Nonetheless, our own interests, trajectories, and subjectivities found their way through this book and its multiple voices. The latter becomes a chorus with the aggregation of our inquiries and the permanent interplay between descriptive and normative approaches.

Across the decades we examine, we deliberately study up and down in an attempt to reach "the most powerful strata" of international and global health, as well as the lives affected by the decisions of the latter (Nader 1972). Such a spectrum of exploration has practical consequences. We follow what Hugh Gusterson calls "polymorphous engagement," which implies "interacting with informants across a number of dispersed sites, not just in local communities, and sometimes individual form; and . . . collecting data eclectically from a disparate array of sources in many different ways" (Gusterson 1997). The characters in this volume are as diverse as clinicians, ministers, hospitals, scientists, bureaucrats, medications, community health workers, reports, economists, DALYs, and WHO experts.

Blurring the disciplinary borders, we try to build bridges between past and present in order to fill two gaps: on the one hand, the chronological lapse left open by the relatively scarce historical inquiries into global health after 1990, and on the other, the scalar breach that anthropologists create when leaving the pre-1990 era to other fields. In so doing, we can rely on archival work of the pre-1970 decades; on archives and personal interviews from the 1970s to the 1990s; and on a combination of comprehensive ethnographies, personal interviews, and archives for the most recent period. In several instances, historians and anthropologists simultaneously conducted fieldwork, allowing for on-the-ground multidisciplinary collection and analysis of data. Their collaborations have collected and interpreted stories new and old about health universalism.

The chapters that follow share insights generated when historians and anthropologists team up to examine the interaction between global health and health globalization as they negotiate change and continuity, standardization, and neoliberalism across shifting spatial and temporal scales. Each chapter takes a critical look at one interaction and invites readers to join in the work of situating global health within and beside broader realms of health globalization, rather than attending to a particular place or malady. The first chapter, "Localization in the Global," considers the ways universalism establishes and problematizes particularity as "local." It uses the term localization to show that health universalism takes particularity as a scalar problem to be addressed through processes such as circulation, experimentality, and community engagement. These processes constantly remake the relationships of the general and the particular across scales, diseases, and times. "Metrics for Development," chapter 2, inverts this theme by recounting the social life of one of global health's central tools, the disability-adjusted life year metric. The chapter shows how metrics are forms of standardization that attempt, but often fail, to render diseases and people comparable and equivalent. By doing so, the metric becomes a social actor that crosses and even constitutes scales. Comparability of diseases allows for a technocratic form of care and policy that is based on the predicted performance of scaled-up interventions and treats all sufferers as similar but for their disease. Chapter 3, "Triage beyond the Clinic," attends to political triage and economic triage to understand shifting ideas about who should create healthcare priorities and how. It reveals that a transformation from state-led to global-health-led prioritization is incomplete, but neoliberal ideas have altered the logic of prioritization to cultivate markets rather than participative citizens.

Chapter 4 on "Markets, Medicines, and Health Globalization" follows pharmaceutical markets out of the field of global health and into health globalization's arenas. The chapter argues that pharmaceuticals are a technical form of health globalization and a condition of global health's possibility. Charting four regimes of market construction, the chapter shows that global health is just one of the many ways that pharmaceutical markets circulate medicines and create arenas of health globalization. Continuing to scrutinize the processes that make health universal, chapter 5, "Tech for All," focuses on technopacks as collections of technologies and techniques that render health technical, transportable, and transferable without major infrastructural inputs. The chapter shows how important globalized flows of know-how and stuff are for global health. This interest in development through technical solutions returns the reader to questions of scale and space. Chapter 6, "Persistent Hospitals," examines three of the crowded clinical spaces where global health technopacks land. This chapter reveals that hospitals, though often silenced in global health's discourses, are a node of articulation between global health and health globalization as they provide, at times with great difficulty, the infrastructure in which global health and health globalization operate. Similarly, the chapter shows that even where global health is strongest, hospitals are often state-created tools to care for populations. As such, they provide an ideal site to trace the state's twenty-first-century attempts to care for the market through caring for populations. Continuing the attention to health at scale as it shifts between global health's field and health globalization's arena, chapter 7 on "Provincializing the WHO" tells the story of the WHO's incomplete transition into the global health field. Arguing that the WHO is both inadequate and indispensable to health universalism, the chapter shows how both global health NGOs and health globalization South-South cooperation pressure the WHO, despite its continued role as health's global clearinghouse and political center. The epilogue discusses how the global COVID-19 pandemic, unfolding as we finalized this book, both reinforces and challenges the book's core message: that global health and health globalization are dynamic interconnected social phenomena and that health in the last eighty years has become an object of management.

CHAPTER 1

Localization in the Global

Andrew McDowell, Lucile Ruault, Olivia Fiorilli, and Laurent Pordié

In October 2017, a major multilateral organization convened twenty experts to evaluate proposals for propagating information technology for health or "e-health"
worldwide. Funding applications—written by large international public-private
consortia proposing multimillion-dollar projects to provide healthcare through
digital and electronic technologies—covered the tables. Each project hoped to
extrapolate on a successful pilot project in a significant way. Scalability was crucial. The proposals, however, did not take into account the historical, sociopolitical, cultural, or linguistic particularities of the milieu in which each pilot was
launched. These were viewed, quite simply, as part of the "local context" that
scalable programs would transcend. Social scientists on the panel raised concerns
about this assumption. Other members seemed to genuinely care about their perspectives, but their votes were outweighed by the collective scoring of medical
doctors, epidemiologists, statisticians, psychologists, economists, and administrators. Ultimately, the process of evaluation and scoring did not allow social science
and its minority position to balance these more unified disciplines and their
numerical strength. This meant that proposals indifferent to the social and cultural complexity of scalability had chances of going through, whatever their potential for success.

While local acceptance was a prime concern in program design, considerations
of what or who comprised "the local" remained undertheorized. A project had to
show local success at some place, among some people, to get a chance to be replicated and disseminated on a large scale—in other words, to become global. In short,
a project needed to speak to the diverse network of global health intervention sites,
fit global actors' priorities, and demonstrate its empirical success as measured by
the medical experts who assessed it. This process begs the question, How did a
diverse set of health interventions across the globe's many locals come to be viewed
as comparable? How were "locals" knitted together to form a "global," and what
happens to local specificity once the global scale becomes thinkable and knowable
as a site of interpretive action?

The group's presumed (or pretended) lack of positionality allows it to act as an objective, universal arbiter and evaluator of situated acts and actors. Developing scalable interventions involves a number of iterative translation processes between the local and the global that are central to the field of global health. This chapter examines such processes. Events like these at a conference table in a European capital are ways of imagining the role of particularity across a whole web of other localization processes. The table is among the few nodes of global health that transcend or lack place. Situated at the center of the global health field's processes, the experts at this table set the rules of commensurability or universality that local or situated actors must follow. For instance, the biological scientists frequently thought of the specific site of a pilot program as a laboratory—a place to test a project before standardizing and extending it. Though these actors are at the end of a long chain of translation processes, they are still busy with the processes of localization that make global commensurability possible. As such, we begin our discussion of localization in global health with the global center of evaluation and assessment. Surprisingly, it is in the middle of localization processes not the end of them. Nonetheless, we cannot stay here for long. Attending to practice, health globalization, and the norms of the field direct us to other processes and other locals that must play by the rules set at this table.

Throughout this chapter, we reconsider the local as a process or emergence rather than a place or a thing, but this is not necessarily how global health uses the term. In this chapter, we first engage the ways that global health produces and reacts to the existence of spaces not fully recognizable to its standardizing, universalizing logics by identifying them as "local." We then study how global health, as a field and apparatus, understands, morphs, twists, and adjusts these spaces, at times imposing global health logics while at other times allowing local knowledge to catalyze a recalibration of its epistemological tools. Next, we search out the places where the global fails to take root in the local. Finally, by taking on the local as process and assemblage within the field, we are able to engage one of global health's material and discursive formations.

Grounding Localization

If the "global" in global health aims to build health universality through techniques of knowledge, comparison, and intervention on a planetary scale, what remains of the local? That "the local" persists—even as "the global" aims to subsume or supersede it—makes for one of global health's central contradictions. How can "the local," as shorthand for specificity, difference, and particularity, continue to flourish in a field that imagines health and bodies as globally standard or standardizable? The contradiction is good to think with and points to some of the contours of global health as it moves in scalar circulations and interprets the success and failure of its interventions on human populations and health.

The local is a *mirage* of perspective and position. Practices, objects, ideas, and interventions that may be local in one context are global when moved to another.

At the same time, those aspects of the global that have become ingrained in a particular context can be lived as local. In this way, localization is a process by which factors outside global health's central tenets or field come to be associated with or inseparable from a particular context.

Locals are global health's boundary objects (Bowker and Star 1999; Huvila 2011). Locals can be hospitals, languages, nation-states, regions, practices, or cities. They can also be cataracts in flows of circulation where a bottleneck or saturation occurs. Indeed, the local, at least in the world formed and framed by global health, comes to be meaningful only in opposition to the global as a discursive space of data, planning, and equivalence while also being the space in which global agendas play out.

Anthropologists often study the local as a point of friction (Tsing 2005), a site that eludes or overflows global health's epistemological techniques (Petryna 2009; Lock and Nguyen 2018), or a space of *bricolage* and the piecing together of globalized resources and community (Livingston 2012; Crane 2013; McKay 2018). Historians, conversely, study the ways in which locals are constituted across time as sites of difference either by the events that transpire there or the effects of larger phenomena on their particularity (Guinzburg, Tedeschi, and Tedeschi 1993). In each case, the local is where action happens, data emerges, cases can be studied, and bodies accessed. The local is also a site of miscommunication, where there are islands of care and slippages flourish.

Localization, we have found, is closely linked to experimentality. Experimentality describes a complex set of processes that make people, bodies, and societies available as objects of experimental intervention by creating populations and people, which are delimited and comparable (Nguyen 2009). As Fouzieyha Towghi and Kalindi Vora (2014, 2) describe experiment: "A signature of modernity, the experiment is a technology of truth making, or in the scientific register producing facts, to test application of 'new' theories through observation. It is a test to demonstrate a known truth, to examine the validity of a hypothesis, or to determine the efficacy and safety of something previously untried." Experimentality, then, is the state of being open to processes of truth making, as well as the forms of power that enable and authorize it through iterative knowledge construction—a process that comes through strongly in global health's discourse of failing forward (Rheinberger 1997). Experimentality, however, plays out in situated local practices where, as Adriana Petryna suggests, risks and rewards are not evenly distributed (2009). The particular constellations of forces that play out in these processes of local experimentality at once identify sites in which novelty can be created and tested and link people through shared risk and responsibility. Moreover, examining localization in global health in relation to experiment helps to contextualize the relationship between the local and the global. If the local is the site of an experiment, then it must have at least some characteristics of a laboratory, particularly those that allow for experiment. The presumption is, of course, that variables can be accounted for, maybe even controlled, in the laboratory local. This controlling or accounting for variation is one localization of global processes.

Localization processes that animate global health include proving a concept, developing a prototype, building evidence of reaching scale, and comparing two treatments. They also include circumscribing and furnishing the places where people—particularly sick people—might be identified, treated, or missed, and where commensurability might be made, aspired, or frustrated. As such, locals are nodes in a global net, but not all nodes are imagined to be local. The World Health Organization (WHO), World Bank, and the Bill and Melinda Gates Foundation might be nodes, but they efface their status as locals. They are imagined, instead, as universal arbiters of the knowledge that local processes create. They constitute global health's fields of action, but they play by different rules. As such, they are both inside and outside global health's constraints of space and money. Local as process thus reveals the rules of global health's game played in health globalization's arenas and what particular places and people must do to be recognized as players. As such, locals are discursive hubs, sites of circulation, and points of interest for traveling experts who knit together a field of global health from arenas of health globalization. By looking to sites of locality here, we help sketch the boundaries of global health as a field and look to the processes that create it. These processes look a lot like those that build the boundaries between the laboratory and the world, but as Hannah Landecker (2013) and Sarah Wylie (2018) show, the poles of experiment and control are shifting in the twenty-first century. The lab is in the world and the world is in the lab, and for global health, with its ethic of action, the whole world has become a space for trial and error (Landecker 2013). It is now necessary to understand how local processes are global and how global processes are local in order to trace the political, economic, and ethical work of global health.

For our purposes, experimentality and localization come together in global health to produce a moving locus of knowledge, originality, and complexity. In each section, we examine how global health concepts play out locally as they are tested, observed, and applied. Localization generates globally standardized health, and it remains the starting point and the final frontier in which the unexpected can happen.

Migrating Locals and Evidence for Scalability

In the mid-1950s, the WHO designated genetics as a high-priority concern. Barely fifteen years later, the Human Genetics Unit was in crisis. Accused of stagnating, it was slated for closure. Beginning in 1979, consultant Anver Kuliev, a geneticist from the USSR, was charged with assessing genetics' potential role in reaching WHO objectives. Kuliev says that the then director general of the WHO, Halfdan Mahler, "challenged me, as a scientist in genetics, to demonstrate if genetics was really important for public health and the WHO."[1] Together with geneticist John Edwards (professor of medical genetics at Oxford), Kuliev came to the conclusion that focusing on endemic genetic conditions affecting specific populations would be a useful starting point for formulating a new hereditary diseases program. A group of WHO experts proclaimed the management and prevention of thalassemia in Cyprus to be the best example of such a program. In this sense, local knowledge and intervention played key roles in rehabilitating genetics within the WHO.

Prior to this intervention, thalassemia, a recessively inherited blood disorder, posed a severe health threat in Cyprus because of the high frequency of an abnormal globin gene in the population. In the early 1970s, about 16 percent of Cypriots carried the thalassemia mutation. This meant a high number of marriages between people who carry but do not express the mutated gene (heterozygotes) and about one in every 135 births having two mutated genes and beta thalassemia disorder (Angastiniotis and Hadjiminas 1981). The Cypriot government had recognized thalassemia as a major public health problem since the 1960s, but its national policy in the 1970s focused on growing medical awareness and better standards of treatment. Intensive treatments with blood transfusions and the pharmaceutical removal of iron from the blood were developed to handle the most severe forms of thalassemia, which is responsible for chronic anemia, slow infant growth, bone deformities, and early death. As curative services improved, clinical management of the disorder raised quality of life and life expectancy. Taking into account the rising survival rate, the estimated costs of treatment and need for blood were identified as an important drain on health resources. In 1971, the Cypriot government sought the support of a WHO adviser, Professor G. Stamatoyiannopoulos, who concurred that continued management of the disorder would be a potentially heavy burden for the community. His report spurred the Ministry of Health to formulate a national prevention program in 1972 as part of the government's five-year development plan. Beyond the goals of more standardized and effective treatments through special thalassemia outpatient clinics, improved blood transfusion regimens, and blood donation campaigns (Angastiniotis, Kyriakidou et al. 1986), recommendations emphasized prevention through public education campaigns and genetic counseling (Cowan 2008). Population screening was enacted in the country from 1973 onward.

Meanwhile, population movements[2] gave this local issue a larger scale. In other words, the needs of "local populations" across the world caught the attention of experts in the Global North, who then dedicated their work to thalassemia and sickle cell disease (hemoglobinopathies), especially in places with considerable Cypriot migration, such as England. This is best illustrated by the case of patients from the Cypriot community in North London whose treatment needs led the clinical geneticist Bernadette Modell to get involved in thalassemia care delivery, epidemiology, and research. Starting in 1977, she also cared for women traveling from Cyprus to London for prenatal diagnosis. As her interest in the issue grew, she began traveling to Cyprus. There, as a result of the Cypriot anti-anemia association efforts, Modell met the minister of health and discussed some of his misconceptions about prevention: "He said that the techniques involved are far too complicated. . . . And I said to the minister of health, 'Well, you know, in my laboratory it's run by Cypriots and our patients are all Cypriots. So if we can do it in London, you can do it here!' And he said, 'Fine, I'll send someone for training.'"[3] The first training in London at the Galton Laboratory was for Michael Angastiniotis, an obstetrician/

pediatrician who came to play a leading role in developing the thalassemia program in Cyprus in the 1980s and 1990s. Through knowledge transmission and the use of equipment, Modell strove to replicate her own diagnostic techniques in Cyprus. This process thus represents a "relocation" of tools and expertise.

Concurrently, Robert Williamson, a biologist who specialized in the application of molecular biology to hemoglobin disorders, became another driving force in the dissemination of knowledge. He organized a meeting in Crete in 1978, gathering "young people from the whole Mediterranean area [so as to] open their eyes to [the] future possibilities"[4] of treating thalassemia. Following this meeting, several Italian, Greek, Cypriot, Portuguese, as well as Indian and Iranian physicians (obstetricians, pediatricians, clinicians, biochemists), received grants for training in England on molecular biology and prenatal diagnosis—sometimes even bringing patients with them. Among themselves, Modell and her colleagues called this project of locally necessary but globally relevant thalassemia treatment the *Club Méditerranée*.[5] The club promoted a global perspective for thalassemia screening, starting from a particular regional local. The construction of an international network and global health interest in a local issue led to strong links between patients' associations and international experts, the circulation of people seeking prenatal diagnosis or scientific training, and also the propagation of educational, diagnostic, and treatment tools.

The emergence of hemoglobin disorders "in areas where they are not endemic" (Angastiniotis, Modell et al. 1995), such as London, paradoxically pushed experts to turn their attention to the Global South, because they realized that their approach could be effective in the context of a large population struggling with the management of a hemoglobinopathy. Simultaneously, the local situation caught the attention of the small WHO team trying to renew the Human Genetics Unit. A confluence of interests between thalassemia specialists and WHO officers, which materialized in Bernadette Modell's collaboration with Anver Kuliev (individuals some interviewees called "the parents of community genetics"), turned Cyprus into a laboratory with the aim of proving the utility of genetics for public health and designing global standards surrounding genetic diagnoses and treatments.

The Cypriot prevention program has changed over the years. In the 1970s, it consisted of public education in order to sensitize the public to the issue. This took the form of mass media reminders, talks in rural community centers, blood donation campaigns, the introduction of the topic into school curriculum, and distribution of information booklets in most endemic areas. In the late 1970s, population screening and genetic counseling were introduced. Population screening rested on the selection of target groups to identify carriers. This changed over the years. At first, priority was given to relatives of people born with two mutated genes called homozygotes and young single people (girls leaving school, men doing their national service). Then, with the advent of fetal diagnosis in the 1980s,[6] the paradigm shifted to focus on "those with the most immediate risk of producing an affected child—those already pregnant."[7] In 1983, the Cypriot Christian-Orthodox church asked couples who sought the church's blessing for engagement to undergo testing for the thalassemia trait to become aware of their carrier status. Even though few couples called off their marriages because of a heterozygosity diagnosis, the advantage of this compulsory test was that people of reproductive age would be made aware of their carrier status and could either refrain from having children or, at the least, perform prenatal diagnosis. As Anver Kuliev recalled in an interview:

> [The] thalassemia control program in Cyprus [was] the first national community program for [the] control of hereditary disease, which ... provided the basis for [the] initiation and development of [the] WHO-model approach for community control of congenital disease.... [As we] discussed in detail during the Second Annual Meeting of the WHO Working Group on Community Control of Hereditary Anemias [in] November 1983, ... it was considered to be a unique experience which might be of great value in initiating a control program in developing countries where congenital anaemias represent a major health problem. (Kuliev 1984)

Thus, the formulation and implementation of this national policy was meant to be a point of departure for community-based control of "congenital diseases." Beyond its disease-based definition, the concept of "community" was, in this context, similar to population-oriented approaches, with a tacit understanding that the target population shared a certain genetic background and cultural traits.

Other pilot studies on hemoglobinopathies were conducted in Greece, Italy, the United Kingdom, and the United States (Boyo, Cao et al. 1983). And yet Cyprus was deemed a model in the struggle for large-scale disease prevention because of its concentration of traits in one demarcated population. This "local" situation combined the features of a population at risk (i.e., a high incidence of thalassemia, said to be the second highest after the Maldives), social visibility of this crippling disease, and the rising burden of treating homozygous people. It also featured the conditions that made disease controllable—a small and isolated landmass[8] and a modest population size (about 600,000 people) with a low birth rate and relatively high standards of living, literacy rates, and standards of healthcare.[9] These features of the local made the population easier "to reach, investigate, and influence" (Angastiniotis and Hadjiminas 1981). As "a small, educated and uniform cultu[ral] community which has inevitably close contact with the homozygous condition," Cypriots were even said to "[respond] well after public and individual counseling."[10] In addition, experts acknowledged the role played by "the collusion between medicine, state and the Church/religion" (Chattoo 2018). Modell outlined the latter institution's role in coercing testing. She noted that "unless you mandate premarital screening, ... it's like everything else! ... Unless you mandate it, it didn't work."[11] But it was mandated, and it did work. Together, these factors made the country a perfect place to launch a local prevention program at a large scale, aiming, ideally, for the eradication of the disease.

According to Kuliev, the Cypriot success in eradicating thalassemia impacted the WHO's priorities as a whole: "Having all the stuff, we formulated for Halfdan

Mahler . . . the program of community control of thalassemia in Cyprus. [He] was impressed by the technique, and he decided to re-establish the programme of genetics." Moreover, this local "archetype" (Beaudevin 2010, 300) directly inspired the community approach advocated by the WHO expert group on human genetics. Kuliev explained:

> You could cover the whole population of Cyprus, which was half a million. . . .
> For this reason, we thought about the approach for community control. . . . So,
> at that point, we thought that it was very easy to overcome and investigate the
> whole community. And to use thalassemia as an example to demonstrate how
> genetics could work. . . . The approach was specifically for Cyprus. . . . In Cyprus,
> all the marriages go in the church, the church would be requested to ask for the
> certificate of testing of thalassemia genes. . . . And because [of that], all the pop-
> ulation was under control and all of them went to the screening, to the Thalas-
> semia center in Cyprus, which was giving them certificates.[12]

The advisory group's early works on the community control of hereditary ane-mia, established at WHO in 1981, mostly emerged from this success story. For instance, two pillars of the community approach—sensitization and the popula-tion's involvement in the WHO experts' recommendations—were rooted in the emphasis, within the Cypriot program, on the local potential for health informa-tion diffusion and the promotion of "community involvement."[13]

In May 1983, a Cypriot delegation reported at the World Health Assembly that their country had "become the first . . . [to be] at the edge of the eradication of thal-assemia," which sounded like "a miracle" to Kuliev. Later, still predicated on the Cypriot testing ground, the head of the Human Genetics Unit "[announced] to the whole world that thalassemia can be prevented," in an eloquent article in *World Health Forum* (Kuliev 1986). Such a visibly effective program of eradication thus provided an ideal basis for continuing to develop preventive strategies and tools and to expand interest in genetic medicine.

In the early 1980s, Kuliev continually supported the Archbishop Makarios III Hospital's Thalassaemia Centre in its application for a WHO technical services agreement to the construction global standards. For instance, he argued in 1984 that "operational research . . . under way in the Institution . . . might be of consid-erable relevance to the WHO Hereditary Diseases Program," notably "on commu-nity knowledge and attitudes to the control of hereditary disease."[14] Throughout the decade, the center received WHO grants to undertake further investigation into "community knowledge and attitude to the control of hereditary diseases" and to "assist in training for population screening and fetal diagnosis of hereditary ane-mia." The Cypriot experience therefore remained a convenient testing ground for eradicating hereditary disorders. Indeed, beyond thalassemia management, the Cypriot model gathered momentum to the point of providing the initial protocol for tackling hemoglobin disorders and even "other genetic disorders on a global basis" (Boyo et al 1983).

However, the idea that a local "laboratory" could incubate global efforts for the control of genetic disorders presumed the transferability of the Cypriot program. WHO experts kept emphasizing the country's community approach as one that should be generalized and incorporated into the health services (preferably the primary care systems) of developing countries with high prevalence of thalassemia (the Mediterranean and Southeast Asia) and hemoglobin disorders more broadly. In 1990, the next head of the WHO Hereditary Disease Program, Victor Boulyjenkov, still assumed that the Cypriot "thalassemia control program deserves the recognition of serving as a model for other such programs which could be established in other countries in the EMRO [Eastern Mediterranean Regional Office]. . . . ."[15] More than a test site, "the local" appeared to be applicable to larger populations, and as such was "advisable for all countries where [hemoglobinopathies] are endemic" (Boyo, Cao et al. 1983).

Simultaneously, Cyprus remained a very special case. Awareness of its limited transferability still stands out in Kuliev's account:

> The idea was community [disease] control . . . because our idea was that you cannot control the conditions without covering the whole community, [when] you have identified everybody who is in the community. And this approach was not possible in bigger countries. Absolutely impossible in the United States, for example, where there is not any community control procedure. It's only family-based. So, . . . it was possible only in some social [health systems] like Greece, UK, France, and so on. But at the same time, in big countries it is impossible to do, as there was not [a] filter, like the church.[16]

Such a dilemma, which is barely perceptible in the debates surrounding community genetics, shows that Cyprus was somehow an illusion, a local constructed by fantasies of an immobile, docile community that extended only as far as social bonds of religions and marriage. To what extent, then, would experimenting at a small scale bear fruit at a global level? Bypassing that question, WHO experts continued to use the Cypriot program as a hybrid reference—that is to say, it was both a matchless case and a replicable model, fostering global standards. It was a local par excellence.

THE LOCAL AS SITE OF INNOVATION

In the late 1980s, tuberculosis (TB)—a life-threatening but treatable airborne, infectious disease—reentered universalized health's sphere of concern. Global health's strategies, values, and epistemics applied particularly well to the disease. Consequently, the globalization of an already-transnational disease involved simultaneous processes of localization and delocalization. To study these processes, we examine two local pilot projects for what would, by 1997, become a global TB intervention. In doing so, we consider the institutions, people, and practices that connected locals in a nascent global web. For instance, laboratories require webs of

connectivity to produce knowledge, and science relies on networks of comparability (Shapin and Schaffer 1985). We consider transformations necessary to move
data, practice, and ideas from a local laboratory in Tanzania to another in India.
Such movement involved standardization and localizations of communication,
comparability, intelligibility, portability, and mutability. The new forms of exchange
between locals are one effect of an imaged global scale of health on particular practices and data. They also create and reshape networks.

The Tanzanian and Indian projects were nodes in 1990s postcolonial networks
of TB expertise, but by the turn of the millennia, the pilots had transformed those
very networks of knowledge. The first project, implemented in Tanzania by the
International Union against TB and Lung Disease, elaborated a novel and draco-
nian approach to TB treatment at a national scale (National Tuberculosis and Leprosy Control Unit 1987). The project used a standardized diagnostic process and
treatment regimen overseen by healthcare workers rather than patients to transcend the local as clinic, nation, and poverty.[17] The second project, run in a TB clinic
in Mumbai, encouraged physicians and technocrats to implement the Tanzanian
protocol and simultaneously transformed the health system and Indian TB science
(Sarin and Dey 1995). Taken together the two projects, or forms of the local, elabo-
rate global health's local laboratories and demonstrate the ways objects and practices accrue a sense of being local through practice, use, and remembering.

These locals, however, were influenced by changes in global institutions like the
WHO and the World Bank. In a situation akin to the Human Genetics Unit, the
WHO's Geneva-based TB Unit struggled and withered in the 1980s (McMillen
2015). Despite the introduction of TB treatment in the 1940s, TB rates seemed to
have increased or stagnated in countries throughout the developing world. There
was—according to the WHO's 1993 declaration of TB as a global emergency—little
interest or capacity to manage the disease outside of Europe and North America
(World Health Organization Global Tuberculosis Programme 1994). TB treatment
at a global scale existed only as pharmaceutical aspiration. Even the TB Unit's two
staff members focused on drug discovery. Aside from the fiscally struggling International Union against Tuberculosis, TB epidemiology and control were the problems of nation-states and bilateral cooperative agreements, not global institutions.

This changed in the late 1980s, when Hiroshi Nakajima became the WHO's
director general. In 1989 he appointed Arata Kochi, a Japanese compatriot, to lead
the TB Unit. As Kochi settled in, he published articles outlining the need for a global
TB control strategy and uniform tools to assess TB programs (Kochi 1990–91; Sudre,
Ten Dam et al. 1992; Raviglione, Snider et al. 1995). The WHO and its officers had
never advocated for such a global standardization before. Kochi hired a young
Italian physician fresh out of the Harvard School of Public Health. The recruit
began increasing the WHO's presence in local TB treatment by providing technical assistance. Ultimately, he led a team that transformed one local program, then
a cluster of replications, and then created a globalized paradigm. In an interview
he explained:

I wrote a protocol based on what I had done in Italy and in Afghanistan, and what I had learned at Harvard. Kochi read it and it is lucky that he did not fire me. Instead he said, "Well, what if we start with a new protocol. We can write it by learning what the Union is doing in Tanzania and Malawi." So, we went to Malawi for several days, and Karel Styblo was there. So were several others who had run the program and we talked it out for several days and we came up with a protocol for the WHO. We started by focusing on what Karel had done in Tanzania. I carried my copy of the "Manual of the National Tuberculosis/Leprosy Program in Tanzania" to Afghanistan even before the meeting, and I used it whenever I had a doubt. So, we sat in Malawi and we discussed the forms they used, and the kinds of diagnosis, and how to do observation and everything. And we transformed it directly—with the help of two women from the CDC [U.S. Centers for Disease Control and Prevention] who know how to do these things—into a set of training modules that we could distribute to countries.[18]

Thus, the group extrapolated a global strategy from a local national program and its guide Karel Styblo, scientific director at International Union against TB. Styblo, as much as the WHO actors, facilitated the globalization of the Tanzanian experiment. He insisted on running a local intervention of drugs known to be effective as if it was a drug trial. He wanted to show quantifiably that his combination of diagnosis, pharmaceuticals, and patient control could cure a high rate of those enrolled. One prerequisite for this outcome was that he enrolled only patients whom he could prove to have TB through sputum-smear microscopy. By enrolling only the verifiably infected, he could use laboratory evidence to show a change of state among patients' smears, from the demonstrated presence to the absence of tuberculosis bacilli. By proving the efficacy of individual cure, Styblo hoped to avoid the need for a population-level effect. Instead of pointing to lower rates of TB throughout the population, he could show the effects of a treatment regimen followed to the letter. Styblo used this careful data collection and analytic process in a particular place and population to make claims about planetary possibilities, just as experimental evidence is used to make arguments about life outside the lab. Despite several years of lobbying by the International Union against Tuberculosis, it was only when Styblo had amassed enough evidence of his project's potential that the WHO and World Bank took interest.

The team then transformed the project from local to global by using it as a pattern for standardizing tools and training. First, they began making Styblo's Tanzanian model portable by creating training materials. The WHO published these training modules as global knowledge, with no specific connection to Tanzania. By erasing the place in which they were created, the training modules transformed what was once a local intervention into a context-independent experiment that was the basis of a globally portable health regime. Nonetheless, this particular local was always already global since the Tanzanian program was originally implemented by another global institution—the International Union against TB and Lung Disease—utilizing the colonial health system's material and knowledge infrastructure (Farmer 2005; Street 2014; McMillen 2015; Packard 2016).

Laboratories are full of training manuals that standardize laboratory practices. These texts provide details about how to stabilize and manipulate objects in order to understand what may happen when a new regimen, tool, or technique is introduced. They also provide a format for inscription techniques (tables, calculi, and reporting sheets) that can be standardized across a larger scientific public to make health global (Latour and Woolgar 1979; Shapin and Schaffer 1985; Haraway 1997). Manuals, inscription techniques, training, and standardized treatment protocols facilitate the sanitization of a local, but they also bring it into scalar processes of comparison and accounting, as Styblo's work prefigured. Nonetheless, attempts to experimentalize the local do not always go smoothly. For instance, when the Tanzania protocol and training materials came to India, they were received as anything but objective and useful.

India had long been a site for testing TB drugs, both because of medical expertise and bioavailability. Managing and documenting this experimentation was a key role of India's TB institutions. Scientists in these institutes carefully monitored field sites and collected long-term epidemiological statistics about them so that the effects of new ways of managing TB could be traced and operations research conducted (Jagota 2000). These projects were led and implemented by Indians from the 1960s until the 1990s, when a new set of TB pilot sites were established to help work out the best ways to organize care and help avoid some of the issues that might occur after scale-up. In late 1992, Indian TB experts suggested that new TB pilots to ready India for a World Bank loan should be run in the existing experimental areas near the three important institutes in Agra, Bangalore, and Chennai. These plans were scrapped by early 1993, however, after an initial review determined that the proposed pilots were too similar to India's existing treatments and incommensurable with the Tanzania project. When finally initiated ten months later, the new pilots would be monitored directly by the Ministry of Health with support from the WHO and frequent appraisal visits by the World Bank. As such, they would need to be in cities and rural areas that were far both from these existing TB institutes and close to routes of international expert circulation. Moreover, in order to predict the projects' outcomes at a national scale "if maximal inputs were given," sites would need to be in those places where the primary health care system functioned well. Thus, global flows and burgeoning asymmetries in expertise worked to limit sites where the local could be meaningful.

Mumbai's municipal corporation hosted one of these pilots. In a rather stark inversion of the local as an unpredictable place with factors like language, culture, community, and infrastructure that make it unamenable to global health, this local was chosen precisely because it was more open to global health intervention. Its medical staff and bureaucracy were largely anglophone and its role as a major economic hub gave it a privileged place in national infrastructures. This local was keyed even into national resources and could be modified by adjusting existing infrastructural settings as needed. One of the pilot administrators linked the kinds of resources provided by the state to particular locals and to a form of experimentation that might predict the future. He said:

> You know we picked those areas where the health system was stronger. Mumbai, Gujarat, Delhi, etcetera, because we knew that all the necessary resources could be there. We really wanted to see what it could do when the program in India was given the very best inputs. Besides, when you do something, you want to do it where it is a best-case scenario, so that you can argue for more resources by saying, "Look, if we put in maximal resources this is the output we will get." That is how you convince people to change.[19]

The Mumbai clinic could mediate the fragility of infrastructures, and extra resources could be given, he suggested, to "see what would happen if everything worked well." This way of identifying a particular place as manageable meant that its connectivities could be modulated and its health resources, particularly those like staff, raw material, and pharmaceuticals that rarely functioned at the same time, could be concentrated. The test here was not of the Indian context but of efficacy in a hypothetically well-functioning Indian health system. The local is a space in which new tasks are measured for their operability rather than population-level effects. Interventions here can occur so as to reveal what may be possible at the global, international, and epidemiological levels. The idea that a particular outcome in a single "local," if given optimal resources, can predict the future of an intervention at larger scale makes for the local as a part of a mosaicked global that is known through specific versions of the local as well as international organizations. The local is a laboratory and an advertisement.

The idea that these locals are controlled and known, however, may suggest a too easy identification between a local and a lab. The local, particularly those local pilot studies that were to reveal the interaction of global priorities and particularly Indian social and spatial configurations, were simultaneously clinics, neighborhoods, train stations, health posts, and social relations. They were the locus of activity, but global health's TB intervention was not the only activity occurring. The pilots were not even the only TB-related activity in these spaces. As one of Mumbai's pilot physicians explained:

> In those days, my clinic served all of the northwest of Mumbai from the Mithi River to the northern boundary of the city, and they came to Mumbai and asked to start the program in one of the areas. They chose the ward that the clinic was in and the health posts near it to implement the project. This was great. We could focus more easily on implementation because it was nearby, but still, I was the only doctor on staff, and still I had to see all the patients from our catchment area. That meant that maybe only one in ten of my patients was from the project and I had to pick which treatments to give the project ones while also using the only treatment available on the non-project ones. At times it was a little delicate.[20]

This was not her only difficulty. She recalled two other serious challenges. The first was the difficulty posed by the inscription devices that she now had to use to document local progress.

> I was terrible at it. Everyone knew when it came near the time to do the monthly reports. I'm not very good at math, and we would have to go through the register for each patient and I had to know what was happening because they would ask. They would see the report and say that two patients were missing and ask what happened to them, so I had to be ready. My husband, he would do all the math and the tables, but I had to know what information to put in.

The physician's local events, a month of "running up and down chasing patients," had to be fit in a table that could circulate from Delhi to Geneva to Washington.

The inscription of local action into a global traveling text was a monthly hurdle, but the pilot physician's colleagues were even more important local challenges. "No one thought it would work. They thought it was not going to be effective with Indian patients. They said it was developed abroad and would never be acceptable to our patients. I said I did not know, but was going to try it." Indeed, Indian physicians from the public system, medical colleges, and even the health bureaucracy criticized the Tanzania protocol, saying that it was from outside India and would not be suited for India's particularities. They hoped to stay with the older, more flexible program developed in India in the 1960s. What was local in Tanzania was viewed in India as global, "WHO," and foreign.

Indeed, the work of the pilots and of WHO's staff in India was to make the protocol developed elsewhere work locally. They were to build standardized projects that could be shown to itinerant experts. These pilots were like acts of comparison in which new evidence is placed in front of an expanded, expert public (Choy 2011). Though we asked each pilot organizer if they had done anything to tailor the project to their context, none could recall doing so.

To make international protocols acceptable to the local, WHO actors looked to the past and to India's TB institutions. They unearthed publications from the 1950s and 1960s to argue that the new protocol did not indeed come from outside but, rather, was based on studies conducted in India. This project led an anthology of Indian science that supported the DOTS (directly observed therapy short-course) model compiled by Tom Frieden—the WHO's technical officer for DOTS oversight who was stationed in India starting in 1994 and would later become head of the U.S. CDC—and called it the "Annotated Bibliography of DOTS." Using several selective reading strategies, the WHO found a way to make Indian science fit with the Tanzanian protocol and argue that the global program was indeed based on Indian science. This historical reconstruction was so effective that many within India's TB milieu were convinced that the new project was simply a reformulation of that old, local project. One of the implementers tasked with convincing skeptical Indian doctors remembered how useful localizing the origins of DOTS to India was. He said, "We showed them studies that had been conducted in Chennai. They were Indian studies and the science was Indian, so it was an Indian program that the WHO was implementing." These processes of remembering allowed proponents of a global program to suggest that it was local and Indian, even though it had been elaborated on the other side of the Indian Ocean.

These two projects are both localized and standardized to link scales and allow for particular epistemological games to play out. Just as a laboratory is still within the world and survives through traffic to and from the world of business, politics, and labor (Latour and Woolgar 1979), local health interventions remain within the global. However, like the controlled space of the laboratory, the local's relations to the global in global health is mediated by imagining, knowing, and controlling "variables." These translations or mediations blur the lines between aspiration and experiment. They create the local as a controlled environment in which to test particular global experimental objects, like human behavior or pharmaceuticals, while adjusting for variables like finances, history, and microbiology (Rheinberger 1997). These locals are sites where variables and people can be documented, at times controlled, and eventually reduced to the manageable; places where global strategies can be developed, tested, incubated, and monitored before entering the world. At the same time, the local exceeds this experimental paradigm; it is a site of complication and lack of fit (Amrith 2006). Indeed, what localizes a place is a set of factors revealing connection to global similarities, dissimilarities, or imagined futures. These contexts come together in contemporary global public health parlance as a "setting."

SkyCare and the Virtual Global

SkyCare is an erstwhile e-health intervention like those covering the European table. A chain of e-health franchises in the Indian state of Uttar Pradesh, SkyCare incorporated global discourses of social entrepreneurship, transnational pharmaceutical and technological flows, satellite communications infrastructure, and ideas of the market as an effective producer of health. Uttar Pradesh is considered one of global health's most challenging "settings." The SkyCare franchise is a stunning example of the localization of global ideas. Franchises like McDonald's have been key to research on localization and globalization because they show how the local is created by unique intersections of global ideas (Watson 2006). Like McDonald's, the SkyCare franchise tapped into global health's core concepts: markets, technology, pharmaceuticals, quality of care, and even a revolving drug fund, while accounting for local health practices.

SkyCare's designers, aptly named World Health Partners, hoped to implement standardized biomedical techniques in a setting where the state-run public health system has historically struggled. They develop a project to connect patients in Uttar Pradesh to medical experts in Delhi. Local franchisee practitioners, most of whom practiced medicine without training, referred patients to these experts via a "sky clinic"—a telemedicine system located in a franchisee's clinic. Patients were connected to World Health Partners' center by video call to be triaged and treated by physicians there. Patients could buy medicine from the franchisee's Sky Pharmacy or be referred to accredited hospitals nearby. The profits from pharmaceutical sales and consultation fees were to pay the local clinic's overhead and the tele-medicine center's maintenance (Lo 2011; Ravindran 2011). A description of the project in the *Bulletin of the World Health Organization* portrayed SkyCare's fran-chise model as an eminently standardizable, self-sustaining, and mobile inter-vention on the front lines of global health. Its authors write:

> The aim is to improve a socially desirable outcome, such as health, while gener-ating sufficient revenue to be self-sustaining. In social franchising, a franchisor offers a standardized, branded set of products [or] services through franchisees who pay a subscription fee to join the franchisor's network. Franchisees, who are typically existing local providers, in turn, receive training and follow ser-vice delivery protocols established by the franchisor. (Mohanan, Giardili et al. 2017, 343)

The system seemed to work well. In 2011, the Gates Foundation was excited to replicate the project in neighboring Bihar. SkyCare, its proponents argued, would help to standardize Bihar's variegated and corrupt medical landscape by training physicians to think in terms of "protocoled" medicine and by habituating patients to expect a high quality of care (Mohanan, Giardili et al. 2017). At the same time, it would address the state's discouraging health indicators without significant infra-structural inputs. In return for approximately $25 million, the Gates Foundation charged SkyCare with improving the diagnosis and treatment of four conditions at the core of global health: tuberculosis, visceral leishmaniasis, childhood pneu-monia, and diarrhea. The collaboration hoped to provide care in over half of Bihar and to make a dent in epidemiological indicators for these locally endemic diseases in three years (World Health Partners n.d.).

They reasoned that Bihar and Uttar Pradesh, with broadly similar linguistic, socioeconomic, and cultural practices, would be commensurable. Furthermore, if the system could work in particularly difficult contexts like Uttar Pradesh and Bihar, it could work anywhere on earth. World Health Partners aimed to build its parallel social profit system just a few hundred kilometers away from its initial location; practitioners reacted with excitement, with several thousand franchised as SkyCare contact points (World Health Partners n.d.). Those who bought in were excited to have access to cutting-edge communication technol-ogy and the incentives they were promised. There was a catch, however. To become a center in which telemedicine services were located, the physician would need to pay a franchise fee of $500, invest $1,000 in equipment, and pay a one-time $17 access fee (Wharton Business School 2014; Mohanan, Giardili et al. 2017). Franchisee practitioners then received training on treatment protocols and how to use the system.

Business schools like Wharton and the Indian School of Business wrote case studies to help inform other social entrepreneurs, and the project won several inter-national awards (Chavali 2011; Chen 2016). A Wharton publication and its man-agement experts lauded the program as follows:

Shane Walker, associate director, consumer medical devices & digital health at IHS, a global information company providing analysis and insights into industries such as health care, believes that WHP [World Health Partners] has devised a strong model for delivering health care to rural populations. Walker, who has been tracking the WHP model closely, says: 'Broadband connectivity issues are being circumvented with cellphones; last-mile supply challenges are being addressed . . . ; reinforcement of quality standards and monitoring patient adherence is being done through mobile phone apps. I find it really interesting that WHP's model is harnessing indigenous informal health providers as village-level franchisees. Fostering entrepreneurship is a good way to achieve sustainability without a reliance on public sector funds. Their approach of integrating preventive care with curative health care services is also forward-thinking." (Wharton Business School 2014)

As the "forward-thinking" World Health Partners expanded the project across contexts, they made changes to franchise terms to increase standardization. World Health Partners reported that "stricter enforcement of norms and standards have been institutionalized to increase adherence to policies and achieve greater credibility" (World Health Partners n.d., 3). The same document goes on to say that patients, physicians, and infrastructures resisted their efforts to standardize: "A cultural challenge is the promotion of long-term behavioral changes that reduce the target population's dependence on ineffective traditional methods of treatment, especially with regard to diarrhea and pneumonia. An operational challenge has been working with lower levels of technology infrastructure than anticipated" (World Health Partners n.d., 4). These were issues associated with the local or "culture," infrastructure, physician behavior, and scaling up.

After three years, the project was only able to reach about 6 percent of the clinics in their catchment area (Mohanan, Babiarz et al. 2016). Local physicians with good reputations did not need the branding or access to expertise in Delhi through the telemedicine system that SkyCare provided. They were less willing to pay the high franchise fee to access the technology and technology-mediated expertise that might undercut their own. Conversely, practitioners who struggled to attract patients were often more interested in training on simple medical protocols.[21]

By the end of the project, a group of international researchers specializing in the evaluation of large programs like this one found that the project had no effect on childhood diarrhea or pneumonia care among franchisees, let alone an epidemiological effect (Mohanan, Giardili et al. 2017). Franchisees too began to revolt. World Health Partners' franchise agreement required that participating physicians send a portion of their consultation fees to the central hub, and local doctors felt that they were given little in return. Delhi, though near Uttar Pradesh, was too far for Bihari patients to travel. By January 2014, most of India's global health players had decided that the project was a massive failure due to an inability to get local buy-in and provide a service that was of value at the ground level. Some of the project's expatriate global health staff left or were asked to leave while World Health

Partners doubled down on its next project with the Gates Foundation in hopes of putting the "SkyCare fiasco" behind it.

The meteoric rise and fall of SkyCare outlines three aspects of localization. First, localization is at times a translation of global health ideas into situated practices (i.e., the making of a franchise, revolving drug funds, digitalization and pharmaceuticalization, and efficiency). Second, localization is the translation of global health ideas to manage existing practices and respond to local ways of dealing with disease. Third, localization is a movement of practices from one place to another (i.e., circulating experts and technologies through flows to reach a resting point somewhere). Together, SkyCare's three facets of localization reveal that localization occurs in concert with the kinds of globalization that knit together global health. At the same time, the global imagination of the local that shaped SkyCare and the way in which global nodes reconstruct local processes reveals localization in texts and transnational institutions.

COMMUNITY: THE DISCURSIVE LOCAL

The local of global health is not only a space but also refers to the people inhabiting it. The concept of "community" is a widespread but particular iteration of the idea of people inhabiting a local. Experts so frequently imagined the local as a community that the two words are nearly synonymous. For instance, development expert and WHO consultant Peter Oakley uses the two words interchangeably in one of the founding texts on community participation in health and development (Oakley 1989). However, this is not always the case. A community need not necessarily occupy a specific geographical unit, and conversely, a group of people who live in the same area does not always compose a community. In this section, we tackle community as a specific iteration of the local by following community participation in health's conceptual trajectory from the 1978 International Conference on Primary Health Care held in Alma-Ata, Kazakhstan, more commonly the Alma Ata conference, through the 1990s, when "participation" became a buzzword. We argue that it was through the institutionalization of community participation that "the local" as imaginary progressively became an element of global health and development.

Convened by the WHO and the United Nations Children's Fund (UNICEF), the Alma-Ata conference launched the primary health care strategy. The strategy developed at the conference officially aimed at making healthcare based on "practical, scientifically sound and socially acceptable methods and technology" accessible to "individuals and families in the community through their full participation and at a cost that the community and country can afford" (Director General of the World Health Organization and Executive Director of the United Nations Children's Fund 1978). Clearly, community participation was one of the key tenets of the strategy. The Alma-Ata Declaration called on governments to "encourage and ensure full community participation through the effective propagation of relevant information, increased literacy, and the development of the necessary institutional arrangements through which individuals, families, and communities can assume responsibility for their health" (World Health Organization 1978).

The concept of community participation emphasized the idea that communities should be actively involved in the identification of their own health needs, as well as in the planning and implementation of the responses to those needs. This idea had surfaced in development discourse well before Alma-Ata, with the emergence in the 1950s of community development, an oft-cited antecedent of community participation in health. But in the 1970s, community participation resonated with a whole set of new ideas: the postcolonial rejection of vertical programs; the Third World critique of top-down international health and development approaches; the emphasis on self-reliance propagated by the New International Economic Order; the critique of biomedicine and medical authority; and the interest in nonprofessional health knowledge and lay perspectives on health and disease (Packard 2016). Community participation was also in line with Alma-Ata's emphasis on developing local strategies to promote health for all, which was embedded in the concept of "acceptable technologies." Community participation in Alma-Ata encapsulated the idea that the local (understood as an alternative to the imperial, Western, high-tech, and costly) had to be taken into account in health development and that this could only happen if communities were allowed to have a say in the determination of health priorities and the design of responses. As a principle of health development, community participation also resonated with a form of political "triage" of health priorities prevalent in the 1970s.

In the decades following the Alma-Ata conference, the WHO actively promoted community participation in various ways. First, the organization endorsed exchanges between member states on this subject. An example is the interregional workshop held in Brioni, Yugoslavia, in 1985, to discuss the progress and limits of the implementation of community participation. Second, through the 1980s and 1990s, the WHO promoted research that aimed at defining and systematizing the concept of community participation, creating metrics to measure it and identify its correlates in order to facilitate implementation and to make it more "effective" (Agudelo 1983; Rifkin, Muller et al. 1988).[22] In 1989, Peter Oakley was commissioned to write a book that summarized critical issues in the implementation of "community involvement in health"—a formula WHO documents used alongside "community participation"—based on the results of the Brioni workshop (Oakley 1989). Subsequently, the WHO and UNICEF commissioned planning expert Susan Rifkin to research factors that facilitated participation in maternal care, childcare, and family planning (Rifkin 1990). In 1989, the Study Group on Community Involvement in Health Development was created to design recommendations and methodologies to implement and evaluate community participation. In all of these projects, community was defined as people living in geographical proximity— despite the variability in size from a cluster of houses to an entire nation; community was a proxy for the local.

The local as community could be modeled through standardized methodologies of intervention. Indeed, from the end of the 1980s through the beginning of the 1990s, a growing amount of research sustained the publication of a number of guidelines for the standardized implementation and assessment of community participation. The proliferation of these new global guidelines testify to the progressive emergence of what Lynn Morgan has called an "overly technocratic view of participation" (Morgan 2001).

In WHO documents and guidelines, the concept of community participation is vast and includes a variety of approaches. For instance, in her WHO-sponsored book on community participation, Rifkin (1990) lists at least five, ranging from passive to active participation. Similarly, in his seminal publication on community involvement in health development, Oakley (1989) situates participation along a scale that goes from "participation as a means" for achieving predetermined health objectives to participation "as an end" in and of itself.

Despite recognizing that these approaches were profoundly different (in the above-mentioned publications), the WHO acknowledged all of them—including the more "utilitarian"—as forms of community participation and thus intrinsically valuable. This legitimacy was further reinforced by the way the WHO framed the objectives of community participation. Indeed, in its documents the WHO framed the objectives of community participation as stressing the efficiency and effectiveness of health programs and ensuring community self-reliance, including economic self-reliance. For instance, the WHO's Study Group on Community Involvement in Health Development listed the advantages of participation as follows: better coverage of services and development projects; improved efficiency and effectiveness of services; better equity among the members of the community; and self-reliance, with people taking responsibility for their health (World Health Organization 1991, 5). This was echoed in WHO-sponsored methodological guidelines for assessing and measuring community participation, which ranked resource mobilization in and by the community, through fees or other methods, as indicators of good participation (Rifkin, Muller et al. 1988).

In the wake of structural adjustment programs in the late 1980s, community participation could also become a mechanism for complying with the imperative of "cost-effectiveness" insisted on in the terms for loans provided by international institutions. Taking the mounting scarcity of public resources after 1985 into account, the WHO actually proposed community participation as a means for improving efficiency and cost-effectiveness despite budgetary constraints.[23] In particular, the WHO's plans for funding primary health care strategy featured *community funding* along with users' fees and private insurance as *alternative sources of finance*. More decisively, the technical discussion on funding national health-for-all programs, held during the Fortieth World Health Assembly in 1987, explicitly proposed community involvement in health development and the decentralization of decision making as tenets of a strategy to respond to increasing budgetary constraints and to maximize effectiveness.[24] Reframing community participation as a tool for facing budgetary constraints is but one example of the way the WHO tried to strategically adapt to a changing context—in this case the ascendance of austerity policies—while maintaining its priorities (Chorev 2012).

It is worth noting, however, that the acceptance of the logic of budgetary constraints and cost recovery was only one phase of this process of strategic adaptation.[25]

In resonance with these overarching discourses, health policymakers often interpreted community participation as meaning that local communities contributed labor, material, and financial resources to the implementation of health measures whose objectives were decided by experts and bureaucrats. This perspective was not unknown to WHO leaders in the field. A WHO report on primary health care implementation issued sixteen years after the Alma-Ata Declaration explained that "while there is a general agreement on the importance of community participation in health development . . . studies carried out in all WHO Regions show that passive participation, in which the public utilizes the health services and contributes money, materials, and labor, is fairly widespread. Yet active community involvement, in terms of the planning and management of health activities, is still uncommon" (Tarimo, Webster et al. 1994, 20).

Indeed, in the 1990s, in a context marked by mounting critiques of structural adjustments, authoritarian initiatives like population control, and "old-style development" (Connelly 2008; Chorev 2012), "community participation" met growing success in international health and development discourse and became a buzzword (Cooke and Kothari 2001; Leal 2010). It was enthusiastically embraced by organizations such as the Organization for Economic Cooperation and Development (OECD), UNICEF, and the World Bank (Kahssay and Oakley 1999). Indeed, at this time community participation as self-reliance resonated with the ascendance of neoliberalism as a style of governance focusing on individuals, costs, and benefits. It is in this decade that the WHO proposed "supporting the empowerment of communities for health development" as one of the key elements of community participation (World Health Organization 1991, 9). It is worth noting that in the 1990s, mainstream development and health experts co-opted the concept of empowerment, which was previously associated with alternative approaches to development, and emptied it of its critical meaning (Al Dahdah 2017). In the 1990s, the new mantra was that empowering individuals—in particular women—and communities was the best way to help them autonomously fulfill their needs and become active contributors to economic development. As many authors have remarked, empowerment became a buzzword in the development jargon of the 1990s because it encapsulated neoliberal critiques of welfare and "dependence" as well as discourses of "human capital enhancement" (Sharma 2008; Baqué and Biewer 2013; Murphy 2017). The association of community participation with empowerment in the WHO discourse could easily be articulated within all of these ideas.

The trajectory of community participation from Alma-Ata through the 1990s provides interesting insights into the place of localization in the emergence of global health. The concept of community participation emerged in the 1970s—a period conventionally framed as preceding the era of global health—from the idea that the local should count in health planning and that local people's voice should be represented in decision making. Nevertheless, while making its way into health governance discourse, community participation was progressively made into a formula through its standardization and translation into a set of methodological packages. In its effort to define methodologies to implement and assess community participation, the WHO participated in the paradoxical tendency in community development to standardize participatory health planning. This tendency was paradoxical because it contradicted the commitment to move away from top-down blueprint approaches to health that were at the basis of the creation of community participation (Morgan 1993; Gujit and Shah 1998). Through the production of research and methodologies, the WHO contributed to transforming community participation from a quintessentially contextual and site-specific (i.e., local) process rooted in the unique history of each place (Morgan 1993, 4) into a transferrable standard package. In this process, the local as community, with its irreducible specificities, became nothing but a slogan or a discursive element in international health jargon.

Once detached from its initial set of ideas and made into a standard package, community participation could easily be aligned with the new logics of austerity and neoliberalism prevalent in the 1980s and 1990s. Neoliberal rationality proposed community participation as a tool for tapping into local resources in times of austerity and making people productive actors in their own development. This transformation granted community participation enduring success during the structural adjustment policies of the 1980s and health sector reform in the 1990s.

The Local as Hub of Global Circulations

Moving beyond global health as a field to examine processes of health globalization reveals localization from a new angle. Health globalization and its arenas highlight the inextricable links existing between localization, circulation, and space. Whether located in the elusive global arena or in an easily identifiable local hospital, everything occupies space. This obvious point provides the backbone to understand processes of localization in health globalization. There must be a ground or tangible space on which localization takes place. Transnational, Asian medical knowledge transmission and patients' international mobility help ground localization.

People, objects, ideas, policies, and institutions circulate through vast and highly heterogeneous networks. They follow circuits, shift direction, change meaning, and get connected and transformed. Claude Markovits and his colleagues put it boldly: "In circulating, things, men, and notions often transform themselves. Circulation is therefore a value-loaded term which implies an incremental aspect and not the simple reproduction across space and time of already formed structures and motions" (Markovits, Pouchepadass et al. 2003, 2–3). Even location itself, writes James Clifford (1997, 11), is "an itinerary rather than a bounded site—a series of encounters and translations." Being mobile and fluid, these people, things or institutions move from one place to the other, but they are always anchored in specific (but changing) grounded spaces that play important roles in defining them. Objects, for example, are context specific, as studies in science and technology have taught us. The status of an Ayurvedic drug is modified when that drug leaves India and arrives in a country with a different legal environment; from being a medicine in India, the drug becomes a health supplement, a functional food, or a nutraceutical elsewhere. In this context, this shift in category (and meaning) is consubstantial with international circulation (Janes 2002; Pordié 2008, 2015). People also experience translocality and transformation when they go across international borders; these changes may bear on their subjectivity (Langford 2002) and on their biology and physiology, subject as they are to transport, jet lag, food intake, medicine, weather, and pathogens. Travel and place help produce distinct corporality: "diverse kinds of travel produce diverse kinds of *re-localized* (i.e., traveling) bodies and biologies" (Roberts and Scheper-Hughes 2011, 21).

While studying networks is central to understanding circulations in global health, examining place highlights the way these networks overlap and collide; thus, the two domains of inquiry should be practiced concomitantly. In order to grasp how a place is socially, culturally, and materially produced, transformed, and inhabited, we need to look at processes. Take the case of an Ayurvedic spa in southern India, belonging to a successful chain of about twenty high-class, standardized centers prominent in the wellness tourism industry and spread across the country and abroad (Pordié 2011). These centers are part of a reputed Indian hotel brand and their clientele is mostly foreign. The average stay of the clients within the spa premises amounts to a couple of hours. However, these clients circulate in a global space that includes the spa as the nodal point of several networks and as a hub for processes of health globalization. What actually brings stability to this hub are the Indians who staff it. Although some may come from states located hundreds of miles away to seize a job opportunity, once at work they become immobile, stabilizing agents. These agents (managers, therapists, cleaners, gardeners, accountants) form the backbone of the global space; they allow for its functioning and sustainability. In this case, the suggested unit of analysis is the spa itself and everything that constitutes it—from the geographically immobile people, institutions, objects, and technologies to the international patients and their means of mobility (such as cars, airplanes, and credit cards). While the dialectical interaction between national territory and global space must be acknowledged and closely examined (Robinson 1998), the significance of the local in health globalization here is exemplary, as it is in general in the medical travel industry: it is a national construct with cross-border appeal and global aspirations.

To be effective and operational, a local hub in health globalization must be embedded in networks that extend beyond borders and must comprise circuits (which may involve new territorial arrangements) that converge within definite places, such as hospitals, clinics, health insurance offices, and international agencies. Such places are situated contexts that house global activities. These locations and networks both result from and produce specific assemblages (Ong and Collier 2005) that crystallize in particular places and moments in time. This does not preclude the fact that these assemblages are fluid; they may change patterns and content while at the same time being prone to a relatively time- and space-bound stability. This merging of places and networks, mobile and immobile agents, technologies and materials plays an instrumental role in the making of health globalization.

A network is qualified by both circulations and linkages, each of which presents different problems. Circulations are plural in form; the nature of the circuits varies according to what or who circulates and where it goes to and comes from. Thus, Chinese drugs follow different circuits than influenza vaccines, pharmaceutical raw materials, Ayurvedic medical knowledge, or Filipino nurses. The same heterogeneity applies to linkages that may be of different intensities depending on whether or not people meet in person, have physical contacts, or communicate through the Internet. Of particular interest for us is that linkages and interactions happen and intensify in specific places that result from the crystallization invoked above, whether it is a hospital, a spa, a teaching center, a multilateral health institution, or specific places connected through cyberspace. These are hubs that allow health globalization to actually take *place*. They localize it.

Spaces in health globalization may take various shapes. In the case of distance education in Ayurveda, linkages are exercised in cyberspace. Ayurvedic therapeutic knowledge is transmitted from India, through the Internet, to international students located anywhere in the world. It is a form of transnationalism that can be described as "virtual migration" (Aneesh 2015), where all human actors are geographically immobile. None of them embodies the transnational the way a migrant would, but all have the possibility of extending into other places and times through their virtual modes of communication. There is an "in-betweenness of social practices linking different local contexts, but not strictly reducible to any of them" (Boccagni 2012, 120). Here virtual contacts within a virtual space—which comprises concrete people and things, such as the teachers, their house, the students and their homes, computers, satellites, physical correspondence, and so on—take a tangible form in knowledge transmission in the granting of certificates and, ultimately, in newly acquired therapeutic practices. Once established and stabilized, a hub in health globalization is characterized by intensifying linkages that foster exchanges. In this case, these exchanges contribute to the production and transformation of therapeutic knowledge and practices; Ayurveda is adjusted and transformed *in order to* become global, for instance, by withdrawing sensory experiences and oral knowledge, two modalities absent from "cyber Ayurveda." These transformations involve creativity and imagination—a social practice characteristic of globalization (Appadurai 1996). However, imagination here is not only affected by the desires of those at great social, cultural, and geographic distance but also by linkages in the form of contacts, discussions, interactions, and frictions between individuals on a planetary scale—be it through the Internet, phone calls, therapeutic interventions, or teachings in a classroom. Medical culture is reorganized across space and time and contributes to the formation of new "translocal cultures" (Gupta and Ferguson 1992; Clifford 1997), albeit in very concrete places.

This is not to say that clinics, hospitals, classrooms, and cyberspatial nodes remain stable indefinitely. In fact, change happens all the time as attempts are made to increase the level of linkages and interactions in a particular place, often with the aim of promoting commercial development. One evident situation is branding and marketing in the medical and wellness travel industry (Crooks, Turner et al. 2011; Pordié 2011). A variety of strategies have been deployed in most Asian countries, from drafting and implementing specific national policies to establishing international accreditations and certifications for health institutions. In general, medical institutions rely on a growing global awareness of the hospital brand and the reputation of the country, such as Singapore for Indonesian patients, or of the city—for example, hospitals in Bangalore, India, are trading on the city's reputation as "India's Silicon Valley" and thus a center for the knowledge-based service economy and scientific expertise. In other places, the context of medical and wellness tourism is significantly different. The Indian state of Kerala has a well-established tourism industry and is a major center for Ayurvedic tourism. This has allowed the Indian state to create the brand "Kerala Ayurveda" in an attempt to attract an increasing number of patients. Given the growing popularity of medical travel worldwide, the success of Ayurvedic tourism and the high volumes of tourists who were already coming to India, various cities and states, such as Kerala, have also sought to expand their "biomedical tourism" industry. This has led to collaboration between entrepreneurs and state governments in many places in India as efforts are made to rebrand the country as a global healthcare destination. Specialized travel agencies and guidebooks, as well as medical structures in the West and health insurance companies in Asia and abroad, work together to reinforce not only circulations but also, and most importantly, linkages in global health networks.

Efforts directed at increasing linkages have entailed a profound reorganization and transformation of medical and wellness infrastructures everywhere. Corporate hospitals have opened specialist accommodation wings, providing rooms equipped with cable television, telephones, sofas, fridges, and air-conditioning and modifying the aesthetics and functionality of medical space (Evans, Crooks et al. 2009). Ideally, medical travel involves the rapid transfer of people from the airport to the hospital—which, interestingly, often shares some characteristics with the new design of airports, such as cleanliness, impersonality, and brisk temperatures—and the provision of foodstuffs from patients' countries or places of origin in order to make them as comfortable as possible. Some of the key staff working in "medical tourist wards" have experience working overseas, are well versed in foreign languages, and consider themselves more aware of cultural considerations. The industry has realized that it needs to adapt and learn from patient responses to intercultural differences and to use this knowledge to minimize cultural frictions in the future.

As far as biomedical travel is concerned, people are realizing that it is necessary to promote a generic, sanitized, pristine medical environment built on international standards and the qualifications, expertise, and international experience of doctors. Biomedical travel is therefore based on a principle of "cultural insulation." Healthcare professionals are trying to create a globalized, culturally neutral space that will be familiar to all, in order to develop a better fit between the visiting patients and the host hospital. Many medical care seekers do not feel comfortable traveling to another country for treatment; some have never traveled abroad before. Therefore, minimizing cultural difference is extremely important to the success of medical travel ventures. Biomedical entrepreneurs are increasingly learning to decouple the word "medical care" from "tourism," preferring to frame their clients as "international patients." These international patients may not be interested in the local culture or place, so providers seek to insulate them as much as possible from it, perhaps offering an optional, one-day trip to a famous and easily accessible temple or monument. Practitioners also appear to prefer to learn and work within the common globalized language and practice of biomedicine, where cultural differences are recognized and removed. Here, universality of therapeutic practice is sought after to ease linkages and interactions.

While local culture is played down in biomedical hospitals, it is emphasized in other forms of therapies. Ayurveda or Thai massage, for example, is perceived to be based on tradition, heritage, and nature, and the corresponding centers or clinics are more often than not located in pleasant, restorative, nurturing, tropical environments. Interior design, furniture, music, and atmosphere are chosen in relation to healing and traditions and form an integral part of the therapeutic service and experience. In these contexts, the visitor's ability to learn about the place and interact with the local culture is of significant importance. However, issues of translation are ever-present in that the "cultural experience" and place are represented, adapted, and translated to meet the needs, demands, and expectations of foreigners, including their cultural conceptions of the body, wellness, "traditional medicines," age, and gender.

In each of these configurations, circuits and circulations congregate at the networks' nodal points, where linkages deepen and interactions intensify. Hospitals, health centers, international organizations' offices, or (virtual) classrooms are such sites of coalescence in global health. They incarnate a type of grounding in health globalization that forms one possible and specific way of localizing.

CONCLUSION

These diverse processes of making sense of something called "the local" within global health are central to the field's mode of understanding and acting in the world. Indeed, the cases presented here reveal a slow and iterative process of making global health scientific. They show the creation of commensurable and portable knowledge that can be deployed at population scale. We then demonstrated how that knowledge can also be created in the periphery, in new locals, by adhering to processes of commensurability and engaging circuits of roving experts who would knit these circuits together and to the metropolis. Next, the chapter established how global ideas condense in particular places as projects, which are tested and, though lauded for their excellent fit with global priorities, are unable to show an effect in the local. We then toggled back in time to consider just one of those ideas, "community," to elucidate how the tenets or formulas required to make locals commensurable came to be. Finally, we considered those zones that, though harboring traces of global health's formulas, fail to engage in processes of localization and commensurability and thus remain outside the scientized field.

Localization as process allows us to highlight how "the local" is simultaneously discursive, material, territorial, and experimental. It is both central and peripheral as a site of knowledge creation and is a process that enables the creation of deterritorialized synthetic knowledge. By looking at these processes, we have made sense of the ways that global health employs methodologies that resemble science to establish the bounds of a field as well as the rules of play.

We have shown how localization is a font of ideas and a foil of commensurability. It is both cause and effect of global health. By considering processes that make the local knowable, representable, and comparable—and thus no longer local—we have looked from the anthropologists' privileged loci of knowledge. We have seen flashes of the global, but more importantly, we have seen how dreams of commensurability grow and swallow up the processes that created them. Perhaps a disciplinary myopia encourages us to recuperate the local within global health, but this is also a project of situating the knowledge that global health aggregates in the name of accountability, evidence-based action, and global science. Whether localization is about community or genes or protocols or pills or commensurability, separating foreground and background and looking at processes of localization shows how global health's knowledge is made from experimentation, movements through space, and the creation of replicable formulas. Its laboratory is simultaneously the world and the village, and people are both the test and the control.

CHAPTER 2

Metrics for Development

Anne M. Lovell, Jean-Paul Gaudillière,
Claudia Lang, and Claire Beaudevin

Global health metrics share with other types of statistics and indicators a certain magical power (Merry 2011, 14), which gives rise to a faith in their objectivity and capacity to replace subjective judgments. This authority of numbers is not new, of course; it emerges with the birth of nation-states in the early nineteenth century and can be traced to earlier eras (Porter 1996; Desrosières 2002). What distinguishes the use of numbers in current neoliberal regimes from earlier periods is their ability to extend the ethos of accountability and the economization of life (Murphy 2017).

No metric more strongly illustrates global health in its institutional and political dimensions than the vast series of numbers gathered in the Global Burden of Disease (GBD). The GBD, a massive data collection enterprise, is currently run and made available by the Institute for Health Metrics and Evaluation (IHME) at the University of Washington with the financial support of the Bill and Melinda Gates Foundation (hereafter Gates Foundation).[1] This metric encompasses something quite different from other numbers circulating within the global health field, such as clinical trial results, statistics for tuberculosis (TB), or the number of people living with human immunodeficiency virus (HIV) worldwide. The GBD belongs to a more complex transformative process than that captured in critiques of counting, "gaming the metrics," "accountability fixation," or "putting numbers before people." Our analysis thus moves beyond these general effects of numbers (Muller 2018) to examine an economized technoscientific imaginary nourished by the comparative capacity built into the GBD.

Social scientists and global health actors alike have analyzed the meaning of the GBD's rise (Arnesen and Nord 1999; Birn 2009; Birn, Pillay et al. 2009; Adams 2016a, 2016b). Frequently, it is approached as the highly visible symbol of the transition from "international public health" to "global health." The resultant political order of nongovernmental organizations (NGOs), transnational corporations, pharmaceutical companies, and influential foundations (Brown, Cueto et al. 2006) also materializes through the diffusion of new tools, standards, programs for

accessing drugs, and technologies—sometimes derived from corporate management and attendant standard procedures, accounting systems, and performance
indicators (Reubi 2018). Private initiative, markets, management, and individual
choice are the keywords of this new world of health, often defined as one more
manifestation of the neoliberal transformation of government originating in the
1980s Washington Consensus on economic policies.[2]

This chapter brings perspectives from medical history, the sociology of metrics,
and medical anthropology to the history of the GBD to tell a larger story about
the economic turn in health and the health turn in the economics of development.
Drawing on reports, archives, interviews with actors from the World Bank and the
World Health Organization (WHO), from networks centered on particular health
conditions, and from national and subnational health administrations, we analyze
the construction and the social and political uses of the GBD. We observe the GBD
retrospectively and in real time to discern how the metric and its institutional
embedding have been achieved, resisted, and transformed.

The history of the GBD can be observed in two seasons, like a TV political
drama. Season 1 covers the construction of this metric through a combination of
health data and an external economic calculus involved in the World Bank's "health
turn": a shift from massive infrastructural development projects to human capital
investments in health and education in the 1990s. This first season, reveals the dis-
junction between how the GBD was conceptualized then and how it was actually
applied in global health policymaking by showing that the World Bank gradually
abandoned national health planning, even as it has continued to invest in global
health projects. After some dormancy, the GBD reappears in Season 2, from the
mid-2000s, as an enterprise of the university-affiliated IHME, funded by the Gates
Foundation. In the hands of think tanks, consulting firms, governmental institutions, NGOs, universities, and the WHO, the GBD moves from development economics to the health arenas of low- and middle-income countries (LMIC). Before
turning to these seasons specifically, let us examine the GBD metric itself.

Metrics, in their simplest form, represent standards of measurement for time,
space, and other dimensions applied through the use of timepieces, yardsticks,
thermometers, and similar instruments. The GBD incorporates a measure of the
relative magnitude of a disease, disorder, injury, or related condition, and its burden, in relation to time (e.g., the duration of a healthy life) and across space (e.g., a
world region). It combines mortality (quantity of life) and disability (quality of life).
Unlike many global governance indicators prevalent today, GBD data never stand
for single diseases; they are of interest only in relation to other diseases (Rottenburg, Merry et al. 2015). These relationships can be expressed through equivalence
in disability, internal to the GBD, and through equivalence in terms of reduced
productivity and economic losses, external to the GBD.

"Burden" is generated algorithmically as summary measures of disease rates
multiplied by disability weights attributed to vastly different diseases, injuries, and
health conditions. As a result, worldwide disease rankings, previously based mainly
on mortality statistics, now include many noncommunicable diseases (NCDs)

absent from earlier indicators. By making "hidden" conditions like mental disorders and substance use visible, the GBD is able to reflect the epidemiological transition in the South, where deaths from infectious disease and malnutrition now converge with lives lived with disability because of NCDs and injuries. GBD developers and its early institutional supporters (the WHO, the World Bank, and the Harvard University School of Public Health) justify their mission to gather data on disease prevalence and treatment effectiveness as crucial to meeting the epidemiological transition challenge (Jamison, Mosley et al. 1993; Murray, Lopez et al. 1996).

The second equivalence depends on the use to which the GBD is put. This equivalence kindled the economic dream behind the World Bank's original "health turn," whereby investment in human capital, including health (e.g., population-wide health interventions), was hypothesized to be as (or more) cost-effective than investments in infrastructure. The economically measured outcome was imagined as productive (i.e., non-ill or disabled) adult bodies. The technoscientific imaginary of development economists thus assumed that health outcomes could be interpreted in the same terms as the results of building roads or educating girls and would therefore be informative for investment decisions across policy sectors.

Furthermore, the GBD's components, when put to use, provide an evaluative dimension linked to broader socioeconomic concerns. In high-income countries in the 1980s, metrics—evaluative, value-laden sets of indicators—spilled over from business and manufacturing into the service sector and ultimately into institutions and domains of everyday life, from policing to schooling to individual psychology (Muller 2018). Metrics contributed to (and expressed) the "corporatization" of public institutions and services, decline in social protection, and privatization of public goods—in short, the end of Keynesian policies that had buttressed a large public sector. This spillover simultaneously produced an audit culture, an evaluative rationality permeating everyday practices and institutional management (Power 1997). Under the governmentality identified with Thatcherism's neoliberalism (source of the first analyses of audit culture), a particular style of management or, more precisely, of standardized accountability became a governing principle of public- and private-sector institutions, with free market norms as the organizing principle of the state (Power 1997; Shore and Wright 2000).

The GBD emerged during this neoliberal turn as part of an array of tools used by development agencies, international organizations, and eventually philanthropic institutions for economic triage (ranking what to invest in) and governance. Like governance indicators (Merry 2011), GBD reduces complex data to single numbers or ranks, allowing comparison and informing prioritization between highly heterogeneous practices and domains in the same way that a common currency allows for the comparison of commodities. The GBD is entrenched in an audit culture, whereby donors demand specific, highly standardized accountability from loan and fund recipients.[3]

For anthropologist Marilyn Strathern, audit itself has become an actant—an agent of a nonhuman kind in the chain of interactions of self-monitoring men and women who have been deemed responsible for carrying out the now-quantifiable work of organizations (Strathern 2000). While directors of global health programs and their local implementers lie behind it, Strathern's actant can be seen in action when frontline workers resist the demands of audits, as malaria nurses did during the three-year health worker strike in Senegal (Tichenor 2016). The GBD's envisioned power as an accountability tool is reflected by Dean T. Jamison, lead author of the World Bank's 1993 *World Development Report*, who "firmly predict[ed]" that by the 2000s, "the official reporting of health outcomes in dozens of countries and globally will embody the approach and the standards described in the [GBD] series" (Murray, Lopez et al. 1996). The extent to which the GBD has been successfully mobilized for decision making and triage in health governance, however, remains an open question.

As evaluative indicator, the GBD is value-laden as an accountability principle that holds policy and program implementers responsible for meeting operationalized objectives and outcomes. The GBD's architects claim that it incorporates democratic values—namely, transparency, egalitarianism, and accountability (Murray, Lopez et al. 1996). The complexity of the whole GBD enterprise rests on the labor of over 3,150 collaborators in 1,100 research centers, universities, and government units, in addition to paid staff and interns.[4] But while apparently transparent, GBD data and the data's construction and uses are often beyond the capacity of even health professionals to fully grasp. Indeed, this work may not be intended for the general public but rather, as David Reubi suggests, for global anti-tobacco initiatives and other global health experts (Reubi 2018).

Whereas GBD Season 1 existed within a particular development economics and technoscientific imaginary, in Season 2, the GBD becomes the tool of health economics that transforms the framing of health agendas for LMICs. We now turn to the Season 1 GBD, its social uses, and its major statistical component, the disability-adjusted life year, or DALY.

GLOBAL BURDEN OF DISEASE, SEASON 1 (GBD 1):
THE WORLD BANK'S TOOL FOR PRIORITIZING HEALTH INVESTMENTS

The publication of the *World Development Report: Investing in Health* (World Bank 1993) justified escalating investments in health as decisive elements of the World Bank's strategy to alleviate poverty. With the *World Development Report* (hereafter 1993 WDR), the Bank officially departed from its decades-long commitment to a vision of development centered on the building of infrastructures, the rise of agriculture productivity, and—when dealing with populations—birth control.

It is not that health had not been among the World Bank's priorities. The Population, Health, and Nutrition division did increase its focus on health throughout the 1980s, but such investments lacked legitimacy, and most economic modeling done at the Bank considered health as an outcome dependent on infrastructural investments and their impact on economic growth. The 1993 WDR reversed the relationship: Health became worthy of investment because it was an economic factor in itself (Kapur, Lewis et al. 1997; Ruger 2005; Staples 2006). In other words, the burden of disease posed an impediment to growth and therefore to poverty alleviation. The change was not a sudden, dramatic event anchored only in the health crises of the moment, such as those associated with the dramatic impact of the AIDS epidemic. Rather, it had deep roots in internal World Bank debates in the 1980s about the meaning and measure of development (see chapter 3, "Triage beyond the Clinic").

Investing in health thus meant first strengthening public national health systems. In the Bank's eyes, however, public management of health was only thinkable if it proved cost-effective, placed performance center stage, carefully accounted for targets, and measured outcomes. The introduction of the DALYs by the World Bank and the WHO was therefore not only a way to take into account health problems neglected when using the usual mortality statistics. More importantly, it constituted a measure that contributed to balancing problems and solutions, such as whether, in a world of limited resources, tuberculosis chemotherapy was putatively more effective than HIV prevention. Even if DALYs did not extend to development in general because they could not contribute to deciding whether states should invest in genetically improved crops versus in health centers, the dream of a general, money-like equivalent was not far away.

DALYs aggregate mortality and morbidity data by combining two different calculations: years of life lost (YLL), or quantity of life, and years lost to disability (YLD), referring to quality of life. To calculate the YLL for a disease category, condition, or injury, the age distribution of mortality numbers is weighted against averaged life expectancy—factoring in the assumed decrease in economic usefulness at a given age. The DALY innovation, however, lies in the second calculation: years lost to disability. The disability weight for any given category is the ratio between one year of life affected by the pathology under consideration and one year of normal life derived through a speculative health investment survey given to a small number of experts. Christopher Murray and Alan Lopez, the GBD's architects, have explicitly stated that quantifying disease burden, far from being a "neutral exercise, entirely free of value choices," involves precisely that: value choices based on the value placed on life (Murray, Lopez et al. 1996, 7).

It is not surprising, then, that the initial DALY calculation method and its use of a "productive life" as a standard against which the disability induced by single diseases, conditions, and injuries is measured has been highly debated. Summarizing a disease's impact in a single indicator based on age, gender, the degree of disability, and the onset of disease was justified as a tool that would allow decision makers to choose interventions by comparing the previously incomparable. They could evaluate, for instance, the difference between the value of one year of life for a child suffering from a vitamin deficiency and the value of one year of survival for a fifty-year-old with cancer. In this way, and in resonance with Morgan's analyses of the metrics economists use (Morgan 2012), the invention of the GBD can be understood as creating "a world of accounting data" in which the data serve governments' needs to monitor the economy under budget constraints, arbitrate between different social investments, and evaluate and optimize returns.

From this perspective, the DALY resembles earlier health economics' quality-adjusted life years (QALY). In fact, discussion around DALYs in the 1990s resembled earlier debates on the advantages and limitations of QALYs. Both indicators were criticized for using coefficients that gave less weight to the deaths of children and the elderly (Yamey 2002); for arbitrarily assessing the value of one year of life lived with disabilities; and for attributing a value to impaired functioning due to a disease, as if "evaluations of the severity and cost" of human misery "[could] be validly standardized across different societies, social classes, age cohorts, genders, ethnicities and occupational groups" (Kleinman and Kleinman 1996, p. 14).

More important for this chapter, however, is the 1993 WDR's connection between DALYs and the measurement of cost-effectiveness. This was a central ingredient in the World Bank valorization of the GBD as the basis for triage among health burdens. Atypically for a major global financial institution deeply involved in the implementation of the Washington Consensus (Chorev 2012), the 1993 WDR approached the central question of what government and the market should do, making a strong plea for action by the former with specific attention to health. This plea for targeted investments was delineated in a much more detailed and prescriptive way with the selection of forty-seven interventions for which the World Bank's panels of economists and health specialists had computed costs and numbers of years of life saved in order to provide a cost-effectiveness ratio. This complex operation actually began in 1988, before the writing of the 1993 WDR, with the establishment of a Disease Control Priorities (DCP) working group within the Bank's Population, Health, and Nutrition (PHN) division, whose initial aim was to develop new tools for measuring the effectiveness (rather than monetary benefits) of health investments.[5]

Indeed, the DCP working group's final document, published as background material to the 1993 WDR, relied on the attempts by panels of epidemiologists and economists to assess legitimate interventions in their field, gather all available economic evidence on their costs and outcomes under optimal conditions, and—when possible—provide numbers for the cost per DALY avoided. These numbers were then used to rank interventions into specific pathologies or health issues according to their effectiveness, thereby blurring the classical divide health economists were making between prevention and treatment. Prevention was considered a "public good" because of its many externalities and the impossibility that a buyer would accrue individual benefits. DALY-based economic legitimacy crossed the divide by favorably ranking highly cost-effective clinical interventions such as tuberculosis chemotherapy, in contrast with poorly cost-effective preventive interventions like water sanitation.

The final outcome of this ranking effort was the proposal of an "essential package of health services" for developing countries. Beyond effectiveness, expressed in terms of the cost for one DALY averted, overall spending was critical to formulating the package. World Bank experts estimated that betting on a massive increase of public expenditures was unrealistic, even if developing countries spent a far smaller percentage of their gross national product on health than developed ones. The essential package was thus limited to doubling what low-income countries were already spending to reach the level of $12 per person per year. The package at once prolonged and provided new legitimacy to existing priorities like immunization, treatment of sexually transmitted diseases, prenatal care, family planning, and HIV prevention. A few items in the categories of noncommunicable disease prevention and clinical treatment, however, proved to be novel: for example, tobacco control; access to medications for pain relief, diabetes, hypertension, and tuberculosis; and a "limited care" cluster focused on the treatment of skin allergies and injuries (Bobadilla, Cowley et al. 1994).

Cost-effectiveness and performance—the values imbedded in GBD 1—as well as the related expectations for an economically rationalized triage partly confirmed the neoliberal scenario, with one caveat: Privatization of health services was only marginally the issue; triage was the fundamental one. As Chris Murray, the man who had pushed so strongly for the creation of the GBD, summarized:

> Decision-makers who allocate resources to competing health programs must choose between the relative importance of different health outcomes such as mortality reduction or disability prevention. Because money is one-dimensional, the allocation of resources between programs defines a set of relative weights for different health outcomes. The only exception to this is in a completely free market for health care where such decisions between competing health programs are not made by a central authority but by individuals, one health problem at a time. (Murray 1994, 429)

This logic of package design typifies the accounting nature of the first calculus of DALYs. Both the comparison of interventions according to their cost-effectiveness and their putative inclusion in a public package of services operated within the framework of an imaginary budget-balancing exercise. This involved the search for the "best" equilibrium between "inputs" (financial resources, most often from states and donors) and "outputs" (the cost of selected interventions) that could include increasing inputs, but most often it meant adjusting outputs to preset levels of inputs (see the example of Bangladesh below). Thus, rather than privatizing, states were now mandated to focus on investment performance, thus entering an audit culture (Power 1997) based on the use of a whole new range of evaluation and ranking instruments (Gaudillière 2016).

PUTTING GBD 1 TO USE: THE REAL BUT PROBLEMATIC "ECONOMIZATION" OF NATIONAL INVESTMENTS IN HEALTH

In the 1990s, despite the World Bank's endorsement of the GBD and its role in the legitimation of health as a new priority for development loans, many general economists entertained the idea that the GBD and DALYs are not economic instruments as such. For these critics, DALYs helped perform a kind of "medical" calculus by allowing for comparison between diseases or between interventions. But they did not provide a rationale for core economic questions like the level of investments in health compared with other economic sectors or the kind of care provision that can be left to the market—all questions central to the management of *national* health systems and budget allocations. Epistemic and political tensions between the public health specialists and health economists working within the PHN division, on the one hand, and the macroeconomists of development at the upper levels of the World Bank, on the other hand, plagued the WDR process. These tensions were less a question of trust or mistrust in GBD data collection and calculus than a matter of broader political issues and epistemic commitments about what constitutes a public good, the specificity of the health sector, and the roles that states and markets should play in the allocation of resources. As a result, after it completed the 1993 WDR, the World Bank stopped investing in the GBD, which was left for Harvard University and the WHO use and for fostering DCP-like evaluations of health interventions.

Moreover, since the late 1990s, in contrast to the initial emphasis placed on ranking and package design, a DALY-based calculus of cost-effectiveness and ranking of interventions has played little role in the Bank's own assessment of health-related loans and package design. The negotiation of health system reform in Bangladesh is a good illustration. The design of a basic package of essential services provided by the state occurred without any ranking of the sort envisioned in the 1993 DCP, even if the process started with the $12 allotment as the exemplar of economic triage.

Local authorities and the donors' mission had to take the Bangladeshi Ministry of Health's annual budget cap of about $3.50 per capita into account. Thus, a group of practitioners, public health specialists, and health authorities met to select interventions in four priority areas: child health, reproductive and population health, communicable diseases, and simple curative care. Costs were computed with the help of an economist paid by the WHO. Assuming that no significant increase in resources was politically feasible, the preparation team's next task was to align the package with the $3.50 ceiling. The technique did not involve cost-effectiveness ranking but rather the scoring of each intervention according to five criteria: cost, feasibility of provision, potential health impact, burden of disease, and economic status (whether the intervention could be considered a public good and the importance of its externalities). The last stage of triage reinforced the dominance of general economic criteria in the process, since eliminating interventions from the package through scoring proved very difficult. It failed to meet the $3.50 target, leaving a deficit in the range of 15 percent. To avoid stalling the negotiations with donors and to secure the help of the World Bank, USAID, and Northern European aid agencies, the preparation team finally agreed to draw up a "contingency plan," which the Bangladeshi team considered a first step. As the World Bank expert participating in the negotiations later explained, this marginal use of cost-effectiveness should not be taken as a surprise: "while [cost-effectiveness] is an economic evaluation tool, public health specialists, much more so than economists, swear by it as a primary prioritization tool" (Yazbeck 2002, 4).

That general economic indicators and criteria prevailed in the management of investments is in line with the World Bank's overall policies. It does not imply that DALYs and DCP ranking are never utilized. Eventually, they played a significant, albeit more political, role in designing of national health system reforms, as the case of Mexico's National Health Program, adopted in 2001, powerfully illustrates. The negotiation of the reform was led by the physician and public health expert Julio Frenk, then minister of health, who had acquired firsthand knowledge of the GBD while a visiting professor at the Harvard Center for Population and Development Studies in 1992 and 1993 and had also contributed to the 1993 Disease Control Priorities chapter on the epidemiological transition. In fact, he had focused on the epidemiological changes in Mexico well before publication of the 1993 WDR stressing the mounting burden of NCDs and profound inequalities in access to care (Frenk, Bobadilla et al. 1989). Back in Mexico, Frenk worked with FUNSALUD, a private think tank advocating for general reform of the nation's health system, and was first author of an ambitious plan presented to the public in 1994 (Frenk, Lozano et al. 1994). That plan, *Economia y Salud*, mobilized the same techniques as the 1993 WDR but attributed a significantly different meaning to their use. In the Mexican context, prioritization was less viewed as the consequence of general economic constraints and effectiveness ranking than a result of differentiated health needs. The plan's general and novel argument for reform was more political than economic and emphasized that the country's health needs originated from two sources: profound inequalities and lack of coverage for the large uninsured segments of the population and the emerging problems associated with chronic disorders and an epidemiological transition. The data documenting this situation had been produced through a GBD-like analysis of Mexico's health statistics, measuring the burden in AVISA (DALYS in Spanish), an indicator deemed necessary for evaluating the effectiveness of interventions and establishing priorities.[6] Unlike the GBD, however, the calculation of AVISAs was strongly linked to the evaluation of inequalities, using data on the distribution of the burden of disease across gender, income level, and territories (the latter reflecting the rural/urban divide as well as the conditions of Indigenous groups). The Mexican GBD was therefore simultaneously quantifying the epidemiological transition and measuring health inequalities and their social roots.

FUNSALUD's recommendations for reform were more socially oriented than any World Bank document addressing issues of coverage and organization. They emphasized the need for a unified health system financed by both taxes and employer/employee contributions, which would ensure universal access to a broader palette of services while allowing users to choose their primary provider. Designing a package of guaranteed interventions was therefore considered necessary for two reasons: first, to meet the economic need for financial sustainability and, second, to foster the political will to redistribute resources and finance significantly increased investments. The inclusion of services targeting "new" chronic disorders was a key element of consensus building. FUNSALUD's study of cost-effectiveness thus mimicked the DCP calculations but for a larger and different range of interventions, with a threshold of inclusion ten times higher than the World Bank's $12 package (Frenk, Lozano et al. 1994, 255).

The tensions between the logic of needs and the logic of costs in this political redefinition of GBD 1 were finally resolved when AVISA-based cost-effectiveness and the ensuing ranking of interventions disappeared during the 2001 national health reform. The 2001 program approved by the Mexican parliament did insist on addressing both chronic disease and inequality, but these issues were documented through traditional national epidemiological statistics on mortality and morbidity prevalence. Priority interventions beyond those targeting the most impoverished segment of the population (malnutrition, tuberculosis, malaria, and dengue) were indeed selected (Secretaría de Salud 2001, 89). But these followed a combination of medical and political motives and were defined in terms of campaigns against diabetes and cardiovascular disorders. Sustainable financing figured prominently in the law with changes that roughly followed FUNSALUD recommendations (Secretaría de Salud 2001, 75). Performance was not approached through cost-effectiveness data but as service output, with the establishment of a data-gathering and evaluation system using WHO criteria for auditing health systems, such as life expectancy, level of inequality, rate of adequate treatment, financial protection, and maternal mortality (Secretaría de Salud 2001, 163).

How can we account for the gap between GBD 1's original objectives and early uses? Since the late 1990s, the global health field has become a world of competing interests and vertical programs, which target one disease or issue and consider health systems marginally, if at all. Although the WHO continues to push for comparisons of interventions across the health sector, the World Bank's policy does not require the comparisons once envisioned across the spectrum of development targets. Even the Bank massively targets vertical programs, mimicking its competing "transnational humanitarianism" partners (Fassin 2011). Of course, state management of health systems has not disappeared, and the World Bank remains a development institution investing in strengthening health systems. But as the Mexico case illustrates, a DCP-like calculus of cost-effectiveness and intervention ranking is of limited value here. At the very least, these measures end up being submitted to broader managerial and/or political criteria. In other words, the global health endeavor at large does not use the GBD metric as it was envisioned. Its actors are more interested in indicators systemized as global and supposedly comparable health data informing a project's symbolic, technical, and political performance (Reubi 2018). This is precisely what the GBD 2, produced by the IHME, provides.

GLOBAL BURDEN OF DISEASE, SEASON 2 (GBD 2): LIMITATIONS AND LEGITIMATION

Although the World Bank commissioned the first iteration of the GBD, its financial support petered out after the release of the 1990 GBD baseline published in

1995 (Murray 1994; Murray, Lopez et al. 1996).[7] The WHO subsequently absorbed the GBD project into the Disease Burden Unit it created in 1998. The unit updated GBD estimates for 2000, 2001, 2002, and 2004 and developed the Risk Factor Burden measure. Alan Lopez remained at the WHO, while Chris Murray, then at the Harvard Center for Population and Development Studies, served as a WHO consultant. By 2000, however, conflict with its member states over the GBD led the WHO to temporarily retreat from the project. After a dry period when the GBD was housed at Harvard, Murray drew the interest of Bill Gates, a strong proponent of accountability and an interlocutor who appreciates complex calculus and the potential benefits of big data (Smith 2015). In 2007, Murray moved the GBD enterprise to the University of Washington where, with Gates Foundation funding and assistance from Julio Frenk and others, he founded the IHME. Similarly, the DCP project, originally established to coordinate expert knowledge in support of the World Bank's 1993 WDR, expanded its mission to include producing knowledge for policymakers. The DCP, also funded primarily by the Gates Foundation, is currently managed by IHME and the University of Washington's Department of Global Health as a joint project of the World Bank, the WHO, and the U.S. National Institutes of Health, among others. In light of these shifts, global health actors have reoriented the GBD vis-à-vis its original rationale in three ways.

First, the GBD in some ways has failed to assume a primary role in determining health policies and outcomes worldwide. According to Murray and colleagues, GBD results have directly impacted health policy worldwide, and they have offered a list of thirty-seven countries and several subnational areas, on every continent, in which GBD research has directly affected the formulation and implementation of policy (Murray, Ezzati et al. 2012, 2063). Descriptions of these cases are difficult to trace, however, even using IHME's publicly available resources. Furthermore, incorporation of the GBD into national programs like Mexico's gave way to decisions based on equity rather than cost-effectiveness and to the use of national epidemiological data rather than global burden measures. Thus, when the GBD did enter national health sectors, it was in ways unintended by its architects.

Nevertheless, since 2000, hundreds of country- and regional-level projects have incorporated GBD data for health planning, much of it intra-sectorial.[8] WHO health economists facilitated this process by developing and applying a model called "Choosing Interventions that are Cost-Effective" (CHOICE) to address avertible burden. Whereas the GBD is limited to cross-sectional information, CHOICE builds in systematic estimations of what the burden of disease might look like over time, given certain assumptions. CHOICE incorporated cost-effectiveness data in a systematic way to make comparisons between targets (e.g., malaria versus maternal and child health). From the early 2000s on, WHO projects brought the model to numerous countries to inform vertical program design and health resource allocation.

Simultaneously, social and institutional actors enrolled the GBD in multiple projects but in different ways than those sought by the WHO. A major figure in the post-2000 promotion of cost-effectiveness in health planning in the

Global South remarked on the multiple non-WHO teams working at the country level:

> In the early 2000s, there were many players capable of doing health economic analyses and very interested in packages of care funded by the World Bank: Abt Associates, USAID, major NGOs, other consultants and groups, all using GBD information. [Their methods were not as] explicit as CHOICE, where you literally take the GBD because it's a population model and see how the epidemiology changes with or without an intervention. People also had other models, more classical ones, like simulation. These models might take some data from GBD, so you can conceivably say those countries were using GBD to inform prioritization and policy discussions. And there are many countries using GBD in [policy] discussions.[9]

Diffusion of the GBD has been accompanied by the steady increase of disease-oriented intervention packages and delivery platforms, promoted in subsequent DCP reports. The WHO has reacted by developing the U.N.-wide ONEHEALTH model, intended to unify the data and methods used to inform country-level prioritization and health system–related decisions. Yet the multiplication of packages and platforms, indicators and actors, and exponential expansion of the applied medical science knowledge base in an already-competitive environment (re)produces silos, exemplified by the expansion of the DCP project from a thin report initially to hundreds of pages in nine volumes presenting a whole palette of specific area packages.

Global financing data collected by IHME, however, provides a second lens on the GBD's use. In short, funding for specific diseases and groups does not follow the GBD logic. To assess whether financing is proportional to burden, expenditure for Development Assistance for Health (DAH) can be "benchmarked" against DALYs.[10] From 1995 to 2015, the three big vertical programs (HIV/AIDS, TB, malaria) and maternal and neonatal care commanded the highest dollars-to-DALY ratio, led by $144/DALY for HIV/AIDS. By comparison, mental health received less than $1/DALY (Charlson, Dieleman et al. 2017). Yet GBD analyses attribute over 10 percent of healthy lives lost and over 25 percent of years lived with disability to the category of mental, neurological, and substance use (MNS) disorders (World Health Organization 2013). NCDs including MNS received only $1/DALY, although the WHO claims that 73 percent of the burden of mortality is attributable to these diseases. Therefore, it seems that DAH allocation follows public health concerns, not the logic of comparative burden. Global mental health actors contend that stigma, discrimination, and abrogation of human rights further reduce the likelihood of such disorders being prioritized.[11]

Finally, we turn to a third characteristic of GBD 2, its reworking by nation-states and rhetorical uses in policymaking. We illustrate them with the India State-Level Disease Burden (ISLDB) initiative and India's National Mental Health Survey (NMHS), both dating from 2015. These studies introduce three innovations. First, compared to pre-GBD era psychiatric epidemiology studies in India that did not use the language of burden, these two studies explicitly measure "burden" but operationalize it differently, the first with GBD methodology, the second with traditional epidemiological methods. The ISLDB measures the burden of all diseases and injuries, expressed in DALYs, while the NMHS restricts burden to prevalence rates of mental, neurological and substance use disorders. Second, both studies aim to provide a statistical evidence base for the magnitude, distribution, and impact of health problems in the country, the first as a public-private partnership, the second as a state and purely public endeavor. Third, both studies are highly visible in the media.

The ISLDB studies are part of IHME's Local Burden of Disease project, which developed in response to internal and external criticism of the GBD as too inaccurate and imprecise to be relevant for local decision making. The project aims instead "to produce estimates of health outcomes and related measures . . . at a very fine, local resolution . . . combining local detail with broad coverage."[12] Such locally scaled estimates, it is hoped, will allow for "precision public health," a more exact targeting of resources and health interventions.[13] However, as for GBD 2 data more generally, its exact relationship to policymaking and prioritization remain fuzzy, unlike in the GBD 1, which linked epidemiology directly to economics.

The ISLDB is a public-private partnership initiative between the Indian Council of Medical Research, the Public Health Foundation of India, and IHME. It receives support from the Ministry of Health and Family Welfare and attempts to answer directly to the goals formulated in a 2017 policy paper on the Three-Year Action Agenda of the National Institution for Transforming India and India's National Health. The ISLDB results have provided statistical evidence for the epidemiological transition and the magnitude of the burden of NCDs while showing large variation in the degree of the transition among the states in India. After launching the ambitious Ayushman Bharat national health protection scheme in 2018—a program that promises universal health coverage and stronger comprehensive primary health care—policymakers hope that "the detailed analysis of the changes in the major NCDs and their risk factors . . . [will] therefore [be] quite useful for [tailoring] the Ayushman Bharat effort according to the need of each state" and to "direct health system resources to maximize impact through early prevention and effective treatment."[14] Planners of the Ayushman Bharat scheme draw on the ISLDB numbers to justify the shift of focus in primary health care from communicable to noncommunicable diseases, including mental health, and to critique the former focus on selective primary health care.

The DALY-based ISLDB reports have therefore become an important resource to talk about problems, justify prioritization, and potentially attract funding for investments in NCDs and mental, neurological, and substance use disorders. Although uncertain, these GBD data are hoped to impact triage in policy decisions. As one of the collaborators of the ISLDB said, "Now we do have numbers. Now at least policymakers know that mental disorders are important, prioritized conditions."[15]

However, contrary to the claims made by the ISLDB initiative, our interviews with state policymakers in Kerala suggest that prioritization in health and the planning of programs either ignore epidemiological data completely and "go by local experience," as a high-level health bureaucrat in Kerala expressed it, or they rely on local or (less frequently) national prevalence studies of the older epidemiological kind. Many state policymakers mistrust DALY-based numbers because they think the calculus relies on poor estimates. Nor do they consider the data as better than that projected and extrapolated from highly diverse classical epidemiological studies in India.

The ISLDB reports assemble data from hundreds of sources. One source of data was none other than the National Mental Health Survey (Gururaj, Varghese et al. 2016), whose background, production, and use of epidemiological numbers we will discuss now.

Commissioned and funded by India's Ministry of Health and Family Welfare, the survey arose out of "recommendations of the Joint Parliamentary Committee, parliamentarians' frequent questions, judicial directives, policy makers' concerns, professionals' needs, and media questions" (Gururaj, Varghese et al. 2016). Three factors led to the survey. First, mental health gained traction as an issue in India following the 1997 Human Rights Commission Report and, shortly thereafter, the 2001 World Health Report on Mental Health (Sayers 2001). Human rights debates in India following the deaths of mentally ill patients who could not escape a fire at a religious healing center in Erwadi in South India because they had been chained to their beds also contributed to this upswing in concern. Second, some officials argued that mental disorders are an important driver of noncommunicable diseases, which are responsible for a large part of the disease burden in India. Third, there was new interest in psychiatric epidemiological data as a way of understanding how broad socioeconomic changes have led to a rise in depression, suicide and other mental health problems.[16] "India as a country," one of the authors of the survey told us, "has moved from larger ad hoc crisis-oriented decision making to more data-driven decision making. In that way, epidemiological data play a very important role." He further stressed that "data become a binding force" in a country "where people scream in fifteen different directions."[17]

There is no dearth of psychiatric epidemiological studies in India; studies have been conducted in the country since the 1960s (Sharan, Mahapatra et al., forthcoming). The novelty of the National Mental Health Survey is its comprehensiveness. Data for the project was collected across twelve states over one year to explore not only prevalence rates but also the treatment gap, healthcare delivery and utilization, forms of disability associated with different conditions, and their direct and indirect economic impact on people's and families' lives. Although the NMHS included the impact of mental health problems, treatment use, and treatment gap, these parameters were not directly subjected to a cost-effectiveness calculus.

The report on mental health consists of two parts: The first focused on prevalence, patterns, and outcomes; the latter on mental health systems, loosely linked to the WHO Assessment Instrument for Mental Health Systems, which was designed to evaluate resources and systems for mental health (Gururaj, Varghese et al. 2016). The survey estimated that 15 percent of Indian adults need treatment for mental health issues, middle-aged working populations are affected most, and urban areas are witnessing growing rates of mental health problems. Based on these findings, the report recommended that "mental health should be given higher priority in the developmental agenda of India. All policies and programs in health and all related sectors of welfare, education, employment, and other programs need to include and integrate mental health in their respective policies, plans and programs" (Gururaj, Varghese et al. 2016). The report also urges the consideration of social determinants of mental health. In addition to completing the survey in the remaining states and megacities, the long-term aim is to repeat the survey every ten years in order to produce long-term comparable data.

Indeed, the idea of facilitating a direct policy impact was built into the design of the survey, and survey coordinators in every participating state were instructed to draft mental health action plans based loosely on the WHO Mental Health Action Plan 2013–2020. The most visible effects so far have been the strengthening of the decades-old District Mental Health Program (DMHP); an increase in DMHP human resources and drug availability; and a new emphasis on common mental disorders such as depression and anxiety.[18]

The case of India provides an on-the-ground example of how one specific nation-state has appropriated, supplemented, and diverted GBD 2 in policy debates. But it also illustrates the ways in which the GBD can be fragmented and modified while being used as a rhetorical device.

CHALLENGING GBD 2

In the real world of interest groups and constituencies, scarcity and competition, a cost-effectiveness analysis (CEA) may inform, but rarely drives, country-level planning and priority-setting. Why, then, has such analysis become a mandatory exercise of the GBD 2 era? As we saw, private and public donors increasingly demand cost and cost-effectiveness data in which the GBD is already embedded. Using CEA pulls noncommunicable diseases like tobacco-related and mental disorders "out of the shadows," to borrow a popular slogan, and onto global agendas.

Surprisingly, the first Disease Control Priorities report included some mental health disorders among the nine diseases presented, but it omitted depression, which three years later would be ranked the fourth most burdensome condition in the world (Murray, Lopez et al. 1996). Instead, the DCP mental health chapter focused on schizophrenia and bipolar disorder, considered then and now among the most severe and disabling mental disorders. The same experts promoting their inclusion as disease priorities noted however that the duration, complexity, and methods of treatment of these disorders lowered their cost-effectiveness compared, for instance, to highly standardized mono-treatments (e.g., for TB). The second DCP report in 2010 compared cost-effectiveness of interventions across disease-burdens. It concluded that treatment for depression, bipolar disorders, and schizophrenia are the least cost-effective of the 319 interventions for high burden diseases covered in DCP2 (Laxminarayan, Chow et al. 2010). Finding themselves in an increasingly competitive intersectoral global environment, WHO and DCP mental health experts have undertaken two major efforts to make the case for mental health investments.

First, to request funding has required, at the very least, arguing that feasible, cost-effective mental health interventions are possible (World Health Organization 2013). Therefore, since 2000, the WHO has invested in health economists. The organization's analysts and DCP experts have amassed a large evidence base for cost-effective mental health interventions (Levin and Chisholm 2013). They especially showcase treatment for alcohol abuse, epilepsy, and depression as "the best value for money" in sub-Saharan Africa and Southeast Asia, areas where data were previously severely lacking (Levin and Chisholm 2013). Second, global actors converged to create the Movement for Global Mental Health, partly modeled on AIDS activism and consolidated through *The Lancet*'s 2017 Global Health Commission and a series of papers published in that journal (Lovell, forthcoming). Yet the same protagonists behind building a data-driven knowledge base lament hospital-centrism in LMICs, arguing that long-term inpatient treatment is not only *not* cost-effective, but it is also often in violation of human rights (Levin and Chisholm 2013, 228, 232). This, of course suggests that health economics alone are not the motor for health systems reform. The attempt to apply objective markers of efficacy is further complicated by social disparities and a lack of parity between mental health and other health areas worldwide and by people's hesitancy to question epidemiological myths, such as the absence of depression in low-income countries (Rosenberg 2019).

WHO economists then embarked on cost-effectiveness studies using a second model, focusing on benefit analyses that, as mentioned above, evoke development economics. Theoretically, the new return-on-investment studies contribute to triaging decisions among different diseases or conditions by comparing both health benefits and wider social and economic benefits, such as productivity lost or gained. Such analyses rely on numerous assumptions and, unlike the CHOICE model, can inform issues relating to equity, especially as global health institutions increasingly promote universal health coverage. In order to speak to equitable forms of intervention, the model breaks down epidemiological and other data by socioeconomic groups. Algorithms generate different scenarios of scaled-up treatment for which "any benefit-to-cost ratio exceeding 1 provides a rationale for investment" (Chisholm, Sweeny et al. 2016).

It is no coincidence that WHO economists conducted a sophisticated "return on investment" analysis for depression and anxiety in time for the first-ever World Bank and WHO summit meeting on global mental health in 2016. The results showed dramatically lower benefits than for malaria and significantly lower benefits than maternal, reproductive, neonatal, and child-health interventions (Chisholm, Sweeny et al. 2016). Such analyses incorporate numerous levels of uncertainty (e.g., whether illness will affect capacity to pay for service and whether treatments exist), but the very existence of an analysis allows mental health to be discussed in the same terms as the targets of big vertical programs. In other words, it emphasizes the importance of mental health interventions, albeit through an abstract exercise whose real-world applications have yet to be shown.

CRISES OF OWNERSHIP AND COUNTING

The privatization of the GBD by the Institute for Health Metrics and Evaluation has spurred much criticism. In particular, analysts consider the private GBD initiative a serious, well-organized, and rapidly expanding challenge to the WHO's public role in generating global health estimates and its mission of promoting health as a public good (Rudan and Chan 2015; Mahajan 2019). Yet IHME has also faced a legitimacy crisis, beginning when the GBD 2010 produced data inconsistent with that of the WHO, which therefore refused to recognize it. IHME was further criticized for the lack of transparency of its methods (Mahajan 2019), which contradicts the proclaimed health democracy values of Murray and Lopez, the GBD's architects.

IHME's extensive collaborations can be seen as both justifying and mollifying such criticisms. The GBD iterations since the IHME's founding (first in 2010, 2012, 2015, 2016, and 2017) have spurred a massive network of collaborators, as we saw above. The GBD enterprise is now so vast that adhering to the ethical principle of disinterested judgment in reviewing its research becomes next to impossible simply because everyone is involved. A senior editor at *The Lancet*, the prestigious journal most avidly promoting the GBD, intimated that finding peer reviewers with GBD competence *outside* the massive collaborative network now poses a challenge for evaluating the hundreds of articles submitted on the topic and its specialty areas.[19] A sociometric analysis of all global health scientific literature since 2008 concludes that the GBD has become its own institution, "with its own core texts, authors and constituencies," at the same time that it constitutes a "boundary object connecting multiple academic and applied areas of global health" (Weisz, Cambrosio et al. 2017, 18).

Notably, IHME's use of the GBD faced fierce criticism for its measure of disability, resulting in a major, though still problematic, modification. The original disability measure had been criticized for excluding and stigmatizing groups according to age, gender, or disability. In 2011, IHME responded to these critiques by bringing together a group of ethicists, philosophers, economists, and researchers. As a result, age group differentiation and discounting were dropped, beginning with GBD 2012. To determine the value attributed to disabilities, medical expert judgments were replaced by multimethod population-based surveys in different countries, albeit mostly high-income countries. The rationale for this last change, some health services researchers hold, is that "in a democratic society the views of the general public are most applicable in comparative appraisal and societal decision-making" (Chen, Jacobsen et al. 2015, 12). However, the change renders comparability between different GBD reports difficult and has failed to simplify an already cumbersome methodology. Thus its usability by national and regional planners and other health professionals, let alone the public, has not been dramatically improved by the change (Chen, Jacobsen et al. 2015). Furthermore, one observer notes, the new valuations sometimes generate counterintuitive weightings:

> [Examples are] the percentage of global burden of disability (in terms of years lost to disability) for acne than each of autism, chronic kidney disease, multiple sclerosis, and HIV in developed countries. This is clearly a question of prevalence compared to severity. Another striking example is the relatively low ranking of cognitive disabilities based on population survey methods. For example, severe intellectual disability has a lower disability weight than distance vision blindness, moderate anxiety disorders, moderate alcohol use disorder, or a long-term knee dislocation (with or without treatment), among others. (McQueston 2014)

The limits of GBD production emerge along both the upstream process of defining, measuring, operationalizing, and standardizing disease burden components, as well as in the social usages made of them downstream. We turn now to the question of definitions and their consequences, and data gathering and its consequences, by drawing again on our anthropological fieldwork and document analysis.

Just before publication of the first GBD, Harvard University presented its World Mental Health Report (Desjarlais, Eisenberg et al. 1995) to the United Nations, calling for a massive investment in and attention to mental health and social suffering. Directed by Harvard University's Arthur Kleinman, the report drew on anthropological case studies of mental health in poor countries around the world and on WHO reports.[20] More importantly and potentially to greater effect, it deliberately harnessed DALYs as a way to communicate the massive loss of productivity due to poor mental health.[21] While widely cited, the report's effect on the uses and legitimacy of the GBD in mental health is unclear, although Kleinman has since become a major global mental health actor, solicited for debates, regularly published in *The Lancet*, and named to expert commissions.

An unexpectedly high burden attributed to depression in the first GBD, coupled with this report, rendered mental health visible but masked the gaps and limitations of GBD analysis of mental disorders from one global region to another. These limitations are especially stark in regions and countries where treatment is least available. For instance, in Africa, the mental health treatment gap, or ratio that measures the difference between prevalence and treated cases, is estimated at 90 percent.

Our own research uncovered a major limitation of GBD data for sub-Saharan Africa, when during fieldwork in Senegal, we were confronted with an absence of statistics and, more importantly, a relative disinterest in them within the Health Ministry's Division of Mental Health.[22] Whereas GBD language and principles are formally used in the health administration of countries like India, in Senegal mention of the GBD before high-level mental health officials and researchers usually drew a blank. It is possible, historically, that Senegal's pioneering psychoanalytically influenced ethno-psychiatry, established during the transition from colony to nation-state, increases disinterest (Bullard 2007; Lovell, forthcoming).

The absence of global mental health metrics in Senegal points to the existence of a persistent epidemiological gap in most of sub-Saharan Africa (Baxter, Patton et al. 2013). Although the WHO, donors, and other global health actors consider epidemiological statistics necessary for formally estimating the treatment gap in those countries, statistics that do exist there are often constructed with "poor numbers"—erroneous, incomplete, approximated, or otherwise problematic (Jerven 2013). To grasp the nature of this gap, it is necessary to recall that calculating the GBD statistics for a given country requires not only associating DALYs with a given cause (disease, disorder, injury, etc.) but also determining prevalence rates, using estimations of the proportion of the population in any one geographical locale that is affected by that condition.

The problem with GBD estimates for severe and common mental disorders begins at the global level, with estimates for aggregate prevalence and burden across all regions and countries. The indicators thus produced are so abstract and disconnected from actual flesh-and-blood populations as to evoke a "posthuman" (Rees 2010). The GBD for these disorders, like all constructions of specific GBD indicators, is built from meta-regression analyses of hundreds of studies. For mental disorders, 77,000 epidemiological surveys on depression, anxiety, bipolar, and eating disorders, as well as schizophrenia, were examined for possible inclusion in the meta-analyses that generated the data used in the 2010 GBD. However, only 1 percent met the researchers' inclusion criteria; hence, over 76,000 studies were omitted from the GBD's epidemiology. The major reasons for noninclusion illustrate long-term shortcomings of psychiatric epidemiology—namely, the difficulty in determining whether a "case" exists (Lovell and Susser 2014; March and Oppenheimer 2014) and the categorical fallacy, whereby culturally specific presentations are diagnosed as mental disorders or else mental disorders are missed because instruments fail to pick up their cultural expression (Baxter, Patton et al. 2013).

The GBD meta-analyses also eliminated studies because samples were nonrepresentative or poorly described. As is also the case in wealthy countries, the majority of people with severe mental disorders in sub-Saharan Africa are not in treatment (Wang, Demler et al. 2002; Fernández, Haro et al. 2007). Thus, identifying mental illness through community or population surveys, rather than from treatment settings, matters. Finally, measures used are often not comparable across studies, and methods and results tend to be incompletely reported.

Finally, the GBD lacks geographical coverage. In meta-analyses, entire world regions go missing. These include parts of Oceania, Central Asia, the Andes, as well as most of sub-Saharan Africa. Yet DALYs and prevalence rates have been produced for all of these countries, as a perusal of the IHME's GBD Compare website tool demonstrates (Baxter, Scott et al. 2014).

The GBD enterprise preempts the problem of missing data by acknowledging it under the broader umbrella of data uncertainty, arguing that summary metrics themselves are approximate or that data may not exist for the most important health problems in a country (Murray, Ezzati et al. 2012, 2064). Beginning with GBD 2010, uncertainty was built into calculations by quantifying "all known sources of uncertainty" in keeping with "the rising standard of analysis in global descriptive epidemiology" (Murray, Ezzati et al. 2012, 2063). More pragmatically, mental health data for Senegal (and other sub-Saharan African nations) are to a great extent generated by substituting data from studies in other countries in Africa that are geographically and socioculturally much different. This form of substitution is justified by a principle that IHME's founder has often hammered home. An IHME technician explained it to us thusly: "[The Global Burden of Disease] operates on the principle that informed estimates are better than no estimates. This is because 'blanks' are often interpreted by decision makers to mean there is no burden due to that cause, which we know is untrue." We might well ask, however, when does a level of abstraction or other built-in assumption undermine the calculations and hence their social uses?

Congenital disorders offer another interesting example of the arbitrariness of the ways in which cases are defined, included, and counted in the GBD. In this domain of health, researchers have proposed an alternative calculation model that could strongly modify the weight of these disorders in the overall indicators. Since the 2000s and in the aftermath of the Global Report on Birth Defects published by the March of Dimes (Christianson, Howson et al. 2006), the international Congenital Disorders Expert Group (CDEG) took interest in the integration of a rather invisible domain within the GBD: genetic congenital disorders (chromosomal and single gene disorders). An independent scientific collective, the nine-member CDEG includes researchers from the United Kingdom (Hannah Blencowe, Bernadette Modell, Joy Lawn,[23] among others), Australia, and Switzerland. According to Bernadette Modell,[24] genetic congenital disorders' absence in the GBD stems from their perceived complexity by "the GBD people [who, in a meeting with her,] said their idea was that you'd have to take every single genetic disease and do a job on it. And they said it's too hard, it's just not realistic." To the CDEG, the main obstacle to the global development of genetic medicine was not complexity but rather "the absence of local epidemiological data on [the] prevalence [of genetic congenital disorders] and the impact of interventions impede policy and service development in many countries" (Moorthie, Blencowe et al. 2017, 347).

Since the early 2010s, the CDEG has strongly criticized the method of integrating congenital disorders into the GBD calculations as a "continuing and self-reinforcing underestimation of the importance of congenital disorders."[25] (For a critique of estimates published by *The Lancet*, see also Modell, Berry et al. 2012.) In their view, in addition to the lack of advanced diagnostic facilities in low-income countries, a second reason for this underestimation lies in the definition of "congenital" used in the GBD (and by the WHO). As Modell puts it, "It means 'anything that happens in utero before birth and is present at birth.' And so this is environmental factors and what I call constitutional factors, which are genetic, chromosomal disorders."[26] Framed in this way, the GBD category aggregates pathologies occurring in utero, with and without a genetic cause, under the heading "congenital" in the "Q chapter" of the *International Classification of Diseases, Tenth Revision* (commonly called ICD-10, 2010). However, this list appears incomplete, as very common congenital genetic disorders are listed elsewhere in the ICD. For example, sickle cell disorders are found in chapter III of the ICD-10, "Diseases of the Blood and Blood-Forming Organs and Certain Disorders Involving the Immune Mechanism," which became "Diseases of the Blood or Blood-Forming Organs" in ICD-11. In both versions, there is therefore no comprehensive determination of genetic congenital disorders but only more specific chapters such as chapter XVII, "Congenital Malformations, Deformations and Chromosomal Abnormalities" in ICD-10 and chapter 20, "Developmental Anomalies" in ICD-11.

Therefore, the CDEG worked on a novel epidemiological approach aiming at a realistic estimation of the number of deaths and new disability cases resulting from these disorders. It is based on a statistical approach of "baseline prevalence of rare single gene disorders" considered as a group. The proposed tool for this new approach, published in 2018 in the *Journal of Community Genetics*, is the "Modell Global Database of Congenital Disorders (MGDb),"[27] which is both an epidemiological tool and an attempt at definitional standardization within a largely shifting public health field (Moorthie, Blencowe et al. 2017; Blencowe, Moorthie et al. 2018; Moorthie, Blencowe et al. 2018). The MGDb is designed to "generate estimates of the birth prevalence and effects of interventions on mortality and disability due to congenital disorders."[28] As a result, the CDEG now claims to "[have] a very simple, basic scientific method for including single gene disorders as a bundle, based on basic principles of genetics."[29]

CONCLUSION

"At the end of the day, GBD is epidemiology, it's not economics," a principal health economist and architect of post-2000 models for allocating health funds told us. "It's not an economic analysis, it's an epidemiological analysis of incidence, prevalence, remission, mortality of different diseases."[30] This remark does not contradict our narrative of the GBD in two seasons. Yet GBD does contribute to the economization of health in at least two ways: by providing a summary metric with indicators to which economic value (e.g., productive bodies) can be attached, and through the social uses to which it is put.

The social usages of GBD 1 and GBD 2, however, contribute to the economization of health in different ways. GBD 1 belongs to a development-oriented genre of technoscientific narrative, in which World Bank economists hoped it could guide triage of health and nonhealth investments. But health, poorly amenable to market-driven policies and infinite in its externalities, proved too unwieldy to capture. Instead, health economists and policymakers harnessed the GBD to develop national-level essential packages of care and inform national health policies. There, the health economist's dream ran up against other values, such as equity, and against the permanence of the political.

The social usages of GBD 2 expanded considerably, but not necessarily in the ways its supporters predicted. Its appropriation by the IHME was in itself a reflection of the neoliberal world, in which international organizations were losing power. The iterations in GBD 2 have revealed the limits of the metric in relation to its architects' goals but also its increasing use in a vastly expanding multi-actor and heterogeneous field of global health. Yet competition, multiple actors, and expanding knowledge bases (re)produce health silos. The recent international push for universal health coverage and the return of primary health care as an intra-sectorial solution to costly silos, while beyond the scope of this chapter, may bring about a third season of GBD.

CHAPTER 3

Triage beyond the Clinic

Jean-Paul Gaudillière, Andrew McDowell, Claudia Lang,
and Claire Beaudevin

One life today cannot be measured by its value tomorrow, and the relief of suffer-
ing "here" cannot legitimize the abandoning of relief "over there." The limitation
of means naturally must mean the making of choice, but the context and the con-
straints of action do not alter the fundamentals of this humanitarian vision. It is
a vision that by definition ignores political choices.
—James Orbinski, President of Médecins Sans Frontières International Council,
Nobel Peace Prize acceptance speech, 1999

Even when accepting a million-dollar Nobel Prize, Médecins Sans Frontières (MSF)
addressed the problem of limited means and the need for choices in humanitarian action. On a global stage, the leader of MSF emphasized what Peter Redfield
calls "the problem of triage"—that is to say, medical prioritization's political nature
and incompatibility with the "humanitarian vision" MSF defends (Redfield 2013, 155).
Triage is, on the one hand, associated with almost every intervention by major
actors in global health. They repeatedly insist on their priorities and the need to
make "tough" choices. Yet, on the other hand, it is difficult to legitimize these decisions because these very same priorities are broadly perceived as opposing a general and comprehensive right to health or, in a less radical vision, the right to have
pressing health needs addressed and effectively treated.

While forming the core of global health, triage is also a common object of
inquiry in social studies of health and medicine. Its treatment in the literature follows two lines of analysis. The first is historical, examining the historiography of
military medicine, on the one hand, and colonial health interventions on the other
(see Lachenal, Lefève et al. 2014 for a review,). Within these contexts, historians
conceptualize triage as a process, a series of choices implemented through authoritative protocols that rationalize and standardize physicians' decisions about what
should be done with impaired or diseased bodies in emergency situations. Triage

as process, for instance, can refer to the transfer of wounded soldiers from the frontlines to various sites of care organized according to a hierarchy of technical capabilities that became typical of modern military health services by World War I. Triage is also used to describe the ways in which colonial authorities managed some epidemics—most obviously in the cases of turn-of-the-century plague epidemics and sleeping sickness during the interwar period—with a procedure of mass screening, isolation and relocation, selective destruction of contaminated personal items, and mass provision of vaccines and other therapeutic agents. The thread linking these ostensibly different configurations is the conjunction of emergency and scarcity, logistics and administration, and discipline and large-scale handling of individual bodies in war or the colony.

The second line of analysis concerning triage originates among anthropologists. They examine triage as an event resulting in the uneven allocation of treatment and resources. This clinical prioritization may also characterize humanitarian medicine, as in the case of MSF that Redfield investigates. Triage may accordingly originate in configurations of "scarcity" where constrains are less linked to the lack of time and the threat of massive deaths than the structural lack of resources, be they financial, material, or human (Nguyen 2010). In the latter case, triage is not only deciding "who will be saved" by being granted access to care, but it is also a political discourse mobilizing numerous actors beyond the individual physician and organizing populations—even if this distributed political dimension is approached as a context for the care relationship. Other scholars examine triage events on the global level, studying the effects of allocation of resources on the daily lives of certain groups. For instance, Kristin Peterson (2014) shows the consequences of prioritization when securing a medicine supply in Nigeria; Alice Street (2014) looks to the outcome of paradigms that privilege treatment over diagnosis on Papua New Guinea, and Julie Livingston (2012) examines the lived effects of decisions not to prioritize cancer care in Botswana. All of these works examine examples of triage to describe "islands of healthcare" (Wendland 2012) in which infrastructures of care are marked by the prioritization of some diseases ahead of others. In each case, triage is an event that occurs either in or out of the clinic but always affects care and individual lives.

Despite differences, historical and anthropological approaches to triage share the centrality of bodies. The act of triage abides in physicians' decisions about individuals and in their ability to perform circumscribed clinical encounters through which people's needs are assessed and weighed against limited means. Within this perspective, although decisions are deemed essential, the collective, population-based, political dimensions of triage become utterly problematic. When discussing MSF's triage, Redfield (2013) recounts how MSF doctors practice triage in what they consider a state of exception, or "temporary suspension of norms," that is not a legitimate course of action and should be considered as the exception rather than the rule. Echoing this, Vinh-Kim Nguyen (2010)—when discussing the access to antiretroviral drugs (ARVs) in West Africa—emphasizes the tensions and controversies that emerge when triage becomes a matter of public debate and a site of mobilization.

Triage's untenable and hidden politics is the point of departure of this chapter. Rather than beginning with decisions in the clinic or the conference room in order to explore the moral and political impossibilities of triage, we start with the structural existence of triage in international and global health and the lack of perceived moral reflection or choice. At stake here is an overt—claimed and implemented—form of biopolitics that turns the management of resources into an instrument for handling populations and sets up abstract investment priorities that are permanent features of health interventions and health systems design in countries called "developing," "emerging," or "low-income."

Systemic prioritization is a form of planning that results in routines. It may operate through diverse and shifting metrics and means. It may be a matter of choosing specific diseases, like organizing tuberculosis (TB) treatment rather than interventions in mental health. It may be a matter of selecting techniques and interventions—for example, establishing a list of "essential" generic drugs. It may be a matter of targeting populations at risk or particular social groups—for instance, excluding migrants or noncitizens from the benefits of programs or general access to care. We want to show that systemic triage is pervasive and that it provides a lens on global health that reveals changes across time and the latter's relations with finance and knowledge.

Considering these general macro-processes of systemic triage, there is an obvious need to shift the gaze from philanthropy and humanitarian action in order to bring focus back to the state. Despite the state's shifting role in recent years, not much has changed vis-à-vis determining health priorities; the identification and definition of national needs and resources remains one of the state's major jurisdictions. Indeed, the state continues to have a role in apportioning resources even as the financial scarcity affecting many states in Africa, Asia, and Latin America aggravates their subordination to donor policies and dependency on donor resources.

Our basic argument is that the transition from international public health to global health has resulted in deep changes in the modes of triage. These changes affect all parts of the process: its core categories, the institutions and experts in charge, the tools involved, as well as the collectives considered. One might say that needs have been replaced by effectiveness or, to be more specific, that political triage has been marginalized for the benefit of economic triage when determining priorities.

In the 1960s and 1970s, when international public health dominated, triage was "political." Postcolonial states, their bureaucratic apparatuses, and their public health experts played a central role in triage because the main goal was to define "basic," "essential" needs through processes that mobilized statistics. These numbers included data about mortality and morbidity and were primarily aimed at creating political legitimacy through providing care and creating a pastoral state. Needs could not become a priority because of their mere existence; there were too many of them. Instead, needs were turned into priorities as a result of their endorsement by legitimate authorities. Even as the global imaginary of health has changed, the strong linkages between prioritization and the construction of political power have endured. This also means that the attribution of priority involves some form of democracy, as the recurring discussions on the specificity of local health needs and the role of communities reveal.

Global health, in contrast, redefined the problem, shifting the basis of authority from the political to the economic and technocratic. One issue that led to this shift was a discourse of weakened states, whose ability to foster development and to act for the population's benefit has been deeply challenged for many reasons, corruption among them. Global donors—from the Gates Foundation to the World Bank to the Global Fund—have taken the lead as investors, with the consequence that priority setting has, to a significant degree, been altered in the course of the negotiations these global actors conduct with their partners, nongovernmental organizations (NGOs), and states. However, there is more at stake in the redefinition of triage than the disempowerment of state bureaucracies. Nowadays, triage is less thought of as a question of prioritized needs than as a management problem, a practice aiming at the selection of cost-effective modes of action in the search for superior performance (Adams 2016a; Gaudillière and Gasnier 2020). An entirely new cadre of personnel has grown out of this change, as well as new data and tools—such as medico-economic evaluation, pilot studies, operationalization trials, and recording and audit processes.

An important qualification of the transition scenario is, however, that the growing role of economic triage does not imply the disappearance or complete erasure of political triage. In this respect, configurations vary widely from one place and one bureaucracy to another. The continuities of political triage must therefore be acknowledged. We also need to interrogate them since political triage has become less centralized, operating against the background of a widely influential neoliberal redefinition of the state's role. The main consequence of this shift—when it comes to health—is less the push for the privatization of care and of its financing than the rise of the audit culture and of the regulation and surveillance of programs and services (Power 1997).

As a consequence, the different sections in this chapter do not simply point to the past of political triage by evoking the primary health care (PHC) strategy and its eclipse or trace the advent of economic triage in the construction of global TB interventions. They also explore the tensions between local political triage and global economic triage in Oman and Kerala, India, revealing a negotiated triaging that define events as well as processes.

Political Triage and Its Economic Alternative: The Primary Health Care Strategy and Its Eclipse

Existing studies of the primary health care strategy adopted by the World Health Organization (WHO) in the mid-1970s tend to insist on the opposition between the "horizontal" and "vertical" approaches to healthcare provision. The horizontal, traditional approach to PHC recommended during the Alma-Ata conference relates to a broad definition of health and emphasizes infrastructures and development. On the other hand, the vertical option (one disease, one technology, one bureaucracy) focuses on maternal–child health and relates to what emerged as an alternative—namely, "selective" primary health care.

Within this perspective, horizontal is synonymous with recognizing health as a right and avoiding hierarchical distinctions between diseases or needs. This interpretation of Alma-Ata, however, is a later construct that emerged within the context of global health. Originally, Alma-Ata was concerned with triage, but a very different form of triage than the logic of the programs that prevailed in the 1950s and returned in the 1990s.

Alma-Ata is renowned as a peculiar moment in international health, the apex of fifteen years (from the late 1960s to the mid-1980s) of rethinking health issues, their relationship to development, and the role and limitations of medicine in providing responses to basic health needs.[1] The Alma-Ata strategy was deemed "horizontal" in relation to four features: (1) the links with development and social planning, (2) the critique of biomedicine and frontier technology, (3) the role of communities, and (4) the emphasis on local (rural) health centers as the basic units of an integrated health system.[2] Let us examine these four points in turn.

The first way in which the primary health care strategy was horizontal was its insistence on understanding health as something broader than the absence of diseases. Rather, it imagined health as a basic human right that could not be isolated from other sectors and, therefore, from the question of development as a whole. This had—in the eyes of the WHO and the United Nations Children's Fund (UNICEF)—two major consequences. The first one was that health should be an object of planning. The primary health care texts endlessly repeat that PHC is a national strategy that presupposes public investments coordinated on a country-wide scale, with a special emphasis on those at the periphery (i.e., the most needy rural populations). The second consequence was that health had to be integrated into general development planning, balancing investments in health and other sectors with an eye on the multiple links between various ingredients of social progress. This perspective gave questions of food and nutrition, water supply and sanitation, and family planning and education policies special importance.

In order to achieve such widespread implementation, primary health care—in contrast to the immediate postwar programs and their excessive reliance on one type of technology—targeted "appropriate, affordable, and acceptable technologies" and the establishment of "local" and "integrated" centers addressing "basic needs" (World Health Organization 1978). Given the broad reach of the proposed intervention, the critical question was, How would basic needs be determined, and what was the best way to meet them? Unsurprisingly, this question provoked conflicting responses.

The first and dominant response was that basic needs should be defined by experts using epidemiological and public health knowledge. That such planning was country-based and therefore associated with specific evaluation and decision-making processes did not imply that the WHO and other development organizations should not consider general priorities. Following a long process of internal consultation involving all the WHO regional offices—and in spite of a lack of transparency regarding the criteria and tools used for selection—the Alma-Ata conference ended with a list of targets without much discussion. Primary health care would include a core set of activities:

> Education concerning prevailing health problems and the methods of identifying, preventing and controlling them; promotion of food supply and proper nutrition; an adequate supply of safe water, and basic sanitation; maternal and child health care, including family planning; immunization against the major infectious diseases; prevention and control of locally endemic diseases; appropriate treatment of common diseases and injuries; promotion of mental health; and a provision of essential drugs. (World Health Organization 1978)

If the priorities did not refer to specific diseases and tended to favor general categories—for instance, "environmental" interventions, population control and reproductive health, and communicable diseases—they nonetheless evidence the strong continuities with international health programs launched after World War II, beginning with malaria and smallpox eradication programs.

The second and soon forgotten response was to admit that the selection of "basic needs" was primarily a political choice and that communities should—at least in this discourse—be granted a say. Primary health care was thus imprinted with some of the 1970s ethos of local management, be it that of the village or neighborhood. In spite of the strong commitment to planning and to the creation of a comprehensive national health system, the *local* in primary health care was at the same time a matter of needs, knowledge, and decision making. Community needs—in whatever way they were defined—resulted in strategies combining specialized (mostly epidemiological and medical) knowledge and local experience with a certain degree of operational autonomy—for instance, the possibility of selecting local personnel or some types of interventions.

Strategy in Practice: The Essential Drugs List and the Rise of the "Selective" Primary Health Care

The trajectory of "essential drugs" at the WHO illustrates the difficulties that Alma-Ata's political triage entailed. The push for an essential drugs list was based on a strong critique of very costly frontier drugs and argued that developing countries should favor the use of a limited number (200 to 400) of generic compounds targeting more pressing disorders—namely, those with the greatest epidemiological impact (Gaudillière 2014a).

Essential drugs were therefore deemed essential because of a tacit balancing of costs and benefits. They tackled "essential needs" at a reasonable price. Moreover, the essential drugs perspective was not a simple matter of drawing up a list. Drug selection was complemented by an overarching development scheme, including state commitments to developing local production of pharmaceuticals and controlling their quality through regulation. In addition, "technologies" were to be evaluated in relation to prevailing inequalities and social fairness. This led to a parallel critique of the hospital and specialized care as costly and benefiting more affluent urban populations.

In practice, the WHO's support for these policies focused on setting up a reference list, a task assigned to a panel of experts made up exclusively of academic pharmacists selected by the organization's pharmacy division. A list of priority drugs for public health policies was not a completely new idea. It had been suggested at the start of the organization, in the late 1940s, during the first discussions of an international pharmacopoeia that would be, for many years, the only WHO initiative in the area of drugs. In deference to European and U.S. insistence on innovative and patented drugs, the idea of a hierarchy of pharmaceuticals based on their usefulness to public health had been quickly dropped. In the middle of the 1970s, the "essential drugs" concept became timely again because the patents on the first generation of products typical of the postwar "therapeutic revolution" had expired, in particular those of many antibiotics, analgesics, and steroids. Most of all, the concept echoed attempts by newly independent states to establish national pharmaceutical markets limited to "generic drugs" (Muller 1982).

The WHO essential drug committee visited twenty-five countries during this period, primarily interviewing physicians and health officials before meeting in Geneva in 1976 and 1977 to decide what would be included in the WHO list. Published in October 1977, the list included only 186 substances, the selection of which was justified by the fact that they were inexpensive (in fact, exclusively generic drugs) and used to treat highly prevalent diseases and symptoms (World Health Organization 1977). Moreover, echoing the European and U.S. controversies on mixtures and fixed-dose combinations, the committee included only simple chemical substances, characterized and designated by their generic (chemical) names with no reference to commercial names. The list was designed as a tool to be available to national administrations, which could add to it and were tasked with deciding what methods would be employed for its use in managing public purchases, writing their national pharmacopoeia, or regulating prescriptions.

The pharmaceutical industry immediately opposed the publication of the list. Opposition took two forms: Individually, manufacturing firms tried to expand the list so that it would include some of their own drugs; collectively, they called the very concept of "essential" drugs into question. The direct, commercial issue at stake was minimal. The list included only products of minor importance for the European and U.S. markets, which focused on patent-protected innovations. For the International Federations of Pharmaceutical Manufacturers Associations (IFPMA), the very idea of the list was the problem, for two reasons: The concept might be extended to developed countries, and innovation policies—the link between proprietary formulas and public health—might be called into question. In addition, by considering the financial constraints specific to developing countries, the WHO list suggested that products should be prioritized based on needs and not on supply. The list suggested that some new therapies were useless and implied that a basic basket would be enough to ensure satisfactory medical coverage from the point of view of public health and national population management. The negotiations that followed highlight the WHO's weak enforcement power and were the starting point of a deep interrogation of its role by the United States. In 1979, the publication of a second list, this time including nearly 300 pharmaceuticals, revealed two major concessions. First, it specified that those drugs not included could be medically useful. Second, and more fundamentally, it referred only to the health needs of the countries of the Global South, explicitly excluding developed countries as it considered basic essential drugs (World Health Organization 1977). In exchange for these concessions, the IFPMA gave up its opposition to the program and its threats to boycott it.

Taking the dynamics of triage within primary health care into account is crucial because it suggests that the controversy about selective PHC that erupted soon after Alma-Ata was not about the mere existence of selection. Rather, it directly echoed the essential drug list debate in that it focused on the political ramifications of the strategy—that is, on the vision of biomedicine, health needs, development, and political economy that was at stake in the concept of prioritization.

This is illustrated by the debates at the famous 1979 meeting in Bellagio, Italy, organized by the Rockefeller Foundation, which brought together leaders from U.S. and Canadian development aid with World Bank President Robert McNamara. The debates built on the same issue of scarce resources, acknowledged at Alma-Ata, but suggested a metric of prioritization different from the politically charged concept of basic needs (Walsh and Warren 1979). Comparison between four forms of triage—total primary health care, basic primary health care, vector-disease control, and categorical or selective disease control—was suggested on the basis of increasing commitment to cost-effectiveness. In order to argue for the potential cost-effectiveness of basic interventions, they highlighted a selective package that combined the DPT (diphtheria, pertussis, tetanus) vaccination for children under six months, encouragement of breast feeding, chloroquine for children in malarial areas, and oral-rehydration against diarrhea, estimating that the cost of preventing one child death from these simple steps would be approximately $200 to $250 (about $760 to $950 in U.S. dollars today). This was, of course, much less than the investments required to create a comprehensive primary health care infrastructure.

THE 1990S AND ITS AFTERMATH: PERFORMANCE-BASED TRIAGE AND THE WORLD BANK

The World Bank's "health turn" of the 1990s is a major landmark in the emergence of global health. The mounting interest in health investments was a genuine change in direction. Until the 1980s, the World Bank dealt mostly with major infrastructure projects, adding agriculture and the green revolution as priority targets under McNamara's presidency (Kapur, Lewis et al. 1997; Staples 2006). Within this framework, health was considered an effect, not a means, of development. More precisely, economic growth was considered the means for developing countries to finance future healthcare and the means to reduce the poverty and living conditions that facilitated the spread of diseases.

Between 1987 and 1993, there was a radical change in the framework. The first World Bank report in 1987 on health services prescribed the need, in the countries of the South, to reduce the financial burden of healthcare on the government through measures such as the highly controversial partial payment of services by users. Then in 1993, the Bank had published its first global report on health. As a result, loan-granting decisions quickly evolved. In 1987, Population, Health, and Nutrition (PHN) loans amounted to $0.3 billion; in 1992, they reached $1.2 billion; and in 1996, $2.5 billion—more than 10 percent of the Bank's total loans (Ruger 2005).

The change was not a sudden event. Rather, it had deep roots in the 1980s and World Bank debates on the meaning and targets of development. For instance, the PHN division's priorities were deeply impacted by contestation of population control programs in the Global South in the 1970s and 1980s, and by the acknowledgment that the demographic transition taking place in many Third World countries was not correlated with the existence or nonexistence of such programs (Connelly 2008; Murphy 2017). One critical aspect of these discussions was the mounting importance of "human capital" as a category of analysis and action, as reflected in a wave of reports issued in the 1980s and 1990s. The economist Gary Becker summed up this position in a seminal World Bank document, stating:

> The importance of human capital to growth is perhaps excessively illustrated by the outstanding records of Japan, Taiwan, Hong Kong, South Korea, and other fast growing Asian economies. But they are obvious examples because they lack natural resource, which is typically greatly overstated as a determinant of economic performance, and face discrimination against their exports in the West. Nevertheless, they have managed to grow extremely rapidly in significant part because they have had a well trained, educated, and hard-working labor force, and dedicated parents. (Becker 1995)

Such theories thus backed a gradual change of focus toward health, education, and women's empowerment, reflected in the growing number of projects the PHN division launched and its transition away from nutrition and population control.

A second characteristic of the World Bank's commitment to health was the complex relationship between this shift and structural adjustment policies. Investing in health did not officially contradict the Bank's conditions—namely, urgent budget balancing and privatization of nationalized industries—for granting loans to states caught in debt crisis. However, structural adjustment programs often resulted in dramatic cuts to public investments in the social sector, even if such cuts were not explicitly among the conditions of loans.[3] Moreover, throughout the 1980s, the idea of "cost recovery" in the health system resonated like a leitmotif throughout the World Bank's reports and memos of understanding. This concept provided the background for the famous 1987 Bamako Declaration, in which African countries expressed their willingness to establish patients' fees for hospital services and drugs.

These fees, the reports argued, would ease the financial burden of health institutions, provide rolling funds to improve supply, and fashion patients-as-clients who would be more responsible for their own health outcomes and more attentive to the quality of service provided. This proposal ultimately backfired, and critiques escalated beyond public health specialists all the way to international organizations, including the WHO and UNICEF (Chorev 2012).

The World Bank's 1993 *World Development Report* (WDR) was a de facto response to this difficulty, as it strongly endorsed, after much revision of preliminary versions, the idea that markets alone cannot provide for healthcare, which is in most instances a public good. Investing in health thus meant strengthening national health systems. This was part of a more general debate throughout the 1980s about the financing and strengthening of health systems in developing countries. In the mid-1980s, World Bank staff recommended reducing public spending and public responsibility for citizens' health.[4] Within a context of budget constraints, it argued, governments should pay only for the services that would benefit society as a whole and let individuals pay for care that would benefit themselves or their families (Akin 1987). Phrased in another way, governments should only provide preventive services while users should pay for healthcare services. As one of the health economists in the World Bank's PHN division explained in a 1985 memo:

> An essential theme of new initiatives should be to have users bear a larger share of health care costs. . . . For most curative services, the arguments for public provision do not, on close inspection, stand up well. In general, developing countries—like most, though not all developed countries—should begin to think about having government do less direct providing of care and more indirect financing and regulating of providers.[5]

Governments should therefore encourage insurance programs and the development of private-sector health services, thus creating and regulating health markets in which patients would act as rational consumers (Akin 1987; Casper and Clarke 1998).

Boiling health down to a single indicator, the disability-adjusted life year (DALY), which measured the global burden of disease (see chapter 2, Metrics for Development), was justified by the need for a comparison tool that allowed decision makers to choose their interventions by planning investments in terms of public health performance (i.e., their cost-effectiveness). Once the framework for the objectification of health needs had been defined by DALY calculations, the central question became deciding which interventions would combine a low level of expenditure with a high level of performance. Forty-seven possible interventions were selected in collaboration with the WHO, and World Bank experts proposed a cost-benefit analysis for each relating annual expenditure to the number of DALYs preserved.

The Bank, in fact, combined DALY calculations with a general evaluation of performance in selected national health systems. For the poorest countries, the Bank recommended an end to financing high-technology hospitals and expensive care infrastructure, which benefited only the middle and upper classes. In their stead it suggested interventions that would meet the needs of the destitute, those populations most "at risk," less because of their exposure to pathogens than because of their social and economic vulnerability. Hence, World Bank experts recommended reorganizing health coverage by creating a publicly offered and freely accessible basic system of care, the only one for which direct, centralized, and evaluable action was possible. In an unusual move for a global financial institution deeply involved in the implementation of the Washington Consensus (Chorev 2007), the 1993 WDR put forward a strong plea for action by national governments:

> Three economic rationales justify and guide a government role in health: The poor cannot always afford health care that would improve their productivity and wellbeing. Publicly financed investment in the health of the poor can reduce poverty or alleviate its consequences. Some actions that promote health are pure public goods or create large positive externalities. Private markets would not produce them at all or would produce too little. Markets failures in health care and health insurances mean that government intervention can raise welfare by improving how these markets function. (World Bank 1993, 53)

The point was not to omit private actors but, on the contrary, to make a critical distinction between basic needs and more individual needs, between countries wealthy enough to cover costs, whatever the mechanism (taxation, insurance, or patient contributions) without drastic triage, and low- and middle-income countries (LMICs) with very limited resources, where most households were not in a position to provide for even their basic health needs. In LMICs, triage was operating de facto, with little rationalization, favoring the urban middle class. In these cases, public provision of an "essential package" of interventions was indispensable. As the Bank noted:

> Perhaps the most fundamental problem facing governments is simply how to make choices about health care. Too often, government policy has concentrated on providing as much health care as possible to as many people as possible, with too little attention to other issues. If governments are to finance a package of public health measures and clinical services, there must be a way to choose which services belong in the package and which will be left out. (World Bank 1993, 59)

The fundamental outcome of these operations was a new performance-based form of triage best illustrated by the proposal to determine an "essential package of health services in developing countries" (Bobadilla, Cowley et al. 1994). The package was limited to approximately double what low-income countries were spending at the time: $12 ($22 today in U.S. dollars) per person per year. The package prolonged and provided new legitimacy to selective primary health care by including existing priorities like immunization, sexually transmitted infection (STI) treatment, prenatal care, family planning, and AIDS prevention. A few new items were also added: tobacco control, for instance, or the more important "limited care" cluster focusing on the treatment of skin allergies and injuries, on the one hand, and access to medications for pain relief, diabetes, hypertension, and TB, on the other.

Although this approach did not result in significant use of the DALY-based technique in planning of health investments at the national level (see chapter 2, Metrics for Development), it did pave the way for the World Bank's massive engagement with global health flagship programs to fight HIV, TB, and malaria from 1995 to 2005.

Triage toward Disease Control: Tuberculosis and "Verticalization" in Global Health

When India's TB treatment program began in 1962, its aim, as one of its creators recalled in an interview, was to treat TB in the communities where it occurred by locating services where patients sought care.[6] The author of the program suggested that the approach was based on patients' "felt need." Because the program located services where patients went when they felt a need for care, it left triage decisions about whom to treat to patients and their families. This emphasis on triage through experienced illness and "felt need" sought to achieve several things, and many of them were clearly political (Banerji 1967, 1971; Nagpaul 1967).

Though selecting who got care seemed in the hands of patients, the decision to build a TB program was overtly political. In the early years of Indian independence, TB gained importance as studies revealed the high numbers of people suffering from the disease (Amrith 2006). The nascent state was constitutionally obliged to respond. Its program to address suffering needed to simultaneously expand a biopolitics that imagined a responsive, pastoral, and democratic state; generate a politics of state planning for modernization; and foster active citizen engagement (Brimnes 2016). Focusing on curing people who had triaged themselves into care, the framers of the National Tuberculosis Program sought to build a TB treatment program rather than a TB control program, another prioritization with political inflections. The priority was to save lives and build relations of state pastoralism and democratic participation while future economic and social development would control the disease (Bhore Committee 1946; Mudaliar Committee 1962).[7] Given these priorities, the program's effects at an epidemiological level were far less important than the physical and political effects the program could have on people who accessed the health system for cure. A focus on patient-guided triage aligned with theories of state building through service provision.

Prioritizing intervention based on patients' willingness to access care rather than their physical condition meant that the program needed to treat TB in its many forms without creating a hierarchy in which some manifestations of the disease[8] were more important than others (Andersen and Banerji 1963; Narain, Nair et al. 1968). Social or political factors rather than biological ones determined triage, and this orientation had system-wide effects. Programmatically diagnosing the many complex manifestations of the disease was not always easy. It often relied on specialized clinical knowledge, x-ray imaging, empirical inspection, and a broad definition of who counted as suffering from TB (Nagpaul 1967; Narain, Nair et al. 1968; Nagpaul 1975; Nagpaul, Naganathan et al. 1979). This was controversial.

In 1968, the scholars from the National TB Institute in Bangalore who led the National TB Program (NTP) refused to limit public health interventions to just one form of TB. Ultimately, they published an article placing India's TB program in conflict with the WHO's global TB directives (Narain, Nair et al. 1968). They argued against the WHO's epidemiology-based system of triage, which privileged contagion, and indicted that system as imperialist and neocolonialist. The Indian scholars wrote, "The main purposed of this paper is to focus attention on the difficulties of defining a case on the basis of bacteriological and x-ray examination and the tuberculin test" (Narain, Nair et al. 1968, 702). The paper emphasizes the need to treat people who have key symptoms, despite their lack of what the WHO called international comparability and bacteriological confirmation (i.e., the tuberculosis bacteria is not visible on slides). In short, the authors argue that patients who cannot be proved contagious and therefore of risk to others still need care. The scholars quote the WHO committee to which they were responding in hopes of revealing the ironic subordination of treatment to knowledge creation:

> The committee believed that it was essential first to agree on a definition of a "case" of tuberculosis. It was decided that, from the epidemiological point of view, a "case" of pulmonary tuberculosis means a person is suffering from bacteriologically confirmed disease. Acceptance of this definition would lead to the provision of statistical information that would be internationally and internationally comparable, and would establish the basis for notification to the public health authorities. All other possible sufferers from tuberculosis, i.e., those in whom the disease has not been confirmed bacteriologically, would be classified as "suspect cases" and would remain so classified unless or until the presence of tubercle bacilli or some other etiology was established. (Narain, Nair et al. 1968, 702)

The Indian group disagreed with this policy, which counted and treated only those with a particular pulmonary form of a disease that can affect the whole body. They rejected the politics of international epistemology and comparability in favor of a national, political policy of giving care to all TB sufferers. After all, "suspect," for those unfamiliar with TB's language games, signals a person who has some TB-like symptoms but is not under treatment by a TB program (Ditiu and Kumar 2012). Their program drew the line between patient and "suspect" differently, and the disagreement concerned triage. It focused on processes of separating patients who should be treated from those who should be monitored and interrogated and the tools by which that decision might be made. By disagreeing on these points, India's TB program deviated from the WHO's international standard. It also rendered patients diagnosed and treated in India incommensurable to those treated on the basis of bacteriological diagnostic criteria around the world. India had developed its own definition of when to treat a case of TB, based on criteria of felt need for care, rather than the presence of bacteria. Thus, one country's system of politically informed triage had international epistemological effects.

As the Indian scholars pointed out, the tools by which diagnoses are made are tools with built-in processes of triage, and they too need to correspond to India's broad political theory of triage. Though the program encouraged physicians to use diagnostic tools to identify and categorize TB sufferers, it did not require any particular method and relied on specialists' expertise. By the 1980s, only 30 percent of patients treated by the project were diagnosed on the basis of observed bacteria or an x-ray (Andersen and Dahlstrom 1983). The remaining 70 percent were diagnosed on the basis of clinical expertise. This flexibility in diagnostic criteria was soon to be embroiled in a dispute over evidence-based medicine and global health. Indeed, by 1988, the lack of "evidence-based treatment" in India led one study to suggest that the program was nearly criminal in its divergence from the WHO's strong emphasis on bacteriological evidence (Institute of Communications, Operations Research, and Community Involvement 1988).

Independent TB and public health experts commissioned by India as well as by donor countries formally reviewed the National TB Program at least five times during these controversial years from 1970 to 1990. Reviewers asked questions about expanding sputum-smear microscopy again and again in hopes that smear, which relied less on infrastructure (x-ray) and expertise (clinical diagnosis), would catalyze broader access to care in the peripheries. Program organizers continued to make gestures toward sputum smear but held tight to programmatic flexibility. This changed in 1992, when the WHO released a scathing review of India's TB program. Among the many faults listed, two are most striking. First, the report claimed that the program seemed not to have had any effect on the TB epidemic, despite thirty years of work; and second, the low percentage of patients diagnosed on the basis of observed bacteria could mean that the project was treating tens of thousands of people who did not have TB at all. Chris Murray, then acting head of the operations research cell of the WHO's TB unit, wrote to the NTP's donor agency, the Swedish International Development Agency (SIDA), suggesting that unchanged incidence and prevalence indicators were perhaps the most damning evidence of programmatic failure.[9] By suggesting that the project spent millions of dollars without reducing the risk of disease, he raised a question of efficiency and answered it by saying that the program was all cost and no effect.

These questions of disease control, comparability, and efficacy—all necessary ingredients for conducting global health's economic triage—were central to the reformulation of whose suffering mattered and who received care. The Indian program was revised to follow more closely the early 1990s global ideology of TB control, and it did so by strongly emphasizing the use of microscopy (Sarin and Dey 1995; Arora and Sarin 2000). During pilot studies, physicians enrolled in treatment only those patients whose sputum revealed bacteria, and it was these patients who were officially counted as cases of TB. This shift to microscopy had two aims. First, by moving from a programmatic emphasis on x-ray to sputum smear, TB diagnosis could be moved out of district hospitals and into primary health centers. Unlike x-ray machines, microscopes were less expensive and more portable. The process of conducting sputum-smear microscopy was simple enough to be conducted by a laboratory technician and its results were far less susceptible to different interpretations by different physicians (Engel 2015). Second, a sputum smear would identify only those patients whose disease was contagious. By focusing programmatic energy on the treatment of contagious patients, officials hoped to limit TB's spread and cause a decline in epidemiological indicators. Microscopy would also generate—as the WHO committee suggested in 1964—"statistical information that would be internationally and intra-nationally comparable" (World Health Organization 1964, 8).

Microscopy as a tool for identifying who needed care involved trade-offs. It would allow the program to reach more people suffering from TB but would diagnose only about 50 percent of actual TB sufferers. It mostly identified people spreading the disease, focused on curing officially diagnosed patients for the purposes of showing a programmatic effect, and identified a standard form of TB that could be compared quantitatively and qualitatively the world over. At the same time, this triage process that made low-cost, community-based, and globally comparable TB control possible meant that some patients would slip under the radar. Despite the urgency HIV brought to TB control, sputum microscopy of people with the HIV virus was less likely to reveal bacteria, even if they were contagious (Perkins 2000; Schutz, Meintjes et al. 2010). Children posed a similar problem. Finally, those afflicted by TB in other parts of the body, once a large proportion of the NTP's patients, would not produce sputum, and if they did, it would not contain bacteria. All three of these groups would fail to meet the threshold of microscopic proof, despite the presence of both bacteria and suffering.

The exclusionary effects of the sputum-smear-based global triage episteme and its statistical comparability did not go unnoticed in India. It caused considerable worry for the first physicians who implemented the revised project in their communities. A World Bank aide-memoire submitted to the WHO writes of the physicians' uneven implementation of sputum-based triage:

> It was noted in several of the visits that the improvement in diagnosis criteria has happened only for cases resident in the area implemented in pilot I, and has not extended to the practice of medical officers regarding other patients. This suggests insufficient orientation and motivation, and still poor use of the laboratory for diagnosis of tuberculosis, with the new strategy being considered a project and not the new program for India.[10]

What the World Bank official points to as an undersupply of orientation and motivation was, in the eyes of physicians involved in pilot I, a concern for this shift in triage. Faced with patients they felt sure—at least using a combination of their clinical expertise, x-ray, and other indicators—to be suffering from TB, the physicians began to set up a parallel system of care. They put those who fit the bacterial model of diagnosis into the new program and placed those who did not into the older program with its less stringent diagnostic criteria. A Delhi-based pilot physician recalled in an interview, "First, we would run the experiment protocol only on those patients who came from the catchment area. Then even those we thought . . . had TB but did not have a positive smear, or those we thought could not manage observation, we would put them on the old treatment. I think probably we had about fifty-fifty in and out."[11] A physician in Mumbai told a similar story and related her difficulty in explaining to patients why some got one treatment while others received a different one. Indeed, only those who revealed bacteria on a smear would be given the new rifampicin-based short course.

> I did it like this until we had no other choice because the other project had ended, and then we had to ask the people we suspected but had no smear to wait a few weeks and come back. Those who had other forms of TB, we put them in a different category or suggested they go to the private sector. It was difficult to tell them that they would need to go to the private sector or that they would need to wait and become sicker.[12]

The shift from diagnosis and treatment on the bases of a more flexible constellation of factors to diagnosis based entirely on sputum smear was dictated by alignment with global health standards. Indeed, the increased use of sputum-smear microscopy was critical for a World Bank loan to finance the program, and rates of patients treated on the basis of sputum smear were included as an indicator of programmatic success. The ability to prove the effectiveness of intervention through documentable cure (a transition from visible TB bacilli on a slide to its absence was the foundation on which cost and effect could be calculated).

The program aimed to manage the epidemic more efficiently by treating only confirmed cases, used appropriate technology that allowed diagnosis to happen in the community with minimal medical expertise, and helped build a community of globally comparable, verifiable, and quantifiable TB sufferers. These patients were given access to different medicines that could cure TB more quickly than the conventional treatment. Even though the drugs had similar effects on all nonresistant TB bacilli, they were reserved only for these patients whose treatment could have a quantifiable epidemiological impact. Though early implementers could choose between modes of diagnosis and triage, when the project scaled up to cover all of India, it included physicians who did not have access to x-ray technology or intensive training in TB medicine. They relied exclusively on the sputum smear. In their clinics, now outnumbering specialized TB clinics by an order of magnitude, those patients deemed to have a suspect case of TB could wait for the disease to reach their lungs or access care in the private sector.

The effects of this change in triage techniques did not occur simply at the level of the patient, but it shaped the idea of what a TB intervention might do, its assessment, and the very nature of what kind of disease matters for global health. Constructing a new triage practice to control TB in India reshaped the biopolitics of TB, adjusting the boundaries of population and disease. At the same time, by separating people suffering from TB into pulmonary and extra-pulmonary cases, it drew Indian pulmonary TB sufferers into a global assembly of people at the root of the TB epidemic. Treating them was cost-effective, for states if not for patients, not just because they would be cured but because they would not infect others. In short, we see triage in its classical state, choosing which forms of illness are of priority status and which individuals, though suffering, can or should wait. Clearly, infectious disease along with cost and comparability are foundational elements of global health, and the effects of such priorities on knowledge and practice are present in both the clinic and in statistical tables. Systematic triage shifts the meaning of health and illness at a global scale, and the case of Indian TB treatment demonstrates the way in which political considerations gave way to economic ones as the impetus to compare and control diseases gained strength.

COMPREHENSIVE PRIMARY HEALTH CARE, MEDICAL GENETICS, AND TASK SHIFTING IN OMAN

Three decades after Alma-Ata, in the World Health Report of 2008, the WHO published a series of country-level case studies focusing on primary health care achievements to bolster continued support for such efforts (World Health Organization 2008a). Oman was among the featured countries. The authors of the report praised the country for being "close to [achieving] universal access to healthcare within a generation" and for having "invested consistently in [the] national health system"—despite the selective primary health care trend in the 1980s. Sharp decreases in under-five mortality and striking increases of life expectancy in Oman backed up the WHO's assessment and its praise of the Omani healthcare system.

The creation of the Omani healthcare system is part of the history of the country's "Renaissance"—that is, the deep social and political changes the late Sultan Qaboos[13] brought to the country during his fifty-year reign (1970–2020). Marcos Cueto writes that "in its more radical [and original] version, primary health care was an adjunct to social revolution" (2004, 1871). Indeed, from its inception in 1970, the Omani regime understood this connection between social change and basic healthcare. However, the scope of the changes was noticeably wider in the health domain than in the political field. Despite timid overtures toward democratization (including after the 2011 Arab Spring), the sultanate remains an authoritarian state with stark inequalities (Valeri 2007). Nonetheless, the Omani approach to primary health care and to the creation of its healthcare system has been radical. The significant financial windfall brought by the relatively recent discovery of oil allows free public healthcare for all Omani citizens (about 60 percent of the population), and biomedical infrastructures have blossomed since Sultan Qaboos's ascent to power in 1970.[14]

Oman's healthcare system grew during the 1970s primary health care moment. In May 1971, Oman joined the WHO. It was the country's first membership in an international organization, and an understanding of internal politics helps contextualize this decision (World Health Organization 1971). As the army was fighting in a civil war against the Dhofar Liberation Front, a separatist communist movement, the healthcare system was one of the strategic pillars of the new regime's legitimacy. Oman's first minister of health explains this period:

We were a new government, so people had high expectations of us; we had to do something, very quickly. . . . Even WHO knew nothing about the area, neither about the Emirates, nor about Oman. We have created a kind of instant Ministry of Health. Rudimentary clinics, but quickly built, that was the important thing. . . . There were political contingencies; people had to trust their leader.[15]

The aim—and challenge—was to swiftly build a network of state-run clinics and hospitals that would both provide care and render the state visible across the country. These twin concerns produced, from the 1970s to the end of the 1990s, a topographical Omani approach to primary health care that did not imply recruiting grassroots doctors or transferring responsibilities to trained villagers but rather an effort to staff small healthcare centers scattered throughout the territory. A majority of non-Omani physicians ran these healthcare centers until the creation of the national Medicine College in the late 1980s. Because the initial yearly budget was the equivalent of only $47 million (in contemporary U.S. dollars),[16] these early years of the Omani healthcare system—which would be ranked first in the world thirty years later for "performance on health level" (together with Cyprus and Iran, for instance; see World Health Organization 2000)[17]—were characterized by effective management of scarce resources. However, one can also consider this peculiar because of the rapid, novel, and ubiquitous way the regime imposed biomedical healthcare on the population. Indeed, the Sultan at the time emphasized the widest possible access through coverage of even the most remote localities. To achieve this, the regime rapidly developed the road network, at times even used military transportation for patients, and created a national patient referral system.

Today, the health system remains mostly state-run. The public sector employs 70 percent of physicians in the country and consists of a relatively dense network of 266 governmental health centers and dispensaries, as well as seventy-four hospitals, including tertiary and specialized centers in the two main urban areas. Other governmental institutions such as the Royal Oman Police or the Ministry of Higher Education administer additional public hospitals. The private sector accounts for 7.5 percent of hospital beds spread among nineteen hospitals and mainly provides nonspecialized care in small private clinics. Their number has, however, doubled since 2000, reaching approximately 1,000 clinics in 2016 (Ministry of Health Oman 2017).

This health infrastructure boom resulted from the careful organization of the Ministry of Health's successive five-year plans and followed the implementation of a primary health care policy "à la Alma-Ata"—that is, a policy centered on a set of activities largely following the conference's definition of basic needs. Nevertheless, the horizontal Omani approach to primary health care differs from WHO recommendations on crucial matters. In fact, it only follows two out of the four key features in the Alma-Ata strategy. First, it strongly connects health to national development goals, such as education, transportation, sanitation, and it treats health as an object of planning. Second, it organizes healthcare availability with a strong emphasis on rural communities and their access to health centers. In contrast, though, the Omani policies did not refer to community participation in the definition of primary health care until the mid-2000s, when "*wilayat* health com-mittees" became responsible for short-term "local supportive plans" (Ministry of Health Oman 2017). Finally, and contrary to Alma-Ata recommendations, the gov-ernmental effort has almost exclusively focused on biomedical approaches and technologies. Although partially in line with the approach initially fostered by the WHO, the Omani version of primary health care nonetheless remains more com-prehensive than package-oriented (for an example, see Ministry of Health Oman 2017, 1.15). This feature is crucial in the official discourse about the healthcare sys-tem, as the 2016 Annual Health Report of the Ministry of Health shows when it calls for "a strong, responsive and sustainable primary health care system as the main entry point and backbone of health care" (Ministry of Health Oman 2017).

Such continuous and unusually strong—though fragmented—adherence to Alma-Ata's main principles is evident in the expansion of the comprehensive pri-mary health care offered, especially concerning noncommunicable disorders (e.g., the availability in primary health care centers for breast cancer screening, diabe-tes consultations, and genetic screening). Oman was one of the rare countries out-side of continental Europe or America (Modell and Kuliev 1998) that reacted to early WHO calls for the integration of medical genetics into primary health care (World Health Organization 1999, 2005, 2006). Though on a small scale, genetic medicine has been part of Oman's healthcare system since the 1990s. Initially, it centered on the diagnosis and management, through community genetics, of inherited blood disorders (IBDs) (Beaudevin 2013, 2015). Local researchers tackled the matter as well, with physicians publishing clinical and epidemiological data about the Omani situation (e.g., White, Christie et al. 1993; Rajab and Patton 1997), hematologists proposing management options (Rajab and Patton 1999), and the Ministry of Health editing a "National Genetic Blood Disorders Survey" (Al-Riyami 2000). Later, the entire spectrum of congenital anomalies entered focus, and Omani clinicians published epidemiological data showing the public health relevance of genetics for the country (e.g., Goud, Al-Harassi et al. 2005; Rajab, Al Salmi et al. 2014). As such, they called for new clinical and research infrastruc-tures. Despite clinical advocacy, screening for IBDs remains limited in the coun-try, as does clinical genetics expertise.

Infrastructures for genetic medicine, however, have grown in major urban areas. In 2010 and 2013, two state-run—though partially privately funded—genetic med-ical centers opened in Muscat, the capital of Oman. Each provides an on-site combination of genetic expertise, diagnostic facilities, and genetic counseling.

Nonetheless, medical genetics in Oman expanded against the backdrop of an increasingly difficult economic situation. The aftermath of the 2008 global financial crisis, combined with a drop in oil prices, created serious budget deficits for the Omani government. Though the state usually absorbs deficits, in 2016, for the first time, it addressed the matter through massive public budget cuts (Oman News Agency 2015, 2016; Reuters 2016; Valeri 2018). Because of these shortfalls, more careful resource allocation in health, or economic triage of health priorities, grew in impor-tance. Although the expansion of medical genetics into primary health care in

Oman continued, the Ministry of Health reduced cost through task shifting.[18] Their revised plan suggests that in regional hospitals specifically, trained nurses can provide genetic counseling and referrals to the capital's genetic centers. It is worth noting that this approach to expanding primary health care remains in line with Oman's historic adherence to the WHO's discourse. In this case, Oman follows the call of Margaret Chan (Director-General of the World Health Organization, 2006–2017) for "task shifting as the vanguard for the renaissance of primary health care" (World Health Organization, PEPFAR et al. 2008, preface, n.p.).

During this time of scarcity of public funds and of trained geneticists and genetic counselors, seven Omani nurses employed in seven different regional public hospitals voluntarily enrolled in the National Genetic Centre's sixteen-month genetic counseling training course. This program involved coursework and role-plays, clinical rotations, laboratory exposure, and visits to local associations and educational institutions. When the program started, Oman had only two formally trained genetic counselors and a third completing her training. The status of the genetic counseling training course and of its graduates, however, remains unclear. Its organizers aim to "train candidates to be able to interface between patients, clinicians and medical geneticists" (Al-Araimi 2016, 4), but explicitly not to "equip [them] to register or practice as genetic counselors or medical geneticists" (Al-Araimi 2016, 7). However, during the training sessions, trainers refer to students as "genetic counselors (under training)," and students also adopted this identification, with the immediate effect of bringing a genetic perspective to regional hospitals where it had formerly been absent. The Ministry of Health's decision to endorse this training program does not, however, account for the reality of task shifting and the practicalities of these nurses' everyday work. For instance, back in her regional hospital, one of the trained nurses struggled to get a dedicated office for her counseling sessions. Once she did, the room had glass walls and no ceiling, which forced her to improvise the privacy she considered necessary to genetic counseling. In practice, she typically asks her office neighbors to leave the building when she conducts a session with patients, and she has glued faux wood stickers on the glass walls. Interestingly, Omani infrastructures not related to health support the attempt to shift genetic counseling from trained counselors to already employed nurses. First, an improved road network and daily domestic flights between various parts of the sultanate allow nurses to commute between their hometowns and the National Genetic Centre for continuing training. Second, fast and reliable Internet access throughout most of the country's urban areas allows their counseling activity to become routine by allowing patient records and referral requests to circulate between trained nurses and Muscat expert centers—albeit often over WhatsApp messaging.

The continuous development of comprehensive primary health care in Oman—in the form of the inclusion of medical genetics—is doubly rooted and shaped. First, the relative wealth of the sultanate, evident in infrastructures, is a material condition of possibility for this development. Second, the lack of trained physicians and counselors and the burdensome economic situation led to the implementation of the task-shifting policy. Economic triage applied to medical staff recruitment and qualification appears here as the price to pay for the sustainability of medical genetics within primary health care. In other words, the parallel practice of economic and political triage is framed as necessary for the preservation of increasingly comprehensive primary health care in Oman.

DISTRIBUTED POLITICAL TRIAGE IN KERALA

A program treating depression in Kerala, India, is evidence of political triage's continuity in Indian healthcare. The program, which is arguably local but shares strategies with global mental health, reveals how policymakers in Kerala prioritize certain conditions over others on the basis of basic needs rather than efficiency, performance, or cost-effectiveness. Experts and communities identify these needs and inform choices made by local and state governments. As in the Alma-Ata Declaration, the selection of prioritized needs is, in the first place, a political choice, involving representation and debate at the local level. By designating certain medical conditions as basic needs, policymakers in Kerala negotiate and align global, national, state, and local political priorities.

In the 1990s, DALY metrics made depression visible to global health. Emphasizing disability alongside morbidity, the DALYs thrust depression into the first ranks of the Global Burden of Disease (GBD) studies. The disorder gained prominence as the global mental health movement and its research consortia and research projects gained momentum. Depression gained even wider attention at a high-level Washington-based meeting of civil society activists, academics, finance ministers, and business leaders held in 2016. This high-level meeting not only consolidated the World Bank's depression-related collaboration with the WHO and the Bank's role as a visible institutional actor in global mental health, but it also moved depression and anxiety "out of the shadow" and into the heart of debates about global health. World Health Day 2017 even further cemented depression in global health. Despite all of this, the portion of national health budgets and donor funds allocated to mental healthcare pale in comparison to that allocated to infectious diseases such as HIV/AIDS, TB, and malaria (see chapter 2, Metrics for Development).

In contrast, political triage based on locally defined basic needs led to the creation of Ashwasam ("Relief" in Sanskrit), Kerala's depression and suicide prevention program. The state strategically launched Ashwasam on World Health Day 2017. Ashwasam aims to integrate the identification and treatment of depression into primary health care. It includes the screening of vulnerable or high-risk groups[19] by trained community health workers, staff nurses, and primary health care physicians; identification of cases of depression; treatment packages of pharmacological and psychosocial care; and referral to clinics run by the staff of the District Mental Health Program, if necessary. A high-level bureaucrat in Kerala emphasized in an interview that policymakers used local experience as the basis of their decision to make screening and treatment of depression one of the state's public health priorities.[20] According to him, policymakers preferred this local knowledge to national and state epidemiological surveys, statewide burden of disease studies in India based on GBD figures, and evidence provided by global-health-oriented research projects. It was not epidemiological or cost-effectiveness data that drove the decision but the experience of mental health experts, he stressed. In other words, policymakers did not employ cost-effectiveness triage based on epidemio-economic numbers but rather a needs-based political triage that relied on local experience, expertise, and planning.

The same experts who designed the Ashwasam program had earlier formulated the mental health–related goals of Kerala's Sustainable Development Goals State Targets for 2030 alongside reproductive, maternal, newborn, and child health and communicable and noncommunicable diseases as a main priority. Thus, although prioritizing depression is consistent with global concerns, its designers emphasized that Ashwasam is a local priority based in a local context. The program provides an example of how globally circulating imperatives or "traveling models" (Behrends, Park et al. 2014)—such as the integration of depression into primary health care; task shifting and sharing; and associated packages of screening and treatment (Funk, Saraceno et al. 2008; Patel, Saxena et al. 2018)—are incorporated into government policies and programs and take new forms during the translation into localities. In a situation of human resources scarcity and "treatment gaps," task shifting or task sharing reallocates certain prioritized interventions from doctors or specialized professionals to nonspecialist health workers. In a hierarchy of providers, general physicians take on tasks triaged as more important, such as pharmacological treatment, while nurses, lay health workers, or teachers carry out psychosocial interventions and mental health promotion.

A team of experts involved in the architecture of the Kerala depression program, discovered a prevalence of depression in nearly one-third of all patients in primary health centers (Indu, Anilkumar et al. 2017). Primary care physicians confirmed these numbers in interviews,[21] some of them claiming a prevalence up to 60 percent in women ages 50–60. More importantly, Kerala's suicide rates rank among India's highest (Halliburton 1998; Münster 2012), and the "suicide crisis" among farmers, students, and the elderly are a matter of public concern. A high proportion of those attempting suicide, a psychiatrist explained in an interview,[22] had had previous contact with the health system for another complaint. Ten out of 150 patients seeking care in a primary health center have a history of suicidal attempt, psychiatrists found in a survey, and most of those who attempt suicide have depression. It is these patients that a suicide prevention training course for physicians and nurses would help to identify. Through the psychiatrization of suicide (and suicide attempts) and the shift of focus from structural causes to individual biochemistry, psychiatrists imagine Ashwasam as a program can literally save lives. Ultimately, it is the suicide risk of depression that aligns depression with other life-threatening diseases and makes triage crucial.

The form of Kerala's primary health care system is as much a matter of needs, knowledge, and decision making as it is of budgeting. Following the shift to decentralized local governance in the late 1990s, localized decision making and budget allocation became a central feature of needs-based political triage in Kerala. Local self-governance[23] and the reallocation of 30 percent of the state's budget to village councils, enabled communities to prioritize, administer, manage, and finance their own healthcare targets based on the felt needs of the people and local development plans. This regime has benefited primary health centers most (Elamon, Franke et al. 2000). Implementing any program on the local level requires aligning local, state, and national priorities. The local self-governance of health reflects the vision of Alma-Ata to define priorities by combining specialized knowledge and local experience. It is the collective interests or distributed political triage of the local assembly, the village council (*panchayat*), the medical officers in the primary health center, and—in the case of mental health programs—specialized psychiatric knowledge that leads to the decision to implement the Ashwasam depression program in these communities. And it is the engagement and the collaboration of the members of the village council, physicians in the primary health center, and community health workers that accounts for the success of this program in a locality. The selection of basic needs here is a political choice in the first place.

In Kerala's political triage, programmatic efficacy is measured in terms of the number of people in the community its interventions touched. This is different from the notion of economic efficacy that characterizes cost-effectiveness triage. While programs such as Ashwasam do produce numbers to demonstrate success, these numbers refer to a stated need in the communities rather than being focused on cost-effective interventions. The political economy of numbers turns individuals taken into the program into achievements, diagnoses into value, and—for community health workers—identified cases into remuneration. In a form of numero-political triage, numbers justify programs by testifying to communities' needs. It is the emotional and existential suffering of people that the newly acquired clinical gaze turns into cases of depression that are counted here. These numbers are important as local evidence for the success of a program, but they do not appear in global health publications since they do not follow standardized research-designs (Adams 2016b). In other words, these numbers legitimize political triage, but they do not provide the basis of cost-effectiveness or performance-based triage.

Political triage that prioritizes depression over other mental disorders is both affected by and affects clinical triage. The Ashwasam program aims to assemble diverse subjectivities into a diagnostic and treatment regime in line with global mental health agendas. Subjectivities in line with international classifications are put into the treatment regime and into statistics, while others with primarily somatic symptoms such as pain, weakness, or heat (Lang 2018)—while still treated—are not categorized as part of the program. In clinical triage, physicians in primary health centers constantly make decisions about who to treat immediately and who to refer (and defer) to the mental health clinic run by the District Mental Health Program. Primary care physicians prefer to treat patients with primarily somatic complaints—turned into symptoms of depression—and milder forms of mental distress and often triage out those who suffer from the more stigmatized psychotic forms of mental disorder.

In the community mental health clinics, on the other hand, patients with milder forms of depression and anxiety are rarely visible for three reasons. First, mental health clinics tend to focus their energy on severe mental disorders. Second, families are reluctant to expose their kin to the psychiatric regime and the stigma associated with it. Third, families in rural Kerala often consider the suffering that psychiatry associates with depression as the effect of socioeconomic adversities or simply as a part of life rather than as a mental health problem. While families attempt to navigate care, cost, and stigma in addressing mental distress, they often lose control of the narrative since the program brings suffering under the purview of the state and turns it into an object of screening and management.

Many community health workers to whom the program assigns the tasks of identifying, recording, surveilling, and counseling depression regard the Ashwasam program as an additional burden in their already packed list of daily duties. In fact, some community health workers refuse the psychiatrization of suffering and continue to focus on their "traditional" tasks of maternal health or infectious diseases. Others comply with the government's efforts to expand Kerala's primary health care system to deal with distress, emotional suffering, and existential despair (Lang 2019). Deciding which households to visit, which patients to attend, and whether or not to include mental health in their agenda depends largely on the priorities of the primary health center and its medical officer as well as the village council's interests and financial considerations. Families are also involved in deciding whether to subject their members to the mental health apparatus of the state, but this choice becomes increasingly difficult as medical staff are urged to identify patients with mental disorders in the hopes of bringing them into treatment or at least counting them among those suffering from such maladies.

The case of Kerala is a case of the continuity of political triage in times of global health. Political triage in Kerala identifies needs on the basis of political participation and is distributed across both state and local bodies. It is deeply interconnected with other forms of triage, specifically in clinical and community settings.

Conclusion

The idea that the rise of global health both enforces and is rooted in a multifaceted process of "economization" of health is a critical ingredient in many scenarios that try to account for the transition from international to global. Broadening the discussion to systematic *triage*—understood as the discourses, decision-making patterns, and practices of resource allocations involved in the field since the late 1970s—this chapter qualifies this process in two important ways.

The first qualification is more historical as it pertains to the Alma-Ata–centered vision of international health as a field of social medicine that relies on the recognition of needs and the understanding of health as right. Of course, primary health care did not, and could not, evade "selection"; like any strategy, it prioritized, planned, assessed, and allocated resources. It was a resolute form of political triage, deeply rooted in the "developmentalist" agenda shared by Third World nation-states and international organizations, including the World Bank. Hence the relative ease with which the selective primary health care perspective won the debate in the 1980s and the continuity in the way in which triage has operated in global health since the 1990s.

The second one concerns the evaluation of triage practices operating at the national or regional level. The cases of Oman and Kerala powerfully demonstrate that political triage can be understood not as the involvement of political/public institutions in the allocation and management of health resources, but as a politics of needs bound to notions of social protection, free access, and community involvement. This politics of needs ignores—if not openly contests—the dominance of economic evaluation and managerial practices, and it remains central in the triaging operations of numerous actors in the field, even if they are less visible than the Global Fund or the Bill and Melinda Gates Foundation. As the recent reemergence of debates about universal healthcare suggest, the presence of political values and assumptions in triage is not merely a lingering reminder of the past, a ruin hoping to inspire nostalgia, but rather a vivid challenge to global definitions of effective healthcare.

CHAPTER 4

Markets, Medicines, and Health Globalization

Caroline Meier zu Biesen, Laurent Pordié, Jessica Pourraz,
and Jean-Paul Gaudillière

On February 25, 1998, the Department of Economic Affairs within India's Ministry of Health and Family Welfare received a fax from the World Bank explaining that it had one month to comply with previous demands regarding the procurement of antituberculosis drugs. These drugs had been paid for by a major loan agreement signed less than a year earlier between the World Bank and the government of India to revamp the National Tuberculosis Program. If, by this deadline, the procurement system was not reorganized to let foreign firms compete, the World Bank threatened, it would suspend the ministry's rights to draw from the approved credit. India failed to meet the deadline, and the Bank suspended the loan. Intense negotiations followed. The World Bank's supervising team reviewed all pending issues concerning the program's organization and declared that payments would not resume unless procurement ceased to be an "in-house" affair, meaning that procurement ought to be transferred to an agency operating on the global market. World Bank officials were concerned about the personnel involved in the ministry's handling of procurement, fearing corruption and kickbacks. Requiring the transfer of purchase to an outside international agency addressed a pressing concern—namely, bringing India more firmly into the global drug market. The World Bank believed that opening Indian markets to global pharmaceuticals would limit the local procurement policy of the National Tuberculosis Program and the government's propensity to favor Indian firms and their generic antibiotics.

Written between the lines of the 1998 ultimatum, therefore, was the fear of bureaucratic inefficiency, faith in market efficiency, and an understanding of how the tuberculosis loan could contribute to reforming Indian economic policies. The World Bank had explicitly stated that the 1997 investment in tuberculosis (TB) control was to operate in parallel with the much bigger structural adjustment loan from the International Monetary Fund that India had accepted under duress in 1993. Two conditions of the latter were particularly important for the TB procurement policy: (1) ending the country's tight import controls and (2) fostering private initiative and the construction of markets by dismantling most publicly owned industrial enterprises.

By 2006, when the final audit of the tuberculosis loan took place, this episode turned out to be little more than a skirmish. The landscape had changed dramatically and procurement of TB drugs had been massively reorganized. The directly observed treatment short-course strategy (DOTS), which the Indian government applied on a grand scale, had become a global standard, sanctioned by the World Health Organization (WHO), for the design of national policies. Procurement was no longer left to nation-states operating in isolation. Instead, the global StopTB Partnership had set up a drug facility bureau under WHO leadership. The facility had a range of functions, from assessing the quality of fixed-dose combinations to granting firms certificates of good practices, and from negotiating bulk pricing to purchasing and distributing drugs for countries that did not wish to build their own procurement infrastructure.

This mundane crisis reveals the massive presence of commercial drugs in one of the most typical global health operations. In fact, one may say that without drugs and their markets, there would be no global health. The global health field is often characterized as having resurrected vertical, disease-oriented, and technologically driven programs while refocusing its goals around access to drugs and proper, standardized uses. The control of HIV, malaria, and TB, the most prominent targets of interventions, are powerful examples associated with the circulation of fixed combinations of antiretroviral treatments (ARVs) for HIV, artemisinin-based combination therapies (ACTs) for malaria, and antibiotics for tuberculosis. These pharmaceutical objects are not only therapeutic agents, however. They are also industrial goods, invented, produced ,and sold by capitalist firms.

Social studies of global health have analyzed the pervasive presence of drugs across the globe in terms of "pharmaceuticalization," even if the term has several other meanings. These studies evoke pharmaceuticalization, for instance, when discussing the globalization of clinical trials (Petryna 2009; Nguyen 2010); the judicialization of access to care (Nichter 1996; Biehl 2007); or the roles of patients' organizations in access to drugs (Robins 2004; Epstein 2007). Although global health and the pharmaceuticalization of interventions in the health of others are often equated, the synonymy remains paradoxical since most studies of global health programs do not focus on the production, circulation, and purchase of drugs while the literature on recent transformations of the drug industry—its financialization and its globalization—does not look at global health.

This chapter aims to examine this paradox not as a deficiency but as a symptom of the problematic status of markets. We argue that understanding the place of pharmaceuticals in the dynamics of globalized health requires distinguishing between global health as a field, on the one hand, and the arenas of health globalization that have nurtured the creation of this field, on the other. As we see in the 1990s Indian tuberculosis story, pharmaceuticals as commercial goods are central to the latter perspective and barely visible in the former. In order to understand this paradox, this chapter focuses on the construction of drug markets—their diversity, changing scales, competing nature, and the modalities of their presence within the field of global health.

Of course, markets are not altogether absent from social and critical studies of global health. On the contrary, they are quite visible but occupy a very specific niche. They are most often discussed in the context of neoliberalism and its post-1980s influence on international health. Markets are thus signposts and outcomes of what is mostly considered a political and ideological reconfiguration of the relationship between public and private, between states and economic actors, in favor of the latter. As a consequence, markets as sites of practical exchange and circulation of goods, as arenas of daily, routine, and social actions, have been left to a different academic genre—namely, the study of pharmaceuticals in the Global South. Recent work in the history and anthropology of pharmaceuticals have thus documented the rise of generics and the migration of their production outside Europe and the United States (Nichter 1996; Hayden 2003; Cassier and Correa 2009); the politics of access and intellectual property rights (Sunder Rajan 2017); the role of regional hubs in the circulation of drugs (Peterson 2014); and the industrialization of poly-herbals originating in Asian traditional medicines (Bode 2008; Banerjee 2009; Pordié and Gaudillière 2014a; Meier zu Biesen 2019).

Following a similar path, our chapter investigates global drug markets as social constructs. But rather than addressing the social life of drugs (Whyte, Van der Geest et al. 2002), our case studies look at the social life of drug markets, following the movement of goods and capital. By doing so, we hope to show the various regimes of market construction (i.e., market regimes) involved in the globalization of health. We are less concerned about how drugs are evaluated and how sales and marketing operate and more interested in understanding the various regimes of market construction involved in the globalization of health. Within this perspective, the notion of regime (Pestre 2003; Lakoff 2010b) is a simple way to signal the diversity of the markets at stake, the multiple ways in which they are constructed, and the regulations that their stabilization and legitimation require (Gaudillière and Hess 2013; Hardon and Sanabria 2017; Dumoulin Kervran, Kleiche-Dray et al. 2018). Central to the notion of regime is also the idea that such social and collective construction of drug markets presupposes coherence in the patterns of action grounding the four major stages in the cycle of goods: invention, appropriation, production, and distribution. The notion thus resonates with the idea of multiple "regimes of capital accumulation" that economists of the regulation school introduced in the 1970s to describe the ways that production patterns, regulatory institutions, and capital investments interacted to "create" the long period of economic growth and capital investment after World War II (Boyer 1990).

The proprietary regime of market construction is one such regime of capital accumulation. Historians of pharmacy in the Global North have, in the past fifteen years, taught us how drug making and the world of pharmaceuticals radically changed after the Second World War, leading to the emergence of "Big Pharma."

The rise of this industry is characterized by five main features: (1) the changing scale of a market increasingly supported by health insurance, thus turning drug purchases into aggregated, collective spending; (2) the mergers or disappearance of vast numbers of small family-run firms that had been established by professional pharmacists; (3) the introduction into the market of new classes of drugs, opening the door to chemotherapy in areas that had either not been working with thera-peutic substances (cancer) or had not been very successful with them (tuberculo-sis); (4) the rising importance of administrative rather than professional or industrial regulations, which led to a significant drop in the number of products sold on the market in industrialized countries; (5) the generalization of chemical-biological-clinical screening as the dominant path to drug invention, which, in the eyes of most firms, enabled the discovery of radically new active substances, rather than the copying, modifying, and combining of those already included in the phar-macopoeia, thus legitimizing massive investments in research and development infrastructures (Chauveau 1999; Hayden 2003; Quirke 2008; Carpenter 2010; Tobell 2011; Gaudillière and Hess 2013).

Scholars less often stress, however, that between 1960 and 1980, this combina-tion of factors radically altered the construction of drug markets, placed the search for "innovations" center stage, and created what we call a proprietary regime of market construction. The idea here is that the advent of structures of pharmaceu-tical capitalism, which combined innovations in pharmaceutical marketing and models of drug development based on screening and randomized clinical trials, changed the nature of market operations (Greene 2007; Dumit 2012; Gaudillière and Thoms 2015). These new structures led to the development of biocapitalist econ-omies that articulated "bio" and "capital" in new ways. Rather than anticipating development and growth on the basis of price competition and organizing short-term management with sales data as the major if not sole market indicator, large postwar pharmaceutical companies increasingly relied on monopolistic practices rooted in patent protection, competition for entire therapeutic classes, and long-term research and development (R&D). Each of these strategies strongly connected with, depended on, and further fed the massive expansion of scientific marketing and of its correlate: the monopolistic control of clinical trials, which increasingly fell to Euro-American firms.

This monopolistic regime of market construction has in the past twenty years been seriously challenged as a consequence of the enlarged consumption of phar-maceuticals in the South, new paths of drug circulation, and—even more decisively—the massive globalization of pharmaceutical production. This chapter, therefore, explores configurations that provide alternatives to the proprietary regime. These alternatives may be described as contrasting and partially compet-ing regimes of market construction, the emergence of which relies on the large-scale circulation of two categories of goods that challenge the hegemony of branded drugs—namely, generics and poly-herbal preparations. However, these new regimes are not the sole markers of crisis for the hegemonic, patent-based regime. This is exemplified in a fourth case study of the market at large, which looks closely at a political economy of drugs that mingles legal and illegal transactions and circumvents institutional power structures.

Our first two case studies consider artemisinin-based combination therapies—hereafter ACTs—in Africa, and the ways in which their global circulation intersects with local practices of market construction. The first case study is based on ethnographic fieldwork in Tanzania and archival research on the WHO's Special Program for Research in Tropical Diseases. It traces the patent and innovation-centered proprietary regime of Big Pharma, which determines the global malaria market through a typical example of chemical-pharmaceutical mass production driven by capitalist logics. The second case study is based on fieldwork conducted in Ghana with global health actors, national drug regulators, policymakers, and local pharmaceutical firms, as well as archival research on pharmaceutical-industry policy adopted by the state of Ghana since independence in 1957. It sheds light on the emergence of local production and distribution capabilities within a broader generic market regime, which aims at reducing dependency on dominant global supply.

In the third case study, we consider how emerging states and regional powers subvert the established order of drug markets and pharmaceutical industries located in the Global North. Empirically grounded in fieldwork in India, this section looks at the industrialization of Asian traditional medicines, in this case, Ayurveda. In particular, we shed light on the heterogeneous political economies that lie beneath what is superficially perceived as a single hegemonic logic of global pharmaceutical capitalism. The regime of market construction represented by this new Indian path to biocapital contrasts with the proprietary regime in two important domains: the creation of intellectual property rights over new herbal drug preparations and the creation of goods by connecting Ayurvedic formulas and biomedical disorders.

The fourth, and last, case study finally opens up the larger question of drug circulation and expands the pharmaceutical nexus by ethnographically showing how a sizable share of drugs circulates through, and overlaps with, official and unofficial drug regulation networks. Taking Cambodia as the place of study, this section sheds light on facets of market construction that may traverse other kinds of regimes, exploring more shadowy circuits of drug production and distribution.

TOWARD A GLOBAL MARKET: BRANDED ARTEMISININ DRUGS REACHING TANZANIA

Tanzania's health policy recommends artemisinin-based combination therapy as the first-line treatment for malaria. The ACT combines synthetic antimalarial drugs with compounds derived from *Artemisia annua*, which yields artemisinin. The Chinese plant, as well as artemisinin-based remedies, circulate transnationally, illustrating new circuits of exchange within the broader scope of drug globalization. In this case study, we examine the proprietary market regime by which ACTs are marketed and circulated to investigate how global health actors (the WHO, national drug regulators, donors), commercial actors (the pharmaceutical industry, private enterprises), and philanthropic institutions have created, controlled, and established their legitimacy. Of course, these categories often interweave, but the main aim here is to provide an example of how the monopolistic proprietary regime, which often provides the very materiality of global health interventions, grounds the global expansion of pharmaceutical markets for ACTs.

Global health ideology follows the logic of scientific discovery, assuming an object can be controlled by the "rational" application of technologies (Chandler and Beisel 2017). Lost in this calculus, however, are the on-the-ground realities and difficulties with which local partners must contend (Lakoff and Collier 2008; Fassin 2012; Gerrets 2012). As such, global malaria eradication is a complex balancing act (Brown 2017), and its oscillations have significant effects on Tanzania's malaria treatment policies and, hence, on access to drugs.

Analyzing the particular regime behind branded antimalarials requires attending to the cultural, scientific, and economic practices that undergird the powerful influence of Euro-U.S. Big Pharma and the markets it dominates (Greene 2011). A complementary and equally important level of investigation is how this influence impacts local health policy and practice (Petryna, Kleinman et al. 2006; van der Geest 2011; Biehl and Petryna 2013). By attending to both, a broad set of political and social transitions taking place within the global circulation of pharmaceuticals comes into view. Seeing ACTs this way demonstrates how global-scale market decisions by pharmaceutical companies influence the health of local populations, both positively and negatively. The standardization of medicines appears, on the one hand, as a necessary condition for the mass production of antimalarials. On the other, it facilitates the development of monopolies on strategic knowledge and drug formulas (Cueto 2013). The wide scale implementation of magic bullets such as ACTs interact with, but also exclude from view, the social and economic factors that affect health systems' capacity to adopt standardized solutions.

Knowledge complexes—like the strategies deployed to market and distribute the traditional Chinese plant—are central to the governance and commercialization of *Artemisia annua*. They require unpacking a complicated story that takes us from the rediscovery of artemisinin in China to commercial *Artemisia* plantations in East Africa and finally to the annual administration of 580 million treatment courses of ACTs across the globe (World Health Organization 2018b).

First, all the basic molecules assembled in ACTs are the products of research programs undertaken by Chinese military, science, and industry (Yu and Zhong 2002). Second, in 2001, the WHO declared artemisinin derivatives to be the most potent antimalarial ingredients ever discovered (World Health Organization 2001). This declaration served as the starting gun in a race between international pharmaceutical companies to purchase and patent artemisinin. From this point onward, the WHO's antimalarial program did not only focus on artemisinin, but specifically recommended the ACT from Novartis, marketed under the name Coartem, as the global standard of malaria care.

Although China owns the intellectual property rights on artemisinin deriva-tives produced in the country (Shen et al. 2010a), it is possible to patent production processes as well as specific products. In the 1980s, Chinese scientists developed an antimalarial combination consisting of two different drugs—artemether and lumefantrine. By the 1990s, Novartis signed a licensing and development agree-ment that allowed the Swiss firm to market the drug outside China. Novartis also signed a collaborative agreement with the Chinese Academy of Military Medical Sciences, Kunming Pharmaceutical Factory, and the China International Trust and Investment Corporation for further development of the combination, eventually leading to international registration of the ACT Coartem.[1] In reality, by gaining the rights to patent the ACT outside China, Novartis secured itself a long-term monopoly on the drug (Maude, Woodrow et al. 2010; World Health Organization 2010a).

Next, as a global consensus emerged around delivering Coartem to resource-poor communities, Novartis turned global health requirements into market oppor-tunities, dispensing the drug to developing countries at "cost" (Novartis 2010). In reality, Novartis, as well as its relationships to and influences on other health policy institutions (via standardization, regulation, and forms of distribution), informs the logic by which ACTs circulate. The firm's evaluation of Coartem mar-kets relies on political and moral estimations of potential malaria threats (van der Geest 2011). As such, the economic interests of the pharmaceutical industry are redefined through the existence of potential threats as validated by the WHO. Both are based on standards developed by the very same actors.

Finally, though production was for many years confined to Southeast Asia, Novartis has since established an industrial partnership with the private German-British-Swiss consortium "Botanical Extracts Limited" (EPZ) to extract artemis-inin from commercial *Artemisia* plantations in East Africa (Bate 2008; Meier zu Biesen 2013). The artemisinin crystals are then transported to Novartis, combined with the additional drug lumefantrine (or benflumentol) in China, India, and the United States, and then find their way back into developing countries as the branded medicine Coartem.

In 2006, the Tanzanian Health Ministry designated Coartem as the country's leading antimalarial treatment. The fact that this ACT was introduced as the first-line treatment, while others failed the WHO prequalification process,[2] fueled sus-picions among Tanzanian pharmaceutical experts that economic interests might have played a role (Kachur, Black et al. 2006). In their opinion, both intellectual property law and treatment policies, which privilege transnational drug compa-nies and the production of their drugs, shut out local producers from the Tanza-nian drug market (Tibandebage, Wangwe et al. 2016).

Market structure is one determinant of a health sector's capacity to produce and/ or consume medicines and to develop local supply. The growth of large-scale donor-funded procurement of ACTs has been the biggest institutional evolution in Tanzania's medicine market. Procurement policies promoted by donors and public-private partnerships that entered the global malaria stage in the early 2000s strongly influence access to ACTs in Tanzania. Such regulatory maneuvers are political and commercial acts heavily influenced by the interests of multinational corporations (see Biehl 2007; Petryna 2009; Sunder Rajan 2017 for this perspective). Countries affected by malaria, such as Tanzania, are forced to import these medicines and secure subventions for them from external donors, such as the Global Fund (Kamat 2013; Khatib, Selemani et al. 2013). No private consumers are in a position to purchase these medicines through their own means.

Accessing Coartem puts countries afflicted by malaria in a position of chronic dependency on external funding bodies. Instead of tackling the conditions facilitating economic dependency (property rights, monopolies), these are further consolidated.[3] Financial dependency on donors leads to a situation in which availability is dependent on a range of unknown factors, such as the future willingness and liquidity of external donors (see Greene 2011). In this sense, current malaria programs with their magic-bullet approach are one-dimensional strategies.

ACTs and their use in Tanzania reveal a powerful proprietary regime characterized by transnational standardization and validation processes, the activities of the big drug corporations, and their monopolies. This regime organizes the largest of global health's pharmaceutical markets. It is made possible by global health institutions, the global health episteme, and global health circuits.

Even in places like Tanzania, where pharmaceutical capitalism is very powerful, people and states persist in creating new local markets and drug circuits. The next case study shows us, through the prism of the supply and distribution policy of ACTs in Ghana, how the generic regime, which has powerfully challenged the dominant proprietary economy, is also built on exclusion, in the sense that generic ACT regimes mainly favor Indian producers and multinationals at the expense of local industries. Norms and standards mobilized for generic market construction have a dual characteristic: they are trusted makers, since they guarantee the quality of medicines, and at the same time they create major barriers to entry into the market for local African firms, which do not have the financial and technical means to comply with these norms (Quet, Pordié et al. 2018).

RETHINKING MEDICINE MAKING: THE LOCAL PRODUCTION OF GENERIC ANTIMALARIALS IN GHANA

The WHO's recommendations for ACTs and the mobilization of international funds for their purchase have stimulated pharmaceutical innovation and industrial production in the Global North and South. These new medicines are far more expensive than older treatments (such as chloroquine) and financing ACTs has become a major challenge for African countries, as shown in the previous case of Tanzania. This is also true in Ghana, which is aid dependent (Whitfield and Jones 2007). In response, transnational actors such as the Global Fund or bilateral programs, like the President's Malaria Initiative in the United States, buy these drugs and subsidize access (Eboko, Bourdier et al. 2011). They are part of a global arena of transnational actors that have developed around the organization of ACT supply to countries where malaria is endemic. Whereas Ghana depends on international grants to import ACTs for public health facilities (and for some parts of the private sector since 2010), the country is also working to strengthen local production of generics as a key to sustainable access to medicine (Hayden 2007). However, as the following case study demonstrates, the emergence in Ghana of local production and distribution capacities in the generic market is impaired by competition from Indian producers and multinationals.

Though Ghana has a long-established pharmaceutical industry, transnational actors that condition their financial assistance on "WHO prequalified" ACTs (Lantenois and Coriat 2014) leave Ghanaian pharmaceutical companies, whose medicines are not "WHO prequalified," outside this market.[4] Ghana began to produce drugs in 1957. At this time, the country embarked on an industrialization program aiming at the substitution of imports in order to support its economic development (Boateng 2009). The Ghanaian pharmaceutical industry initially included European and American multinationals, local private initiatives, and GIHOC Pharmaceuticals Ltd.—a public firm established in 1967 as a partnership between Ghana and Hungary (Pourraz 2019). Responding to technological and financial limitations, the Ghanaian government adopted an industrial policy favorable to the establishment of pharmaceutical factories on its territory. This policy consisted of financial and fiscal incentives, administrative support, and measures to protect locally produced medicines against imports. Because of this investment, the local production of drugs in Ghana was for decades able to satisfy the country's growing health needs and combine public health interests with the imperatives of industrial and economic development (Mackintosh, Banda et al. 2015; Pourraz 2019).

Today, Ghana has thirty-six local pharmaceutical companies. Even faced with strong foreign competition, local industries still supply 30 percent of the medicines sold on the private domestic market, including 5 percent of prescription drugs and 25 percent of over-the-counter medicines, such as tonics, ACTs, and analgesics (Harper and Gyansa-Lutterodt 2007; Chaudhuri 2015). While imports from Asia, Europe, and America meet 70 percent of national pharmaceutical needs, Ghana does manage to export some of its local products to the region. Nonetheless, the Ghanaian private market is largely saturated with cheap generics, imported mostly from India, against which local firms have difficulties competing.

When Ghana officially adopted ACTs in 2004, it had to choose between different combination therapies recommended by the WHO. At that time, Novartis was the only firm to produce the artemether-lumefantrine combination Coartem, and Ghanaian officials worried that the medicine was too expensive[5] and that production would not be sufficient to meet African demand. These access and cost concerns were considered scrupulously. Ultimately, the possibility that Ghanaian firms could produce the alternative artesunate-amodiaquine combination—they were already producing monotherapies of artesunate and amodiaquine—pushed the Ministry of Health (MoH) into choosing the latter as the first-line treatment. Furthermore, the private sector in Ghana occupies a dominant position, accounting for more than 60 percent of the supply of medicines (Jacquemot 2012), and about two-thirds of drug purchases are paid for by patients themselves. The MoH thus tried to have local producers supply the private market for ACTs. To this end, three Ghanaian companies embarked on the production of artesunate-amodiaquine, even though it required significant investments in terms of equipment, supply of raw materials, and R&D.

The introduction of an artesunate-amodiaquine combination led to significant adverse drug reactions, and local manufacturers were quickly accused of producing pills with the wrong dosage. As damage control strategy, the MoH decided to intervene by forbidding Ghanaian firms from manufacturing artesunate-amodiaquine and recalling locally made batches. Ghanaian firms ceased production at great financial losses. Then, in 2007, as a response to this crisis of confidence, the MoH decided to revise the national malaria treatment policy and to add artemether-lumefantrine as the second-line treatment. Since then, it has been Ghana's most widely used ACT combination.

Following the "artesunate-amodiaquine crisis," Ghanaian firms gradually moved toward the production of artemether-lumefantrine, hoping to capture a share of that market (Pourraz 2019). At the same time, the Ministry of Health, which relies entirely on international grants for the purchase of ACTs, partnered with the Global Fund for the pilot phase of the Affordable Medicines Facility-malaria (AMF-m) program to supply part of the Ghanaian private sector with subsidized "WHO-prequalified" ACTs. This program is designed as a manufacturer-level co-payment system intended to reduce the prices of high-quality ACTs in order to increase their accessibility and affordability in both public and private sectors. It favors market-based solutions that rely on private actors to sell ACTs cheaply enough to compete with alternatives such as monotherapies (Chorev 2012). Through this mechanism, the Global Fund purchases the WHO-prequalified ACTs of the six companies (Ajanta Pharma, Cipla, Guilin, Ipca, Novartis, and Sanofi-Aventis) with whom the Clinton Health Access Initiative has negotiated an 80 percent price reduction (Davis, Ladner et al. 2013). The Global Fund pays 95% of procured ACT costs and sets a maximum price that manufacturers must not exceed when selling ACTs to private intermediaries for distribution (Davis, Ladner et al. 2013). This system favors retailers, who only pay 5 percent of the total cost of the drugs that they distribute, over small-scale manufacturers, who would not benefit from the Global Fund subsidy. In this sense, the AMF-m program constitutes a very important subsidy for private-sector distribution as well as for multinational and Asian generic producers.

This new mechanism makes it possible to introduce higher-quality, subsidized ACTs on the Ghanaian private market, which had been partly reserved for local manufacturers. The MoH encourages Ghanaian manufacturers whose ACTs are not "WHO-prequalified" and who are also mostly wholesalers and retailers to participate in the AMF-m pilot project as retailers rather than producers. Therefore, public health interest can be used to justify Ghana's decision to join the program in spite of the fact that local industrial interests are at stake. Joining the program was also an opportunity for the government to respond to the country's ACT crisis of confidence by distributing quality-assured and affordable medicines to the private sector. As a result, however, the open market is now saturated with subsidized ACTs, and local producers cannot compete. The AMF-m project thus led Ghanaian manufacturers to end their production and R&D of ACTs because of limited market returns.

As a response, in 2013, the Food and Drugs Authority of Ghana started to work on a road map that aims to help local firms comply with Current Good Manufacturing Practices (CGMP) and thus meet the WHO prequalification criteria by 2020. This effort has been supported by the United Nations Industrial Development Organization (UNIDO), which has offered technical expertise in drawing up the road map. The objective is twofold: to guarantee the quality of drugs distributed on the local private market and to support Ghanaian firms in their quest for prequalification and subsidized markets. But the process of industrial standardization is long and requires significant investments, and to date none of the drug plants in Ghana have met the standards required for prequalification (Pourraz 2019). Access to the required capital remains a constraint for Ghanaian firms, and no transnational actors are ready to provide financing.

Analysis of the introduction of ACTs in Ghana and the effects of the implementation of the AMF-m pilot project on local production reveals how the Indian and multinational dominated generic regime is built on a form of exclusion. By conditioning drug purchases on WHO prequalification, markets for transnational generics create a hierarchy between global and local manufacturers. Attempts to create a local generic ACT market regime, decrease dependency on dominant global markets, and align industrial and health policy goals are all the more difficult given that the implementation of global health norms and standards excludes local producers (Mackintosh, Banda et al. 2015). The regulatory system, which originally legitimized and strengthened the generic regime as an alternative to the proprietary regime, has become an opportunity for multinational and Indian generics producers to dominate the market.

The Reformulation Regime: Industrial Ayurveda Goes Global

The radical transformation of Indian Ayurvedic medicine over the past twenty years is a complex process of industrialization and unequal but significant integration into the world of global pharmaceuticals, if not global health as a whole. Ayurveda is one of several traditional medical systems currently recognized by the state of India as an autonomous system of knowledge and practice. As such, it is regulated and officially integrated into the country's health infrastructure.

The modernization of Ayurveda has gone through several waves since the early twentieth century: professionalization before independence; institutionalization after 1947 with the gradual creation of an infrastructure (diplomas, medical schools, hospitals, and dispensaries) juxtaposed to the dominant biomedical health system; and integration into primary health care in the 1980s following state recognition (Attewell 2007; Bode 2008; Banerjee 2009). The most recent wave began in the 1990s and represents the industrialization of the tradition with the rise of a pharmaceutical sector that is mass-producing ready-made therapeutic combinations of plants, which are "reformulated" (often radically simplified) versions of recipes from the official corpus of Ayurvedic treatises (Pordié and Gaudillière 2014b). The firms trading in these remedies range from local family ventures to global players with thousands of employees that market products throughout Asia using "scientific marketing" tools like those of any large, industrialized drug company. Their preparations are mostly purchased by consumers in the new urban middle-class as part of a self-management of health, risks, and bodies that resembles what Western users critical of biomedicine do when looking for alternative forms of care. Reformulation of Ayurvedic recipes means simultaneously simplifying and standardizing poly-herbal combinations in order to adapt them to mass and mechanized industrial processing, draw on elements of biomedical experimentation in order to provide evidence of medical value, and combine Ayurvedic and biomedical categories in order to address the health needs of cosmopolitan consumers. The specificity of the regime underlying the industrialization of Ayurveda is especially visible in two domains: (1) the creation of intellectual property rights over the new preparations and (2) the creation of global markets through the coupling of Ayurvedic formulas and biomedical disorders.

Intellectual property rights play a peculiar role in Ayurvedic firms' reformulation strategies because traditional formulas are viewed differently from biomedical drugs. On the one hand, when they closely replicate classical combinations, they are viewed as collective resources that must be protected from private ownership. On the other hand, when they significantly differ in ingredients or proportions from the preparations represented in classical treatises, they are handled as innovative products that can be appropriated through trademarks and patents. The status and operations of the Traditional Knowledge Digital Library (TKDL), established by the Indian government in 2000 to oppose the patenting of traditional poly-herbal therapeutic preparations, powerfully illustrates this conundrum. The TKDL simultaneously acknowledges firms' desire to prevent biopiracy and also works to prevent the global patenting of Indian traditional remedies (Gaudillière 2014b).

Unlike many databases in biological and medical research, TKDL headquarters house not only computers and software run by highly qualified IT experts but also a library in the conventional sense of the term—a space filled with ancient books and manuscripts, handwritten notes, and darkened photocopies that are carefully examined by teams made up of young, mostly female practitioners of Ayurveda, Unani, Siddha, or Yoga—traditional medical systems officially recognized in India. A typical formulation sheet in the database provides the following information: the name of the formula; the list and quantities of plants included, with their official botanical names; a broad description of the preparation mode (basically a Galenic equivalent for Ayurvedic groups of drugs); its directions for use; and the sources documenting the formulation (in other words, its traditional authority).

Yet TKDL documents do more than simply provide an inventory of tens of thousands of recorded recipes, which in practice correspond to a much smaller number of clinically different formulations. By arranging the knowledge according to composition, production process, and usage, the TKDL format closely follows the structure of patents, focusing on the combination of medicinal materials rather than on the medical context and the clinical meaning of the original texts. In fact, this alignment with the structure of patents is necessary to ensure the usability of the database. As a resource in intellectual property disputes, the TKDL formulas are read by patent examiners working in Europe, the United States, and China. They need to be easy to grasp, and the whole corpus must be searchable on the basis of intellectual property law categories. It is therefore not surprising that at the TKDL, traditional Indian medical knowledge is reformulated according to the chemical ontology of patents—that is, in terms of composition and preparation process. The major adjustment to this framework, however, is the fact that TKDL information relies strongly on plants and botanical categories.

By borrowing the patent-derived notion of the "composition of matter," the digital library is not only a tool in intellectual property disputes but also a powerful instrument in the pharmaceuticalization of Ayurveda. It tacitly suggests that therapeutic efficacy originates in the self-contained assemblage of plant extracts, in the *materia medica* of Ayurveda, rather than in a clinical process that assesses the humoral status of the body, considers the patient's way of life, and designs ad hoc preparations that take context into account.

Given the TKDL's official aim of resisting biopiracy, contractual access agreements have been signed only with national partners (i.e., the dominant intellectual property agencies of relevant countries). The European Patent Office (EPO) has been authorized to consult the TKDL since February 2009. An access agreement with the United States Patent and Trademark Office (USPTO) was reached a year later. The impact of this access on intellectual property practices seems to be significant, at least in the European context. Since 2009, dozens of patent applications have been denied on the basis of "prior art" information provided by the TKDL and its lawyers.

However, not all contested patents are canceled. The tensions between the logic of the TKDL and an emerging EPO regime of patentability focusing on the innovative value of reformulation are best illustrated by patents for which the claims have been modified following examiners' demands. In other words, the EPO recognizes not only the prior art status of traditional knowledge but also its value as a resource to be mined. Legitimate innovation with medicinal plants is no longer addressed in terms of isolation and characterization of active ingredients but, rather, takes up the logic of invention through reformulation: newly defined polyherbals are deemed patentable when associated with standardization and the scientific evaluation of their effects. EPO examiners thus use and help reinforce the translation of Ayurvedic medicine into identifiable botanical compounds, a tendency that is already present in the TKDL documents. So, the price paid by TKDL managers for their success at the international level is the juxtaposition of two contradictory results: reinforced protection of classical formulas through a national inventory and increased industrial appropriation of reformulated compositions.

On the one hand, tradition is stabilized through the composition and translation of a reference library; on the other, the path is open for its "pharmaceuticalization" and inscription into the drug-knowledge economy.

Although widespread, the viewpoint that "traditional" Ayurveda and "modern" biomedicine are two mutually incompatible medical systems, and that the former is gradually disappearing through its alignment with the latter, is unable to render the complexities of the contemporary reinvention and globalization of these medicines. Such a dichotomy misses how the reformulation practices which facilitate the industrialization of Ayurvedic formulations borrow from heterogeneous medical knowledge, combine bits and pieces from various bodies of practice, and invent previously unknown preparations to create modes of (pharmaceutical) intervention irreducible to biomedicine (Pordié and Gaudillière 2014b).

An essential dimension of this reformulation is its industrial nature. Industrialization means that the core actors are Indian, Ayurvedic, drug-producing companies, some of them large enough to operate as global players. Industrialization also relates to the manufacturing process—that is, the search for productivity and economies of scale through mechanized processing, automated machinery, standardization, and possibly laboratory-based quality control. Like pharmaceutical capitalism in the Global North, the Indian Ayurvedic industry engages in processes of market construction that mingle experimentation, sales, and prescriptions. However, the work of reformulation entails specific contradictions stemming from its unique way of combining epistemic tradition and capitalistic modernity.

This may be illustrated with the process of developing a neotraditional, polyherbal remedy to treat symptoms of menopause. Menopause is an unusual category in Western medicine. Although its heritage is as ancient as that of reproductive physiology, it remained a marginal medical category until World War II, largely because it was associated with normal changes in a woman's reproductive life. It could cause undesirable symptoms, but these had no pathological dimensions and were deemed to be transitory. As recounted by historians of medicine like Elisabeth Watkins, the medicalization of menopause is deeply rooted in a process that took place during the therapeutic revolution of the twentieth century: namely, the transformation of women's sex hormones—estrogen and progesterone—into pharmaceuticals, which are chemicals purified and produced in bulk. By the late 1950s, this process resulted in the invention of a vast palette of molecules bearing common structural features with natural hormones but acting either as catalysts or as antagonists (Watkins 2007). Symptoms that had been medically untreatable and uninteresting suddenly became sites of intervention.

By the early 2000s, however, biomedical hormonal replacement therapy (HRT) faced a dramatic crisis. In the mid-1990s, the U.S. women's health movement successfully lobbied the National Institutes of Health (NIH) to fund a large epidemiological study of HRT called the Women's Health Initiative study. When the first results were made public in 2002, they dramatically opposed the claims that HRT was safe. Rather, the Women's Health Initiative study found that women in HRT showed an increased risk of breast cancer and cardiovascular disorders. This news triggered a major crisis of confidence in HRT, which resulted in many women choosing to go off the treatment. By 2004, prescriptions had dropped by 30 to 50 percent, not only in the United States but also in most European countries.

The Indian Ayurvedic industry was quick to take advantage of this opportunity, as Menosan, a preparation invented by the Himalaya Drug Company in Bangalore, shows. Himalaya began to market Menosan in 2002 as a safe and natural alternative to the problems identified with biomedical HRT. Like the promoters of HRT, Himalaya advocates pharmaceutical intervention to remedy the hormonal "deficiency" that renders menopause a quasi-pathology. Himalaya thus markets Menosan as a natural therapy for menopause since it is a plant-derived product. In other words, it is an industrial poly-herbal whose complex composition is defined in terms of wholesome plant ingredients and whose multi-herbal combination allows for critical synergies between the qualities and effects of each individual plant.

However, to understand Menosan's "multiple ontology," one must look beyond Himalaya's public discourse stressing its botanical composition, a discourse ostensibly rooted in the world of traditional medicine. When discussing the reformulation practices involved in the invention of the new preparation, the Ayurvedic physicians at the Himalaya Drug Company reveal another world—one strongly committed to the mining of Ayurvedic classical texts.

The firm's mining of Ayurveda rests on a feedback loop between the texts and the laboratory, sites that obey two different logics. The first is a logic of translation and *materia medica*, focusing on the supposedly stable composition of plants and a series of equivalences between botanical designations, on the one hand, and vernacular and Sanskrit names on the other, that have been worked out over two centuries of interactions between pharmacists, botanists, and Ayurvedic practitioners. This logic hopes to find *shastric* combinations containing plants whose ingredients have been linked by biomedical (as well as Ayurvedic) pharmacology to biological processes that cause menopausal symptoms—for instance, neurological regulation of the vascular system. The second logic is one of commonalities and clinical knowledge. It assumes that pathologies have stable symptoms that will have been described in ways that can be made to correspond with contemporary diagnoses. This logic makes it possible to look for classical formulations targeting the components of the menopausal syndrome. Given the flexibility of equivalencies and combinations, it is not surprising that Himalaya Drug Company scientists explored the properties of more than forty formulations in the early stages of Menosan research, and that this poly-herbal was actually created through the testing of many possible combinations, a process not unlike the development of a pharmaceutical drug.

The trajectory of this neotraditional remedy is not only the making and commercialization of a new product for a known pathology but also the making of a new medical problem, since there was at the time of development no menopause problem in India for which Menosan could be presented as a solution.[6] This is a decisive component of Himalaya's market construction. The company actively works to pathologize menopause among Indian physicians and Indian women, borrowing many practices from multinational firms, scientific marketing included. As with biomedical drugs, scientific marketing at Himalaya tends to target physicians rather than patients, through direct lobbying and the design of clinical trials. The scientific marketing of Menosan is nonetheless particular in one major respect. Given the lack of concern over menopause, Himalaya must not only promote Menosan as an excellent solution but also menopause as a risky condition. The Indian Menopause Society (IMS), founded in 1995, is an important partner in this work. Himalaya regularly supports IMS events, and it also collaborates with the society in the production of flyers and posters on the potential dangers of menopause—without any mention of Menosan—to be posted in physicians' waiting rooms.

The limitations of this enterprise are, however, undeniable. They are rooted in the problematic relations that the dialectics of bio and capital maintain with the dialectics of modernity and tradition. After fifteen years of marketing, the sales of Menosan are significant but limited. For many women, menopause simply isn't a problem for which they need a solution. Equally as difficult is convincing the biomedical practitioners who treat menopause symptoms of the neotraditional remedies' efficacy. In spite of a certain rhetoric of "liberalization," the Indian path to biocapital is just as institutional and political as the generic regime of market construction.

Transactions at the Interstices: The Licit and Illicit Circulation of Drugs in Cambodia

Examinations of patented drugs, generics, and poly-herbals presented thus far have unpacked the patterns of market construction underlying global health deployment. However, the markets for pharmaceuticals are not always entirely official, legal, and institutionalized. Hidden transactions, unofficial modes of regulation, smuggling, corruption, and other ways of circumventing laws and formal authorities do take place. Markets themselves make no distinctions. Taking the case of Cambodia, we now consider illicit practices that are in many ways co-constitutive of pharmaceutical markets, varying in degree but present in all regimes of market construction.

For this purpose, we will take a look at Kimly's drug outlet. Located on a dusty road in Phnom Penh, Kimly organizes her store by therapeutic family on open shelves fixed to three walls. In the middle of the room stands a small mobile shelf that holds more medicines. Kimly is unqualified. She rents the license that legalizes her outlet from a pharmacist who is otherwise busy with her work for a UN agency. Kimly sometimes works with the help of her husband and young daughter. In Cambodia, drug outlets and pharmacies are often treated like any other form of family businesses.

One afternoon in September 2015, Kimly stood up and suddenly kicked the mobile shelf toward the back of the room. Inspectors from the Department of Drugs and Food (DDF) had arrived on two small motorbikes. The men asked the usual questions, presented papers to be signed, and quickly checked the expiration dates on random medicines and counterfeit drugs. They left after a cup of coffee. This event reveals that the mobile shelf contained antimalarial pills supposedly only distributed in hospitals, as well as drugs imported without taxes, such as antibiotics made in France and a number of mass-produced poly-herbal drugs from India. They were illicit drugs. Kimly had stored them there so that they could disappear from sight with a single kick.

The flexible nature of state-directed pharmaceutical regulation in Cambodia, a country which is prone to high levels of corruption,[7] means that a sizable share of imported drugs end up being distributed illegally. These are either legitimate pharmaceuticals that have been hijacked from hospitals and sold elsewhere or legitimate pharmaceuticals that enter the country without passing through the official market channels. This latter option can be much more cost-effective; there are ways for importers to pay taxes on only a part of their shipment and pay bribes for the rest. These drugs end up in stores such as Kimly's, following a trajectory that goes through both licit and illicit environments. The market is thus composed of goods that change status as they go along. They may be legal at a certain point (bought abroad and imported, or sold in licensed pharmacies) and illegal elsewhere (entering into the country without paying import duties, made using expired ingredients, or distributed by unqualified retailers). This kind of situation, where both licit and illicit circuits collide, characterizes each and every sector of the pharmaceutical market in Cambodia, from production to distribution to sale. In other words, to understand market construction in the real world, we need to look at the intersections and entanglements of licit and illicit circulations and practices.

Although they might be viewed as a way to circumvent the hegemonic ACT regime discussed in the first half of the chapter, these practices also reveal an omnipresent form of political economy. In Cambodia, as in many other places, the making of the pharmaceutical market occurs inside and outside official regulation, legal practices, and sanctioned public health regimes. Its configuration goes far beyond industries, policies, and standards and thus expands what the "pharmaceutical nexus" (Petryna and Kleinman 2006) actually is. An in-between universe of social relations and material arrangements, which intertwine legal and illegal spheres of transactions, forms the breeding ground for creative and sometimes risky behaviors and ways of getting-by.

The dialectic relationship between pharmaceuticals and money is key in justifying all kinds of practices, but this situation is more than just a material economy. State logics, private undertakings, alternative strategies in the import and distribution of drugs, the appetites of business professionals, and the ambitions of prescribers all shed light on the gray zones that form pharmaceutical markets. They constitute a liminal political economy that is not subject to a standard set of categories or rules. This kind of political economy is interstitial, multivalent, and sensitive to circumstances; it opens up avenues for creative agency and arrangements, social innovation, and material heterodoxies. This gray political economy is not marginal in Cambodia. It is pervasive and present at all levels of society. Thus, the

Cambodian example not only helps to unpack crucial aspects of market construction in the globalization of health, but it also provides a unique perspective on the role and functioning of the state at its margins (Das and Poole 2004).

Apart from a half dozen Cambodian firms that produce a handful of different generics, most drugs present in the country are imported (Bureau-Point, To et al. 2016). For instance, antimalarial drugs paid for by the Global Fund and distributed by U.N. agencies come by air from Italy. Before the drugs enter the Cambodian market, a sample of each Italian shipment is sent to a certified laboratory in Nepal for quality testing. Drugs produced in France, partly made from raw materials imported from India or elsewhere, follow sea or air routes, as do Korean or Chinese pharmaceuticals. Thai and Vietnamese health products follow land routes and may pass through wholesale drug markets located at the borders. The percentage of these latter products is expected to increase following the recent economic integration of the Association of Southeast Asian Nations (ASEAN). Currently, India is the main provider of drugs to Cambodia, with more than 60 percent of market share. In 2012, Dinesh Patnaik, the then Indian ambassador to Cambodia, stated that over $100 million worth of Indian pharmaceuticals were sold in the country, an amount thought to have doubled by 2016. However, only half of these products come directly to Cambodia from India; the remainder moves through intermediate countries such as Thailand, Singapore, or Malaysia (Ma 2013). Such forms of transnational business relations, whether they involve a direct Indian–Cambodia relationship or go through intermediaries, form a part of market construction in Cambodia.

There are several legal ways for pharmaceuticals to enter Cambodia by sea, by air, or overland: the port of Sihanoukville in the south, the airport of the capital Phnom Penh, and some entry points across the borders with Thailand to the west and Vietnam to the east. It is in these transitional spaces, supposedly under the scrutiny of DDF inspectors, that the imports are subject to taxes and to inspections for quality assurance. However, in a country where law enforcement remains weak—and this is especially true in the realm of pharmaceuticals—these requirements are not systematically implemented, as Kimly's case shows.

When shipped, pharmaceuticals usually travel in refrigerated containers to guarantee the safety and quality of drugs. After being stored in the importers' warehouses, the vast majority of pharmaceuticals end up at the Olympic Market in Phnom Penh, a nodal point of private distribution. There, dozens of wholesale pharmacies provide goods to smaller retailers of varying sizes who distribute medicines throughout the country. Drugs are often transported from Phnom Penh using the distributors' own vehicles, as well as by private pickup trucks or minibuses, which transport goods along with their clientele. Further away from the capital and other urban centers, distribution methods become more diverse: Vans from drugs suppliers pass regularly through the villages, but drugs can also be found on the roofs of minibuses, on the back of a motorcycle, or being pulled on a trailer. When the situation allows, medical representatives are also involved in the supply. As shown elsewhere (Quet, Pordié et al. 2018), these alternate supply routes contribute to regulating pharmaceutical flows; they form the logistical backbone of unofficial coordination. They also provide a solution to the problem of pharmaceutical distributors offering large quantities that do not suit small-scale pharmacies. This also applies to workers of nongovernmental organizations involved in health programs who might order their supply by phone and have it transported to their province by the private minibus networks. Drugs end up in rural pharmacies by following heterogeneous routes.

These routes move in and out of legal environments, transforming the drug's status. Several illustrations will make this clear. A few years ago, in a dark alley of Rong Klua Market in Aranyaprathet, Thailand, Cambodian drug traffickers arranged for two trucks to be loaded with biomedical and poly-herbal pharmaceuticals and cosmetics. The road to Phnom Penh, which goes through the former Khmer Rouge bastion of Poipet, is risky since there are still many checkpoints where vehicles may be searched and drivers interrogated. Although completely legal in Thailand, these pharmaceuticals gained a new (illegal) status by crossing the border. Mobility along a transnational route plays a significant role in transforming these objects' legal status. The context in which the object is situated brings about a shift in category: from being a legal pharmaceutical it becomes illegal, in a movement that signals the "fragility of objecthood itself" (Appadurai 2006). However, having close relations with high-ranking authorities, the traffickers arranged for two army trucks driven by military personnel to ensure that they would not be stopped at the checkpoints. By taking an alternative route and avoiding formal taxation, the shipment also gained significant value before the drugs were reinjected in the market.

Storage temperature also demonstrates how pharmaceuticals can cross legal boundaries. Until 2015, there were no specific regulations on the temperature at which drugs should be transported and stored. Then a bill was passed that stipulates that storage temperatures should be respected and special equipment, such as refrigerated vehicles, used. However, while some importers do use temperature-controlled warehouses, several others explained that storage temperature is not considered to be important since most drugs will end in nonrefrigerated pharmacies and outlets. Similarly, although outside observers may see refrigerated vehicles on the roads—such as the small *remok*, a two-wheeled refrigerated trailer attached to a motorbike and used to transport drugs and cosmetics in urban centers—this does not mean that the refrigeration is turned on, as we noted on many occasions. The operators frequently turn the system off to save gas. Hence, legal drugs go through illegal environments before reaching legality again, at the pharmacy. The drug's status (licit and/or illicit) thus fluctuates according to the type of circuit taken, the actors involved, and the nature of the transactions and negotiations.

The situation can, however, be more dramatic. Local importers and manufacturers have developed strong links with Indian counterparts over the years. Indian companies have representatives in Cambodia who facilitate and negotiate commercial transactions. Many firms in the kingdom import raw materials from India, including active compounds and drug additives, and they try to obtain them as cheaply as they can. This applies even if it means buying expired active ingredients. In such a case, the Cambodian firm produces new drugs from old materials, ascribing them a new identity (as generics) and, most importantly, a new expiration date. "This is how a drug can live five years longer than it should," explained a former DDF officer. This dangerous situation illustrates another way by which drugs move from illegality to legality, through the machinations of criminal businesspeople familiar with the intricacies of quality inspections and the idiosyncrasies of inspectors themselves. These cases exemplify the complex social and political mechanics that animate the relationship between businesspeople and the state, driven by their respective interests (Bourdier, Man et al. 2014). It is not uncommon for inspectors to receive cash or presents, in the form of travel or five-star dinners, from international firms under the guise of "good friendship." Nonfinancial transactions must also be considered as an integral part of market construction.

Such liminal political economies are ubiquitous, inescapable realities. In Nigeria, speculative networks and practices also help stock the country with pharmaceuticals (Peterson 2014). Similarly, in the Congo, the overlap between legal and illegal spheres has made some small traders new figures of economic success, while others have succeeded as intermediaries (Ayimpam 2014). Examples may be found in literally every part of the planet. The gray political economy of drugs is a site of social creativity that affects market construction and functioning. This has consequences for global health. As we noted at the outset of this chapter, without drugs and their markets, there would be no global health. This means that the very fabric of global health ought to be examined not only through the lens of institutions and official/legal markets and transactions but also through the myriad dubious networks and practices that help to construct the pharmaceutical market.

In this market regime, like in the others, drugs move through circuits that traverse many locations and are deployed on several scales—from countries in Asia and Europe to manufacturers in India, ASEAN regulators' offices in Jakarta, warehouses in Phnom Penh, and small outlets in the heart of Cambodia. This complex configuration highlights the fact that circulating pharmaceuticals often cross boundaries between legality and illegality. Ways of operating in the market work as a messy assemblage of practices. They interact, complement each other, and coexist in opposition. In some instances, drugs are stored under controlled temperatures, while in others they travel freely on random minibuses, ignoring the law and indulging in risky behaviors. Ultimately, the global pharmaceutical market involves a much larger universe than that composed by government authorities, international agencies, honest manufacturers and dealers, and qualified health personnel.

Conclusion

This chapter highlights the critical role pharmaceuticals have acquired in the dynamics of health at a global scale. It has investigated the social life of drug markets and the "regimes of market construction" involved in global health as a field and the arenas of health globalization. From this perspective, our notion of regime emphasizes the coherence and patterns of action grounding a pharmaceutical market's four major stages: invention, appropriation, production, and drug distribution.

The trajectory of artemisinin-based combination therapy in Tanzania highlights the patent and innovation-centered proprietary regime of "Big Pharma." A typical example of chemical-pharmaceutical mass production shows how this regime frames the global malaria market. Growing pharmaceutical consumption in the South and the massive globalization of pharmaceutical production since the 1990s, however, have challenged the monopolistic Big Pharma regime of market construction. A broad generic market regime has emerged and led to the global distribution of WHO-certified artemisinin-based combinations made in India. Based on fieldwork in Ghana, our second case study shed light on the links between this global circulation of generics and the emergence of local production and distribution capabilities. It revealed alliances that connect drug regulation agencies, policymakers, and local pharmaceutical firms.

Competition with branded drugs often relies on alternative goods. The large-scale circulation of poly-herbal preparations, originating in the industrialization of Asian medicines, exemplifies this reliance. Fieldwork in India shows how the invention of neotraditional Ayurveda drugs established reformulation as a novel regime of market construction. This regime contrasts the proprietary model in two important domains: defending herbal mixtures as alternatives to the chemical paradigm for understanding drug novelty and efficacy, and creating goods by connecting Ayurvedic formulas and biomedical disorders.

By stressing health globalization in practice, the chapter also shows that making pharmaceutical markets in countries of Asia or Africa relies on a myriad of (at times dubious) networks on several scales. Our final case powerfully exemplifies these markets by following pharmaceuticals in Southeast Asia, where a sizable share of drugs circulate through, and overlap with, official and unofficial drug regulation networks, revealing a political economy that enmeshes legal and illegal transactions to actively alter global health agendas for local ends.

CHAPTER 5

Tech for All

Andrew McDowell, Claudia Lang, Mandy Geise,
Sameea Ahmed Hassim, and Vegard Traavik Sture

New technologies are the targets of multiple debates about global health's potential for social, political, and economic changes in the lives of those it seeks to affect (Farmer 2005; Street 2014; McMillen 2015; Brimnes 2016; Packard 2016). Global health's critics (and some of its proponents) argue that technical solutions, such as pharmaceuticals, mosquito nets, and vaccines, cannot solve the broader problems of inequity, (post)colonial resource extraction, and environmental precarity that cause high and unevenly distributed rates of disease across the planet (Farmer 2005). They note that these technologies tend to be oriented toward a specific disease and that they facilitate vertical programs. Critics describe interventions as technological fixes (Latour, Mauguin et al. 1992; T. M. Li 2011) or, even more dramatically, as Band-Aids on corpses that pile up on decayed or broken health infrastructure (Banerjee, Duflo et al. 2008; Stoler 2009; Koch 2013; Street 2014; Chabrol 2018). Finally, many question the ways that innovative technologies redistribute financial, biological, and informational resources between the countries where they are used and those that produce them (Ferguson 2006; Sunder Rajan 2006; McGoey 2015).

Proponents of global health's high-tech strategies, however, see technologies as potential shortcuts to development, health, and prosperity (Sen 1998). They hope that technology can bridge gaps left in the health system (Kwankam 2004). Finally, those who encourage technological global health and development view such interventions as a source of national productivity (Chorev 2015, 2016). They argue that technologies are motors of development because they provide increased health and human capital; catalyze trade as their material parts are sold in international and domestic exchange; shape new pools of skilled and semi-skilled labor; and finally preserve and enhance existing pharmaceutical markets (Cassier and Correa 2003, Quet 2017). What is striking is that despite their differences in approach, both sides of the debate share global health's confidence in the connection between vitality and development.

Despite their role at the center of critical reflection on global health, few scholars examine global health's technical objects and processes. Although accounting technologies and metrics have been well studied, they are only a small part of the massive technical apparatus of objects and epistemes that make up global health and render health technical. Our goal here is to describe a selection of global health technologies, parse their use and meaning, and consider their effects on health and development at a global scale. We do so by focusing on several modular combinations of technology and technique that we call *technopacks*. For us, technopacks are the packages of devices and methods that travel along global health's circuits of intervention and knowledge. Technologies are tools (e.g., scales, screens, sequencing machines, pharmaceuticals) that are deeply connected to scientific rationality, ideas of reason, and the ability to reveal and impact something about the person or phenomena on which they are used (Ingold 1997). Techniques, on the other hand, are the practices that put these tools into action and make them meaningful (Foucault 1984). Technique and technology are inseparable. They come in packs precisely because the use or "affordance" of a tool in global health is often an appeal to a particular action such as care or counting or development (Hutchby 2001). In short, global health's ethic of intervention requires that tools be used and that we study them in the context of practice.

Indeed, the integration of technology and technique, tool and application, structure and practice has allowed health to go global. While technoscience uses the concept of "frame technologies" to study people, places, things, and activities coming together around one tool or technical object (Clarke and Casper 1996), we suggest instead the notion of technopacks to signify the coming together of technology, technique, and infrastructure. The technopacks we describe here are similar to what Redfield (2008) calls a humanitarian kit. They are premade modules of objects and capacities that claim to include everything necessary to "'work' under all circumstances" (Akrich 1992, 211) and have limits built in to safeguard against nonstandard use. Technopacks integrate multiple forms of technology that include tests, trials, and pharmaceuticals as well as technologies of the self that make and remake subjects who use them and who they are used on (Nguyen 2009).

The "technical" aspects of technopacks, their integration of mechanisms and actions deemed both specialized and industrial, are essential for our understanding of global health since technology enables particular forms of expertise and opens health to technical knowledge (Foucault 1973). Thus, technology marks nearly every part of global health knowledge production and intervention. For example, the use of screening tools to transform the emotional consequences of rapid social and economic change into the globally recognizable category of "depression" demonstrates how the technical transforms the exclusions and pains of globalization into an object of global health intervention. The creation of corroborating data also renders information and action technical. "Technical assessments" and "technical profiles" often spell out the needs, markets, and potentialities of innovations long before the material specifications of global health's new tools have even been imagined. Moreover, technical advice and assistance are key preoccupations of institutions like the World Health Organization, the World Bank, and philanthropic foundations but often go unconsidered and undefined.

Interestingly, technologies themselves are viewed as inert material wholes in circuits of global health, while the techniques to put them to use tend to be understood as obstacles, localizations, or experiments (Friedman 1990; van der Geest, Reynolds Whyte et al. 1996; Escobar 2001; Inda and Rosaldo 2002; Janes and Corbett 2009). Understanding these components as part of a technopack reveals new ways of thinking through circulation. Though technopacks undoubtedly travel, they move much like anthropologist Anna Tsing's "traveling packages." Tsing describes traveling packages as bundles of significance or narratives that become "unmoored" from the symbolic and political system in which they emerged to travel across space and time (2005, 234). In the process, they are written over with new meanings and uses. We borrow from this idea to suggest that technopacks similarly become unmoored from their initial site of innovation or invention. We show that when assembled as technopacks, the dialogical relationship between object and practice transforms in its travels through globalized health. Contrary to the idea that technology might be an "immutable mobile," an object that remains the same despite being employed in numerous contexts through tinkering or improvisation (de Laet and Mol 2000), technopacks are consummately mutable mobiles. They change and reconfigure themselves and their surroundings through their movement and use, encouraging design tinkering and improvisation. Technopacks are put into action to solve a particular problem and, in the process, they and the health system to which they are applied change. We consider how this movement is made possible and what it does to these seemingly globalized forms that hope to bring both standardization and development at once. We find that indeed keeping technology and technique together is a challenge that is not always met.

As such, technopacks are simultaneously fact, artifact, action, and aspiration. They are instantiations of epistemes and discourses that come to act on their own and on behalf of global health planners and mediators. They transform discourse into object, but they often slip out of the tight grasp of global health actors to have myriad unintended but important consequences. Despite these subversive tendencies, thinking with global health's amalgams of tools and techniques, which we call technopacks, helps to make sense of processes that are recognizable and applicable across space and time while highlighting the differences that acts of rendering technical cannot efface. Moreover, when examined in their mobile form, technopacks reveal themselves as inflecting new technologies, techniques, and sociotechnical imaginaries, sprouting new technopacks that include forms of deeply context-specific relatedness within them.

Engaging globalized technopacks like depression-screening tools, microscopy, DNA amplifiers, prenatal screening, and genetic profiling of diabetes, we document the complex combinations of technologies and techniques that render health technical, including the intermingling of pathology and technopacks and the effects of technologies on health systems. Our considerations of technopacks do not put an end to debates about the role of technology in global health. Rather, they lay bare the connections between global health's logics and practices.

Indeed, ideas about health universalism and what it is are written into the technopacks themselves, but so are experimentality, the state, and deep anxieties about pharmaceuticals.

Technopacks often include pharmaceuticals, while pharmaceuticals are always and already technopacks. The technical aspects of pharmaceuticals have been so effectively distilled, integrated, made portable, and standardized that they move across the world with seemingly little regard to technique. Nonetheless, pharmaceuticals do not travel as smoothly as this story suggests, and their techniques of use are not always shared across contexts (Nichter and Vuckovic 1994; Peterson 2014). Vastly different patterns of antibiotic resistance throughout the world make the importance of pharmaceutical technique clear. Indeed, innovations to improve the impact of pharmaceutical technopacks abound in global health and may be one of its defining features. In fact, global health's skeptics and proponents alike worry that new technologies are superficial fixes attempting to stave off an impending bacterial Armageddon caused by growing antibiotic resistance. The difference between the two camps rests on optimism or skepticism and is centered on whether or not a techno-centered race for new molecules is sufficient.

Global health funders and institutions often provide drugs within larger technopacks of diagnostic, prescription, and adherence tools that emphasize pharmaceutical stewardship through standardization and efficient use. Pharmaceuticals as technopacks within other technopacks reveal that technopacks are both aggregative and segmented. They shift aims and outcomes in the presence of new forms. A directly observed treatment short-course (DOTS) strategy for tuberculosis (TB) is an excellent example. TB treatment before DOTS was a pharmaceutical technopack that combined several pharmaceuticals and diagnostic technologies. It did not, however, include directions that specified how to use those technologies. For example, it gave no specific instructions about how to assess x-rays, how to determine the quantity of bacteria in a sputum sample, or how patients should take the medicine. However, as global consensus grew concerning the value of efficient adherence to a pharmaceutical regime, this technopack was broadened, including surveillance and governance technology focusing on standardizing diagnostic criteria and practice, guiding patients in drug use, and observing them to guarantee adherence to protocols. Today, countries all over the world implement this technopack, and it shapes interventions, bacteria, and people in globally similar ways.

Finally, technologies cannot be separated from the healthcare systems within which they are used, administered, and organized. At the same time, technopacks are more than just technological fixes in broken systems. These are technical rather than structural innovations, but that does not mean that they cannot change the health system. In fact, they often reconfigure health systems, bolstering some aspects, weighing down others, and amputating many. Put another way, technopacks allow certain kinds of systemic and technological innovations and foreclose others that mold health to look, feel, and unfold in globally intelligible ways, despite diverse health system contexts. One such technopack is a genetic test in the clinic or at "the point of care" that aims to avoid any technical inputs. When introduced to a Tanzanian hospital, this pack changed flows of work and expertise throughout the institution and altered the skills needed by laboratory technicians across the country to diagnose TB. Another example is a depression-screening technopack in Kerala, India, that led to the enhancement of the skills of local health workers. Our data show that, throughout the world, technopacks and their integration into health systems remake what it is to be sick or suffering, to be a citizen, and how practitioners and policymakers identify which issues are worthy of intervention. By changing definitions of who, where, and how to intervene, technopacks change health systems. They affect the ways these systems react to new technologies, manage people, and prioritize diseases. In short, making health technical means relocating technology in social relations and practices—in other words, resocializing it—and this process transforms ideas of health, society, and social action in new and unexpected, although not always unpredictable, ways.

The depression technopack that we describe in the next section is a case of rendering mental health technical, but not *merely* technical. Its integration into primary health care affects not only health workers' tasks, skills, and priorities but also how people think about and intervene in emotional and physical suffering. At the same time, its resocialization in Kerala mobilizes local biologies and moralities.

The Launching of a Depression Technopack

The depression relief program, Ashwasam ("Relief" in Sanskrit), integrates depression treatment in the Indian state of Kerala into primary health care. It centers on a technopack of screening and care for depression. It renders sadness and globalization's growing pains technical, standard, and manageable by global health interventions. The depression technopack reshapes suffering into a mental health problem and folds it, along with other noncommunicable diseases, into a broader narrative of epidemiological transition and primary health care priorities. It promises development by enhancing human capital through better mental health. At the same time, it tweaks global mental health's packages of screening and care by expanding depression as a category and localizing screening tools. More importantly, the depression technopack changes the health system by expanding the skills of health workers, and it remakes what it means to suffer from mental illness, who suffers, and how to intervene. A more dispersed bundle of depression technologies and techniques has existed in Kerala for the last three decades, but the cluster of specific screening technologies initiated by the Ashwasam program produced the specific depression technopack in primary health care we describe here (Lang 2019).

The Ashwasam technopack resembles globalized "packages of care" for depression that are promoted by the World Health Organization (WHO) and the Movement for Global Mental Health. These globalized packages of care are "evidence-based interventions" combining drug therapy and psychosocial interventions (Patel, Simon et al. 2009; Patel and Thornicroft 2009). They are developed by research teams financed by international donors and run by mental health non-governmental organizations (NGOs)—islands of care that often come to stand in for state-provided mental health treatment. In Kerala, however, the depression package is engaged with the state. In the hands of the administrators of the Ashwasam program, the more abstract depression technopack stretches to incorporate Kerala-specific forms of suffering and health governance. Moreover, the injection of the reconfigured technopack expands Kerala's primary care system of community-based health surveillance and treatment, training multipurpose health workers to target inner feelings, suffering, and existential despair.

This depression technopack also assembles local epidemiological numbers. One of the architects of Ashwasam began his training classes for the program by quantifying the problem: 10 percent prevalence of depression in the community, 27 percent prevalence among patients in primary care (Indu, Anilkumar et al. 2017). These figures came neither from global statistics nor from India's National Mental Health Survey. They were local but no less urgent. It is these sufferers who previously slipped through the psychiatric gaze that the Ashwasam program aims to detect, and it is this technopack of identification, surveillance, and care that is offered to do so.

Mental health professionals, epidemiological surveys, and media reports in Kerala link the ostensible rise in depression that these numbers indicate to larger sociocultural transformations, usually narrated as cultural decline or crisis. High rates of depression, as with suicide, expose the flipside of the "Kerala model of development"[1] and index the disappointment of unfulfilled political and social promises. Kerala's international reputation rests on a strong primary health care system and a citizenry of notably good health. As such, depression represents a particularly pernicious threat to the state's reputation and its powerful, if overwhelmingly positive, narrative of development and progress (Lang 2018).

For many critics, mental health professionals and laypeople alike, depression boils down to an admission that the quest for and achievement of development comes at the cost of the well-being of the people. If Kerala is depicted as a "society in distress," a crisis produced by a host of sociocultural changes in recent decades, then solutions are sought in a technopack as a form of psychosocial engineering or governance intended to produce mentally resilient subjects and remake dilapidated familial care relations.

Ashwasam is a vertical program to address depression in primary care. Although program designers and policymakers stressed Ashwasam's alignment with global agendas, they framed the package it offers as a local, Kerala-specific solution to depression, deeply embedded in the state's model of health governance. One way in which they adapted the screening tool to a local context is by reducing the number of questions. This is supposed to speed up the screening process and be compatible with the hectic workday of community health workers in Kerala.[2] General physicians in primary health centers then align diagnoses of mild, moderate, and severe depression with specific packages of pharmacological treatment—and ideally counseling—that mirror the WHO Mental Health Gap Action Program (mhGAP) intervention guide (World Health Organization 2010b), although program designers and policymakers in Kerala did not explicitly mention this global health resource.[3]

While the depression technopack aspires to shift health workers' gaze and to reconfigure distress in line with a globally standardized symptom catalog for depression, the screening technologies and techniques that are intended to work to change subjectivities often fail to do so. Aching and overheated bodies, anger, and lack of mental control feature prominently in patients' articulations of distress, and a localized depression technopack asks healthcare workers and physicians to turn these experiences into standard symptoms of depression and offer care. Aware of the reality of stigmatization, the technopack holds the promise that everyone should be able to talk about emotional suffering without being ostracized because of mental illness. This promise, however, often fails to materialize in practice as mental illness and its treatment continue to be viewed as threats to social integration and reputation.

The depression technopack used by the Ashwasam program also organizes counseling arrangements and technologies in a novel way. Packages of care often come with new ideas, modes of relating, and notions of privacy and confidentiality, a kind of globalized discourse of psychology. But arranging such privacy in the context of long queues forming outside open doors and consultations, which may include a patient's entire family, can prove difficult. Arrangements are often hasty and improvised. Another aspect of the technopack, the ideal of nonjudgmental listening and nondirective counseling, is often impossible given the busy schedule of unsettled nurses and is simply omitted in many cases, along with an entire apparatus of psychosocial interventions. These kinds of pragmatic adjustments mean that the depression technopack in practice is relying almost exclusively on psychopharmacological treatments. In their busy outpatient departments, doctors quickly match narratives of social suffering, difficult life situations, and "unspecifically" aching bodies with a prescription for a selective serotonin reuptake inhibitor (SSRI) or a tricyclic antidepressant, thus turning suffering into a mental and pharmacologically fixable pathology. In Ashwasam, as much as in India's District Mental Health Program, pills take priority over not only psychosocial interventions but also more inclusive forms of policy (Jain and Jadhav 2009).

Meanwhile, the medicalization and pharmaceuticalization of social distress, poverty, and broken families, enabled by the depression technopack, also serve as a powerful tool for governing and surveilling populations and mobilizing care. While in clinical encounters, symptoms of socioeconomic adversities and difficult lives are turned into symptoms of depression, but back in patients' homes, community health workers often reinterpret symptoms of depression as the effects of disrupted family relations. Depression is portrayed as a consequence of deteriorating ties of care and dismantled moral obligations; unhealthy bodies and minds reflect bad families, and patients' symptoms of depression may then express fraying or severed bonds of love and lack of care. Here, medicalization through a depression technopack becomes productive in providing an idiom to critique a family's moral economy and mobilize care for the recovery of afflicted persons at the level of individual families. Drugs as technologies of care not only lead to novel pharmaceutical forms of care for previously nonmedicalized suffering but also to the mobilization of support in the context of familial marginalization and neglect.

The depression pack with its technology (screening tools, diagnostic categories, psychopharmaceuticals) and techniques (training, screening, counseling, counting) thus brought about a change in thinking about, intervening in, and surveilling emotional suffering. Assembled within Kerala's restructured primary health infrastructure, this depression technopack not only reveals imaginaries of development and health but also brings into relief the processes of localization, experimentality, and triage in global mental health. As we will see in the next section, just as the depression technopack shifted what it meant to be a mental health patient, DOTS as a novel TB technopack changed what it meant to be a TB patient.

A Sliding Scale: TB

In the 1990s, India's tuberculosis treatment and control program centered on two technopacks that combine diverse pharmaceuticals, technologies, knowledge formations, practices, and imaginaries of development in the same setting. The nationwide shift from a technopack centered on x-ray technology to one centered on the microscope shows how bundles of technology and technique are more than the sum of their parts. The transition from one technopack to another tracked changes in the ways global health understood itself and its interventions as funders began to assess efficacy as the epidemiological impact of whole packages rather than constituent parts like a pharmaceutical, a technology, or a technique (Reubi 2018). Simultaneously, the transition shifted what it meant to be an "Indian" TB patient and a TB patient in general.

Small changes in India's TB's technopack allowed for a wholesale technical shift and helped it to persist for more than two decades. India's shift was a move away from a more flexible diagnostic and treatment approach using bulky technology to a verticalized program implemented by general physicians in primary health centers (Agarwal and Chauhan 2005; Koch 2011). The shift from a diffuse set of resources to a protocolized program, however, happened through a series of technological, practical, and policy changes. India's changed TB technopack had two effects. First, it changed the parameters that defined the normal and pathological for TB in India. Second, these epistemological changes rippled through global health intervention and TB science.

In the 1960s, India's TB program was primary-health-oriented and, at least aspirationally, patient-friendly. It was integrated into the broader health system, run by its staff, and linked to multifunctional technologies (Banerji 1967, 1971; Nagpaul, Naganathan et al. 1979; Jagota 2000). The program gave physicians ample diagnostic and treatment flexibility in order to meet patients' needs. To achieve such flexibility, however, the program relied heavily on x-ray or mass miniature radiography (MMR) to diagnose and guide outpatient treatment using available drugs.

Treatments often included eighteen to twenty-four months of isoniazid, paraami-
nosalicyclic acid (PAS), and/or thiacetazone on an outpatient basis, and patients
returned to their physician monthly for refills and consultations (Brimnes 2016).
X-rays could be read directly by physicians and, over time, multiple x-rays could
show the progression or regression of disease. X-ray and MMR machines were
expensive and often located in district-level health centers, so patients who sought
care at village health centers would need to be referred to them. The limited number of x-ray machines made moving TB diagnosis to the community challenging,
and TB services relied on community health centers to refer patients to the district hospital (Jagota 2000). Reports from the 1980s show that referral was difficult
in part because of weak links between health system actors.

X-ray, however, was not the only technology for diagnosing tuberculosis. Technicians can often see bacteria in a smear of infected sputum when scrutinized under
a microscope. This technique, called sputum-smear microscopy, has been an
accepted TB diagnostic method since the 1880s. Unlike X-ray, smear provides information only about TB. It requires reagents, a microscope, a laboratory technician,
and, unfortunately, exposure to potentially TB-infected sputum. For these reasons,
and perhaps others, physicians preferred diagnosis by x-ray, which could give a
broader sense of lung health, clinical signs, and patient history without relying on
a laboratory technician and with less exposure to TB bacteria.[4] X-ray was so essential in India that only a few months before a major shift in the technopack used for
the public management of TB, the government of India asked the Swedish International Development Agency to purchase an additional batch of x-ray machines
for the TB program.[5]

In the opening years of the 1990s, however, the WHO shifted its perspective on
x-ray technology and the diagnostic technopack it stood for (Caminero 2003). A
new worry had emerged; perhaps x-ray-based diagnosis—owing to inter-reader
variations and its reliance on the correlative evidence provided by hazy shadows
that are often, but not exclusively, made by TB—was misdiagnosing people sick
with other lung issues as TB patients and subjecting them to years of unnecessary
antibiotics (Nagpaul, Naganathan et al. 1979). Of equal importance was a desire to
avoid the unnecessary cost, in time and medicines, that each of these overtreated
patients represented to the health system, state, and bilateral funders. To avoid real
and fantasied overtreatment, the WHO, drawing on data from East Africa, promoted its recommendation to redesign public health interventions for TB around
microscopy alone (Caminero 2003).

In India, worries about overtreatment opened a Pandora's box of difficulties,
some known, some unconsidered, and some fabricated. Anxiety about overtreatment brought with it questions about the number of people actually being treated
in the first place, and a 1992 review conducted by a diverse group of multinational
actors reported what it called "irrational" and "unstandardized" treatment, as well
as a lack of clarity about what happened to patients after their years of treatment.
When patients disappeared from the records, what happened to them? Were they
cured? Were they still sick? Were they in treatment somewhere else? Were they

dead? This was no small question; 70 percent of the patients who had begun treatment since the 1960s had disappeared. Many assumed that they had been cured, but there was no way to be sure.

The ocular, x-ray-based technopack did not just fall victim to diagnostic failure. It was incompatible with the rise of an evidence-based, standardized, and epidemiologically oriented way of managing TB that would soon come to be known as DOTS and the drugs on which it relied. DOTS would be based on sputum-smear microscopy because of (1) the relative ease with which microscopes could be purchased and maintained, (2) the smear's clear demonstration of a causal agent for TB symptoms, (3) lower rates of inter-reader variation for smear, and (4) the relative certainty it could give against false positives. With this new protocol, the discussion around what constituted a "case" of TB, once open for interpretation, was now closed; it was a patient whose sputum revealed bacteria. All others were patients in waiting, regardless of TB-like symptoms.

At the same time, examining smears of sputum for the little red, rod-shaped bacteria is not an easy task. Shifting from x-ray to smear required a new intermediary—the lab technician. It was now the technician who provided a crucial piece of evidence not accessible to the clinician's interpretive gaze. One could, of course, suggest that smear was a clear choice. It was a less expensive technology with less interpretive margin, it could reach rural health centers, and it could be argued to be more effective since it would target for treatment patients who could spread the disease. Still, the switch was controversial among Indian physicians. Ultimately, the promise of comparability turned the tide. Unlike X-ray or clinical acumen, smear made TB patients diagnosed by its methods comparable and verifiable over space and time. It created a pool of people within and outside India's borders whose data could be grouped together in "cohort analysis" in order to understand predictors of treatment success or failure. At the same time, global health actors were now able to set a baseline of epidemiological data for DOTS and its combined new molecules, technologies, and patient observation techniques. In this way, DOTS is a total technopack in which clinical expertise and patient desires, politics writ large, are rendered globally modular and comparable. Indeed, the pharmaceutical molecules were only one part of a much larger process of rendering bacterial and human life technical.

The need to convince physicians and India's health technocracy to adjust their TB technopack—not just to prioritize sputum smear but also to include accounting procedures, standardized drug regimens, and observation—was crucial. It was not, however, easy. Clinicians and public health experts in India made a threefold argument against this new technopack. First, the pharmaceutical regimen that made observation feasible was untested in Indian bodies. Second, patients would not have the will to visit the health center every other day for months on end. Third, the technical capacity to perform a quality sputum smear and analyze it was not present in the public system. At the same time, both inside and outside India, there were questions about Indian experts' ability to conduct the kinds of statistical analysis that would make meaning from the data that the DOTS system aimed to produce. Still, smear's propensity to identify infectious TB sufferers and ensure comparability across cases of TB was viewed as a way to focus resources on those who most needed them. This focused approach, proponents argued, would make DOTS effective, despite barriers.

Proponents eventually convinced Indian authorities to launch a trial of the program. The technology and techniques for DOTS arrived as a technopack and needed to be tested as a whole in a new setting. The results of these pilots, however, were difficult to engage. Indian TB experts had the knowledge to question the efficacy of parts of the program but did not have access to data that would allow them to question the whole package. To test the whole technopack, the government and the WHO, acting as a technical and policy adviser, set up what at the time were called pilot projects. These projects would be at first located in three sites—Delhi, Mumbai, and rural Gujarat—and later would expand to include Calcutta, Bangalore, rural Kerala, and another site each in Delhi and Mumbai. In these special sites, the new project could be implemented, observed, and used to generate baseline data for the technopack in India.

This idea of testing and questioning a technopack as a whole, greater than the sum of its parts, is essential for an understanding of technical packages in global health. Sullivan (2011) and Geissler (2013a) suggest that global health generates islands of care, and we add that technopacks make these islands possible. These pilot areas were global health islands in a sea of primary-health-oriented care. They were chosen because the health infrastructure in those locations was solid. "We chose places that already had a strong system, so we could show what the rest of the system could do if given enough resources and attention. They were a best-case scenario," one of the organizers said.[6] These clinics were equipped with a physician willing to treat only those patients whose sputum revealed bacteria, a laboratory technician, a microscope, slides, reagents, several fieldworkers who would administer medications in neighborhood health clinics, and pharmaceuticals. Clinicians were also furnished with a bundle of forms to be completed each month in order to report their findings. On those forms, they reported the patients whose sputum revealed bacteria and their treatment outcomes. They showed considerable success in curing patients they diagnosed and treated in this way.

The WHO's TB unit was heartened and asked Karel Styblo—the clinical epidemiologist who developed the project that would be elaborated into DOTS—to come and visit.[7] His visit was to assess using these pilots as a new epidemiological baseline for India before these islands were expanded to cover the whole country. The question of an epidemiological baseline had been a key factor in the move away from an x-ray-based project to one using smear, and one of the earliest documented sources that presages the shift was a note from Chris Murray (of the WHO's TB unit) wondering how the TB intervention in India, at work since 1968, could have had no epidemiological effect.[8] The initial figures had been generated during the 1955 prevalence survey as a by-product of a UNESCO push for Bacillus Calmette-Guérin (BCG) vaccination in India. Murray wrote that these numbers must have changed after twenty years of TB intervention. Thus, Murray argued, a new prevalence survey was a top priority. Funding such a study, however, ended up being less of a priority for the WHO than shifting the technopack toward DOTS.

By sending Styblo to scrutinize the data created in these islands of DOTS technopacks, a new incidence and prevalence rate could be calculated based on bacteria present in sputum. Analysts found that the number of people whose sputum smear registered as TB positive was indeed lower than the number of people predicted to have become sick with TB that year according to the 1955 study. The new TB incidence, as calculated by Styblo, was now the incidence of TB that could be found by smear rather than by other technopacks for TB, like x-ray or bacterial culture.

At the same time, the new pack could be proved effective since it could show the changed status of sputum on slides from bacteria-laden to bacteria-free. In fact, the islands of implementation for the DOTS technopack showed a success rate of between 80 and 90 percent, depending on location. By doing so, it could make a claim to be cheaper, accessible, and epidemiologically effective. The DOTS packet with its technology (microscopes, pharmaceuticals, forms, and statistical instruments) and techniques (microscopy, observation, cohort analysis, and cost-effectiveness calculation) was a wholesale change. Its implementation was a shift in technology whose goals were to protect a resistance-prone drug from overuse and to enhance Indian labor capacity by reducing the prevalence of TB. Ultimately, the technopack aimed at promoting state efficiency and its ability to bring about development. In short, the bundling of technologies and techniques were part of the coming together of global health in the 1990s, and attending to technopacks allows us to interpret some of global health's contemporary forms, like global comparison, global epidemiology, and healthcare islands. In the case of this particular TB technopack, we see a continued shift that accommodates new technology and real worries about rising rates of drug resistance. The newest technology no longer looks for visible bacteria but rather its RNA in a polymerase chain reaction (PCR) reaction, in what has been called "a lab in a box" or "GeneXpert."

GENEXPERT: OF GENES AND EXPERTS

In 2011, the WHO announced that it would endorse a large-scale rollout of Xpert MTB/RIF or GeneXpert, a fully automated and integrated real-time PCR test for TB-diagnostics and detection of rifampicin (Rif) resistance (World Health Organization 2011). Global health technology tends to provide lofty, universalistic promises of far-reaching impact on implementation. GeneXpert's promises are no different, and in the WHO's initial policy recommendations, it is presented as an easy-to-use, safe, and accurate device that can be used in district and subdistrict healthcare facilities with limited infrastructure and minimal training. With assurances of saved time and increased accuracy, GeneXpert addresses two of the major challenges for global TB control: diagnostic delay and increasing rates of drug resistance. It is the technological center of a diagnostics strategy that speaks directly to U.N. Sustainable Development Goal 3, which includes ending the global

TB epidemic by the year 2030. Furthermore, GeneXpert policy aims to quickly identify those patients for whom standard TB drug regimens will be ineffective, thereby avoiding the misuse of pharmaceuticals and extreme or total drug resistance. This promise, however, is left only partially fulfilled by its ability to provide information about rifampicin resistance but not the thirteen other drugs used in first- and second-line TB treatment.

When trying to make sense of globally distributed biomedical technologies, it is useful to address how their mobility affects and is affected by localized clinical settings (Appadurai 1996; Petryna 2009; Harper 2014). We will do so from the vantage point of the GeneXpert technopack, which compiles numerous actors and techniques, and using evidence from Tanzania. Temeke Regional Referral Hospital in Dar-es-Salaam is one of an increasing number of GeneXpert sites in Tanzania, and it provides a sound example of how a technopack can be rife with gaps and cracks in everyday clinical practice—gaps and cracks whose oversight allows promises to be made but whose existence prevents them from being kept.

GeneXpert was introduced in Tanzania in 2012, and Temeke was one of the first clinical sites to implement it. The hospital received two devices through an initiative coordinated by the Foundation for Innovative New Diagnostics (FIND), and the organization planned to run a training and monitoring project through the first year of GeneXpert implementation in Tanzania. However, due to difficulties in some of the implementation sites (including Temeke), the pilot project continued until 2015. For the first three years, GeneXpert performance was monitored by a team in the Central Tuberculosis Reference Laboratory in Muhimbili Central Referral Hospital, led by a Tanzanian microbiologist and a British FIND consultant. The core difficulties they identified and tried to address were GeneXpert underutilization, unregistered devices, and severed lines of cartridge distribution.

In a July 2017 interview, a FIND consultant explained that she could not understand why Temeke's machine performed as poorly as it did when her experience showed that other, similar hospital setups were able to efficiently implement the technology. She wondered why the hospital failed to use GeneXpert's forty-tests-per-day capacity when there were no major issues with cartridge procurement. One potential answer to her question, however, can be found in a national site assessment report in which she writes that Temeke was the only site that could not be assessed since no operator was available at the time of the visit.

As of 2017, the rate of GeneXpert tests in Temeke had increased, but still there were several gaps related to the stability of outputs. Sometimes, thirty tests would be performed in a single day, while at other times, there were periods as long as a week with no activity at all. In other words, the core promise of the global GeneXpert rollout, to decrease diagnostic delay and ultimately provide better access to treatment, regularly failed to materialize in Temeke.

GeneXpert is swift and accurate in detecting TB and Rif resistance if an optimal sputum sample has been properly processed and entered into the device, but for the technology to do its job, it needs to be connected to broader structures of diagnostics, treatment, and care. When we consider GeneXpert not as a singular technology but as an assemblage of technologies, patients, healthcare professionals, and bureaucrats interacting through techniques of clinical assessment, coughing/spitting, registration, sputum processing, analysis, reporting, and treatment initiation, it becomes clear that the technology cannot fulfill its promises on its own. Indeed, technopacks rarely function smoothly. In Temeke, it is difficult to think of GeneXpert as a technopack comprised entirely of smoothly functioning and properly intercommunicating single components. Addressing the technology's relationship with one specific technician can further exemplify this, as the following extract from field notes at Temeke hospital shows:

> [I] went over to the lab around eleven as usual. What struck me today was the large number of filled sputum cups and [diagnostic] request forms sitting on the wooden table [outside the laboratory, in the patients' waiting area]. Entering the laboratory, I noticed that Patrick was missing, and only one of the students [doing internships in laboratory technology] was present in the microbiology room. He was struggling with registering the incoming samples, and had yet to initiate the first [Gene]Xpert cycle of the day.

Patrick is one of two GeneXpert managers in the Temeke laboratory, and throughout it was clear how much the technology's everyday success or failure relied on his presence and the techniques he embodied. A laboratory technician, Patrick started working with GeneXpert in Temeke in 2015, and he was designated as a national super-user in August 2017 because of his high test-output and low error rates. Patrick is dedicated to his work, but he also struggles to make ends meet. Currently, he works full-time in Temeke, takes extra shifts in a private diagnostics laboratory, and runs a small-scale loan operation. Ma, the other technician, is a medical microbiologist and has a broader set of responsibilities in the laboratory. He would only sporadically be assigned to work with GeneXpert, and Patrick had the strongest relationship with the technology. Through his relationship with the GeneXpert technology and techniques that made it run, Patrick also had the strongest links to the TB clinicians in the hospital, the district TB and leprosy coordinator and the regional TB and leprosy coordinator of Temeke, as well as the GeneXpert team in the central TB reference laboratory.

On this particular day, Patrick had taken an extra night shift. He would not come back to the lab until the following day. Despite his absence, there was an ongoing TB-screening project for secondary school students in the municipality. The project resulted in a higher load of incoming samples than usual. Ma was assigned to the blood bank, and the only person available to operate GeneXpert was a student with limited experience. The result was a backlog of samples that would take almost a week to process. With smear microscopy, an experienced laboratory technician could have prepared up to fifty slides simultaneously and then taken several hours to investigate them all, providing a more time-efficient diagnosis than GeneXpert. Patrick frequently emphasized this issue; seemingly minor delays or hiccups in the interaction between GeneXpert and its surroundings could have huge implications for the technology's performance. On several occasions, he found himself turning to microscopy in order to process samples, which would otherwise have piled up indefinitely.

While instrumental challenges such as temperature and dust control, stable electricity, and limited cartridge shelf life are acknowledged and well documented in GeneXpert policy and evaluation papers (Theron et al. 2014), they overlook the human factor in the operation of the technology. No matter how easy and quick the technology is in its immediate operations, it cannot work without a whole set of human skills that have a strong effect on its functioning and temporality and potential effect at clinical and epidemiological scales.

Technopacking Genomics, Mestizaje, and Diabetes in Mexico

In Mexican genomics research, blood samples move from syringe to tube to centrifuge to microarray and then through a sequencer in order to generate a transcribed rendering of genetic variation and disease risk. In the process, their contents are written over with new meanings and uses through techniques and technologies guided by ideas about origin, treatment, and the priority of diseases.

Mexican scientists and policymakers began promoting genomic medicine in the early 2000s as a solution to noncommunicable diseases that were burdening public health and economic resources. They hoped that genomics could help analyze and treat common diseases, boost Mexican biomedical research, and make a contribution to international genomic medicine by factoring in Amerindian genetic variation. This goal generated a specific set of actions and rationalities—a genomics research technopack—affecting how Mexican scientists use technological devices to analyze and treat diseases such as diabetes. The techniques that interpret and move technologies such as genome sequencing machines rely on understandings of the inheritance of genetic variation and disease, informed by identity politics and one of its central ideas, mestizaje. The use of mestizaje in understanding diabetes informs the genomic research technopack in Mexico, exhibiting Madeleine Akrich's concept of "de-scription" and her claim that one can find inscribed in a technological device many of the assumptions, aspirations, and values of those who designed it (Akrich 1992).

The genomics research technopack Mexican scientists use brings together aspiration, action, and artifact. The technologies that genomics researchers use do not (yet) have pharmaceutical or therapeutic applications. In this sense, the Mexican diabetes genome technopack is aspirational. However, this aspiration mobilizes discourses and objects, technological devices, and techniques. In order to translate genomic knowledge into therapeutic and preventive applications, scientists design and carry out studies, recruit certain kinds of participants, and process biological samples through DNA extraction and genome sequencing, for which they need test tubes, pipets, microarrays, centrifugal extractors, sequencing machines, computers with program interfaces, electricity, and a building in which their research can be based. In Mexico, the National Institute of Genomic Medicine (INMEGEN) serves as this hub. It houses the technologies, techniques, and infrastructure, as well as the aspirations that catalyze their use.

The particularly high prevalence of diabetes in Mexico led to the hypothesis that an inheritable origin, traceable to ancestry, makes Mexicans more vulnerable to developing the disease. There is a history of genetic research linked to specific population groups in an attempt to connect different biological makeups to disease outcomes in Mexico, starting with studies on genetic hematologic traits in Indigenous groups in the 1960s (Lisker, Loria et al. 1965; Lisker, Zárate et al. 1966). In the early 2000s, as the Human Genome Project completed the first sequencing of the human genome, Mexican scientists saw opportunities for more precise inquiries into the Mexican population's genetic diversity and possible linkages to diseases such as diabetes (Jiménez-Sánchez 2003). In addition to this new reservoir of data, new DNA sequencing technologies offered the means of identifying and mapping large numbers of genomic markers. The International HapMap Project began to study genetic variation among selected populations worldwide by identifying, cataloging, and mapping single nucleotide polymorphisms (SNPs).[9] This reduced the number of genomic markers needed for determining patterns of genetic variation. Using just the tag SNPs, researchers were able to find chromosome regions with different haplotype distributions in two groups of people—for example, those with a disease and those without (International HapMap Consortium 2005). The HapMap Project and its study of SNPs were technical resources in uncovering genetic diversity, and a haplotype maps an object they produced. Thus, scientists interested in understanding the implications of genetic diversity for health research explicitly connected haplotype maps to disease as the source of reference for genetic association studies. Such studies work on the hypothesis that inherited genetic variation plays an important role in the pathogenesis of disease. As such studies proliferated, the interest in sampling and characterizing the genetic diversity of more worldwide populations grew. This is the context in which researchers used sequencing technologies to create connections between population groups and disease. The output from the sequencing machines became information on both ancestral identity and disease.

In Mexico, INMEGEN advocates proposed studies to identify variation among the population that could create useful information for health and science in Mexico and internationally. Its researchers undertook a large-scale study of Mexican genomic diversity, categorizing haplotypes common in the Mexican population—later presented as the "Mexican genome"—that could be traced back to ancestral lineage. These genetic variants would be linked to knowledge about common variants associated with diseases such as diabetes. Proponents further envisioned preventive and individualized medicine "based on a person's genetic factors of protection or risk" (Jiménez-Sánchez 2003; Silva-Zolezzi, Hidalgo-Miranda et al. 2009). A form of medicine that determined if a population-specific genetic cause existed for diseases like diabetes was an aspiration connected to fixing a public health problem. At the same time, it fed into hopes of stimulating innovative scientific research leading to development and growth. Genomic medicine would save health expenses and boost Mexico's scientific, medical, and economic profile based on the unique genomic contribution INMEGEN researchers claimed their work would make (Jiménez-Sánchez 2003; Taylor-Alexander and Schwartz-Marín 2013).

INMEGEN researchers attributed the unique genomic profile at the root of this genomic research technopack to the country's history of *mestizaje*, the result of 500 years of genetic mixing of European, Amerindian, and African populations. Mestizaje is a central node of identity politics in Mexico. Pushed by the government after the Mexican Revolution to forge different population groups into a common Mexican national identity, today the mestizo figures as a political, social, and biological representation (Wade 2017). The Indigenous population today is simultaneously set apart from the homogenized mestizo population and included as a contributor of unique genetic variants. The Indigenous component has made the mestizo's genetic profile a valuable biological resource, complementing what researchers found in populations of the Global North.[10] The figure of the mestizo as a cultural and scientific idea and the ancestrally based genetic vulnerability to diabetes work together as techniques in the genomics technopack. Genomics research manifests the figure of the mestizo through DNA sequencing and data analysis as a variable combination of biogeographical genetic ancestries.

Both DNA extraction and sequencing on the basis of variants are heavily regulated steps in which technopacks are instantiations of their epistemes. The socially informed mestizo narrative and the genetic screening and disease prevention narrative rely on genomic technologies, and the technologies loop back into these different narratives. Sequencing machines are one way to get and create genomic knowledge through techniques such as the creation of mestizo identity and different ancestral groups materialized through genetic markers, choosing people for sampling, and interpreting the results into maps.

To render legible, categorizable, and analyzable the diversity in the Mexican genome, INMEGEN's flagship study, the Mexican Genome Diversity Project recruited 300 Mexicans with mixed ancestral backgrounds—mestizos—from six different states and thirty Indigenous participants from a Zapotec community to give blood samples. The sampling technique shows how "mestizo" and "Indigenous" functioned as organizing categories. When identifying participants for sampling, mestizo identity was taken for granted whereas the Zapotec participants had to testify that they and their ancestors had been born in the state where the sample was taken (Silva-Zolezzi, Hidalgo-Miranda et al. 2009). The distinction appeared in the barcodes labeling the blood samples, which had different numbers for mestizo and Indigenous participants (García-Deister 2014). Categorizing the samples at the moment just after taking blood transformed their meaning before they traveled to the lab where they would be sequenced. Narratives about population variation and Mexican identity fed into the techniques of extracting and sequencing so that even before being extracted, DNA is not a raw bodily extract. Blood samples in the Mexican Genome Diversity Project already existed as fraught objects.

The Mexican project used SNP methodology to analyze the samples of the six mestizo populations and the Zapotecs and compare them to data from populations included in the International HapMap Project. In an entanglement of technologies and techniques situating the SNP-based methodology, DNA was extracted from these blood samples with the help of solvents and a centrifuge to separate blood plasma from the red and white blood cells, to extract DNA from the plasma, and to purify it to make it accessible and legible. After this, DNA was placed on a small biochip known as a microarray. This microarray went into an automated sequencing machine and was then computationally analyzed. The machines surveyed each genome for markers of genetic variation, the tag SNPs. Researchers depicted these ancestrally informative markers schematically in diagrams and maps showing the frequency distribution of SNPs in the different states where samples were taken (Silva-Zolezzi, Hidalgo-Miranda et al. 2009). This process shows all the technical work that goes into maps of human variation, and a technopack determines the specific use of blood samples, the markers that define their interpretation, and how they create information. A sequencing machine relies on the actions that prepare DNA for reading. Then, researchers of the Mexican Genome Diversity Project determined what genetic markers the machines looked for based on previous population studies, such as the International HapMap Project.

In the extraction and sequencing chain, blood samples go through various regulated steps of meaning-making through the use of a DNA extractor, a microarray, and a sequencing machine. Then the interpretation of the machine's output relies on identifying indicators of genetic variation that genomics researchers deem meaningful, such as tag SNPs. Without these, it would not be possible to create maps of genetic variation to construe ancestry and disease vulnerability. And through these indicators, this research pack performs the category of mestizo and produces the mestizo's disease vulnerability.

The Mexican Genome Diversity Project's first study ended with a presentation of the "Mexican genome map" to the public in May 2009.[11] During this presentation, INMEGEN's director estimated that the study would allow for concrete health applications within five to ten years. In a study tying genetic variants to diabetes risk some years later, INMEGEN researchers claimed that "now, through the development of genetic risk exams, the contraction of diabetes by millions of people will be delayed or prevented" (SIGMA Type 2 Diabetes Consortium 2014). Therapeutic or pharmaceutical interventions would bring standardization and efficient use as part of a larger technopack of diagnostic and intervention tools. The researchers did not mention how such a genetic risk exam would be embedded in care or what would happen after undergoing such an exam. In fact, while INMEGEN researchers proposed the use of genomic technologies to analyze and treat common diseases several years ago, the knowledge acquired through genomic research has not yet been channeled into therapeutic interventions. Therefore, this technopack does not reconfigure care around pharmaceuticals or therapeutic interventions in the way that technopacks do in the other cases discussed in this chapter.

The therapeutic genomics technopack, one that uses genomic knowledge and/ or technologies to treat or prevent diabetes, is stuck in the research-toward-care stage, while diabetes continues to grow as public health issue and genetic, ancestry-based categories are being (re)created and further biologically embedded. These activities change the very meaning of what genomic medicine entails. The Mexican genomic-diabetic research technopack feeds into local categories configured around genetic knowledge, disease etiology, and ancestral markers. Yet, as researchers continue to work on new technologies and techniques—such as new sequencing machines, new ways to read and act on genomes, and new extraction methods—the research technopack might one day include therapeutic and preventive technologies and techniques.

Cuba's Prenatal Screening Technopack

In Cuba, primary health care services form the core of the health system and foreground a public health approach based on health promotion and disease prevention. Prenatal screening to detect genetic disorders is organized across the health system's three-tiered infrastructure. All three of these tiers coordinate to form Cuba's "medical genetics network." Genetics services in Cuba were originally organized around pregnant women. The idea to focus the management of genetic disorders on pregnant women was tested at the initiation of the medical genetics program in 1982. For local genetics experts, high prenatal care attendance rates make pregnant women a good focal group; 98 percent of pregnant women receive regular prenatal care, and as part of this care, they have access to genetic services. In this context, analysis of a "screening-pack" develops a perspective on the ways and means through which technologies and techniques suffuse medical genetics' activities and transform them.

In primary care, obstetric consultations with pregnant women and family physicians combine physical examinations with information about family medical histories to determine possible genetic risks. They then advise pregnant women on the risks of common and detectable genetic conditions that might affect the baby. The family physician organizes the collection of blood and urine samples, which are sent to tertiary laboratories for testing. In addition, women have routine ultrasound examinations throughout the course of the pregnancy. Women experiencing low-risk pregnancies usually receive ultrasound services that allow health practitioners to monitor the development of the fetus, but these women do not usually undergo other tests. High-risk pregnant mothers are usually examined at a municipal polyclinic, and, if an ultrasound shows any abnormalities, they are sent to a provincial medical genetics center where they undergo a further, specialized ultrasound. In cases where a genetic cause is suspected, expectant mothers are given the choice of undergoing more invasive procedures in order to collect fetal genetic material. These samples—fetal blood from the umbilical cord and amniotic fluid or tissue samples with the same embryological origin as the fetus—are then sent to laboratories. At both the municipal and the provincial centers, couples are offered counseling by trained genetic counselors. Cuba's National Medical Genetics Center located in Havana "coordinates the medical genetics network, human resource training, research and health services" of the country (Marcheco-Teruel 2009). The national center also hosts five laboratories specializing in genetic analysis. The aim of genetic screening is said to be so that "the child's care can be planned in advance, leading in many cases to greater possibilities for survival and better quality of life; it provides families the choice of interrupting pregnancy where this is legally permissible; and offers reassurance to the majority of couples who have normal results" (Méndez-Rosado, Quiñones et al. 2018).

Thus, the technopack presented here consists of prenatal screening technologies, the techniques with which they are used, and the patient bodies that are acted on. The Cuban screening-pack is laden with the language of global health methods and goals in that it "targets," "renders neutral," and "rationalizes" the most basic workings of human difference in the name of "health" and "development." Moreover, the narrative of the technopack is pervasive and strong; women in Havana seem keenly aware of the risks of genetic disorders and take their genetic consultations seriously.

Pregnant women attending a genetic consultation at a municipal polyclinic revealed the enthusiasm and seriousness with which mothers regard these state-provided health services. Internet access and printed materials are limited in Cuba, and health information relies on oral communications between patients and health practitioners, television and radio broadcasts, and discussions among the general public, such as we see taking place in this waiting room. Couples attend their prenatal consultations as advised, gathering in lines and waiting rooms to see specialists. The women were observant of what seemed to be unwritten triage rules, giving priority to women with babies and to women pregnant with twins. While waiting, women struck up conversations easily with one another, exchanging information and experiences.

We accompanied a friend, Dayana, to her local polyclinic for her sixth genetic consultation. She chatted with another young pregnant woman carrying twins and recounted how they had met at an earlier genetic consultation. They talked about the health issues they faced, their visits to the provincial genetic center, and more generally about where to buy affordable baby products. Dayana had documents with her, which included a UNICEF-provided pregnancy card, some prescription slips, and a genetic consultation form. The pregnancy card lacked space to record all her prenatal clinic visits—one every two weeks—and an additional piece of paper had to be glued onto it. The genetic consultation form also required additional papers for recording the visits. The genetic form records first- and second-trimester ultrasound examination results as well as the genetics program ultrasound examination results. In Dayana's case, there were three follow-up ultrasounds recorded. The form also contains information about the risks of malformations, consanguinity, genetic diseases in the family, and the exposure of the fetus to alcohol, smoking, and radiation, as well as blood and urine test results (including alpha-fetoprotein), an entry for recording the intake of folic acid, and a genetic risk category score.

The ultrasound was conducted in a room kept at a low temperature by an air conditioner. According to Dayana, the ultrasound machine often overheats and is dependent on the air conditioner for its accuracy. She was eight months pregnant and concerned because her previous ultrasounds showed the fetus was underweight and had a mark along the digestive track. She had visited the Provincial Center for Medical Genetics in Havana a week before. Doctors there had done further tests to determine if there was a problem. The tests confirmed that the mark they saw on the ultrasound was an air bubble and not an indication of any malformation. Still, Dayana, worried about the weight issue, decided to go for a follow-up ultrasound at the polyclinic. She had already had five ultrasounds. During the consultation, the geneticist told Dayana that the ultrasound did not show anything new, and she did not mention the weight issue. As a nurse noted something on what looked like a handwritten spreadsheet drawn across two pages of a notebook, Dayana insisted on the weight issue and asked for clarification. She was determined to get a definitive answer. The medical practitioner responded by reiterating that the clinic took this issue seriously, but she need not worry because she did not have a high-risk pregnancy. To the contrary, Dayana had been through weeks of stress and had been diagnosed with high blood pressure by her family physician, and she insisted that she had been regarded as high-risk all along.

Dayana's experience demonstrates the ambiguities that exist in standardized screening in Cuba. The technologies and practices involved in screening reveal the disjointed configuration necessary for accuracy and the unmatched parts that come together along a series of different tests, diagnoses, and follow-ups. The genetic markers can be clinically unclear, as well as poorly communicated between medical practitioners and patient. The technopack comes together and falls apart, succeeds and fails. This Cuban genetic-screening technopack is a linkage of necessary parts. Without the air conditioner, the machine can overheat and create false results. The machine is not independent of the local context; it is placed in an existing structure, the polyclinic and the relatively new genetic consultation office indicated by a sign on the door. The machines also cannot function when there is no gel to use for the ultrasound, as Dayana learned when one of her visits was canceled because this necessity was lacking. Different health practitioners, including genetic specialists, are found along the chain of linked services across the city. When a test is unclear, pregnant women are sent to the main maternity hospital that houses the Provincial Center for Medical Genetics. There, a group of genetic specialists performs further tests using more advanced—some say more accurate—machines. The health practitioner tries to assuage the concerns of the patient by insisting on risk classifications—although different practitioners can of course disagree on these classifications—and the importance of the woman and her baby in the national "development" program.

Through the lens of a technopack, one can see medical genetics applied to the experience of life's "natural" events as revealing the "possibility for further care," a "reassurance" in the absence of a disorder, or a way to sidestep an "avoidable burden" if one is present. These are all ways of making screening meaningful. Cuba's sociopolitical and economic milieu is particular. The lack of material resources in the health system is compensated for with a robust cadre of health professionals. It is much like a kaleidoscope; the parts are constantly shifting, but every once in a while, they come together to show purpose and give clarity. This, of course, belies the story about the efficacy of the medical genetics technology that global health actors are so eager to tell.

Conclusion

The complex mobile apparatuses that we have called "technopacks" are some of global health's moving parts. They certainly circulate both in the global health field and in health globalization arenas as machines, medicines, and epistemological practices. They are also tools, techniques, and people that undergo transformations as they circulate. Though technical, our explorations show that technopacks rarely succeed in rendering health mechanically technical. Instead, they are modular, aggregated, and segmented material and discursive entanglements that integrate technology and its implementation toward a health-related if not always treatment-oriented goal. As such, health globalization and global health's technopacks shape, are shaped by, and rely on the health systems within which they are activated. This reliance comes in the form of infrastructure, staff, and techniques, and at times a technopack stretches health systems thin or reorganizes the forms of knowledge it creates. This means that as technopacks circulate, they bring with them their own ways of creating and contesting knowledge about health and illness. As such, they can and do effect disease categories and epistemes, as the TB and depression case studies showed. However, as GeneXpert makes clear, technopacks also rely heavily on tacitly held techniques or those persisting from older technopacks that are as often left out of their instruction manuals as included.

Alongside this combination of technology and techniques, technopacks bring a very particular connection between technology and development. In each case, technopacks are imagined as catalysts for development, either by increasing labor force partition, or potential discovery, or by preventing costly life. In this system, they have the potential to reveal neoliberal rationality at work in global health interventions. At the same time, we have shown that a technopack's logic need not necessarily be neoliberal, and at times that logic can and is subverted by users like Dayana in Cuba. What is clear, in any case, is that technologies are wrapped up in health at a global scale as mobile packets that respond to both a hope for development and an impetus to act, whether motivated by market capture, neoliberalism, or health for all.

Technopacks like those described here in India, Tanzania, Mexico, and Cuba might easily be maligned as technical fixes to systemic or social problems, but their influence is far more than that of Band-Aids. They change health systems, ideas about risk and security, and even the kinds of people subjected to medical intervention. To write of technopacks means showing how technologies and their affordances are dynamic in the same moment that they create and document comparability. They can and do make some aspects of health comparable, but in the process, they transform the illness experience and are transformed themselves by global health's rules of the game, circulations in arenas of health globalization, and the processes of localization replete in interventions across scales. Finally, technopacks are, as Latour and Woolgar (1979), among many others, have argued, a distillation of history. More precisely, they are bio-logistical tools that combine logics of efficiency, human capital, labor, accounting, and action to make human health modular and perhaps even global.

CHAPTER 6

Persistent Hospitals

Claire Beaudevin, Fanny Chabrol, and Claudia Lang

Global health's ethic of action is based on an assumption that functioning healthcare—public hospitals, health infrastructure, and expertise—does not exist in the spaces where global health is most active. Yet many public hospitals exist in sites of global health intervention. Thus, in the context of global health, state-run hospitals are paradoxical objects of mistrust and investment: They are bypassed and criticized on the grounds of inefficiency but are nonetheless continuously funded and invested with social and political value. They are necessary components in numerous health interventions, which ironically often include global health programs designed to make up for their shortfalls. In other words, hospitals remain important, but they are often unacknowledged loci of care, training, and research, as well as sites of larger processes of health globalization. This paradoxical status places hospitals in a central position within the field of global health and the arenas of health globalization.

In this chapter, we ask: How do novel diseases, techniques, and tools enter these hospitals, and how does global health change the hospital as a site of care, affecting—or not—its infrastructure, human resources, supply chains, and position in the health system? To answer these questions, we examine three hospitals—in East Africa, the Middle East, and Asia—in light of three globalized domains of health: medical genetics, tuberculosis, and mental health.

Recent scholarship shows how global health both reconfigures hospitals and encourages innovation within them. Novel global health targets, such as cancer in Botswana (Livingston 2012) or HIV/AIDS in Tanzania (Sullivan 2011), do indeed transform hospital spaces and infrastructures. Moreover, global health generates highly funded "enclaves" of healthcare and medical research characterized by large flows of knowledge, material, and resources, within often largely dysfunctional state hospitals (Sullivan 2011; Crane 2013; Geissler 2013b). Prestigious research universities of the Global North "scramble" for African university hospitals to accommodate their global health research and programs (Crane 2013). In doing so, they produce forms of inequality, exclusion, and unknowing (Crane 2013;

Geissler 2013b). In such contexts, improvisation and experimentation prevail (Livingston 2012). Moving beyond the narrative of state hospitals as ruined buildings, decayed institutions, and playgrounds for global health actors (Street 2012), our cases show both the persistent but invisibilized presence of hospitals in the global health era and their reconfigurations when novel global health diseases and technologies enter—and sometimes tear down—their walls. After all, hospitals have been targets of international health programs long before the primary health care movement.

Debates about health equity within socialist and Third World circles in the 1960s and 1970s tended to criticize the hospital. The 1978 Alma-Ata Declaration does not mention hospitals, but the World Health Organization (WHO) report on the event shifts the hospital's dominant position within the healthcare system to that of a necessary support structure for primary health care, which should be the locus of health interventions (International Conference on Primary Health Care, World Health Organization et al. 1978). The rapid shrinking scope of primary health care policies in the decade following Alma-Ata, however, from comprehensive to selective, affected hospital-related activities by prioritizing certain targets, but it did not trigger a thorough rethinking of the role of hospitals in health systems. Several WHO reports from the 1980s bear the mark of debates that promote the district hospital as the best institution for supporting primary health care, on the grounds of its efficiency and moderate operational costs. Similarly, the World Bank's *World Development Report: Investing in Health* (World Bank 1993) balanced the presence and absence of the hospital. It advocated against *hospitalocentrism*, targeting the hospital as too expensive and not serving the needs of the poor. Nonetheless, the report acknowledged the hospital as an important part of the three-tier structure of the health system and the referral pyramid and gave the district hospital a prominent place. Again in 2008 and in 2018, while celebrating the thirtieth and fortieth Alma-Ata anniversaries, WHO reports acknowledged the limits of hospitalocentrism—when hospitals have a prominent and organizing role within health systems—and a focus on specialist, tertiary care (World Health Organization 2008b, 2018). The most recent report states, "Hospitals can play a powerful role in supporting and amplifying the benefits of primary health care. This requires building on hospitals' unique strengths while dissolving the walls that separate them from the rest of health systems—and from the people they exist to serve" (World Health Organization 2018, 1). The report describes hospitals as "key contributors to primary health care development" and an "essential setting for healthcare workers' education," but it acknowledged a need to move "from isolated institutions to . . . community and person-centred" networks (World Health Organization 2018, 2). However, few reports provide concrete alternatives to hospitalocentrism.

The debates around de-hospitalization, in the case of specific domains of global health such as tuberculosis (TB) and mental health, evolved as a reaction to this primacy of the hospital. Experts challenged the hospital as the primary locus of care and a crucial health infrastructure. De-hospitalization movements advocated for minimizing hospital stays in order to limit costs and bring care closer to communities while maintaining access to pharmacological treatments.

In the global fight against TB, the necessity of hospitalization is a recurring question, especially since the directly observed treatment short-course (DOTS) strategy entered the picture as a first-line intervention. When chemotherapy treatment arrived in the 1950s, full hospitalization in Europe and North America was the norm. However, in developing countries, the cost of hospitalization and the lack of hospital beds were important obstacles. In Tanzania, initial hospitalization was not implemented in the 1970s, despite the prevalent WHO policies of the time. Instead, the International Union Against Tuberculosis and Lung Disease (IUATLD) helped to build the National TB and Leprosy Program, which also promoted the implementation of shorter regimens without hospitalization. Nevertheless, medical teams at Kibong'oto National TB hospital practiced hospitalization, and Tanzanian authorities proposed it in 1977 as the official policy, although it was rejected by the IUATLD (Gradmann 2019). Notwithstanding the fact that international proponents of short course treatment for Tanzania went so far as denying Kibong'oto the designation of "specialized TB hospital," this institution played a key role in legitimizing the hospitalization of TB patients, especially in the initial phase of treatment. Recently, multidrug-resistant TB epidemics have reopened the debate on hospitalization globally. The severity of clinical cases has led to rehospitalizing patients for long periods, in order to foster recovery and prevent contagion. However, many clinical and public health experts warn about infection risks in hospitals—because they see hospitalization as more risky for patients and providers—and recommend more ambulatory and community-based care and treatment. Advocates of care outside the hospital also frequently and successfully use the argument of lower costs compared to inpatient treatment (Schnippel, Rosen et al. 2013; Loveday, Wallengren et al. 2015).

In mental healthcare, the role of the hospital has been a central question, which predates global health. In this context, the term "deinstitutionalization" refers to the process of, first, closing large psychiatric hospitals where persons with suspected mental illnesses were confined indefinitely, and second, opening clinics to offer care within communities (Brodwin 2013; Thornicroft, Deb et al. 2016). Worldwide, this double movement has been promoted as the way forward for modern mental health services (Kohrt, Asher et al. 2018; World Health Organization 2019). Such deinstitutionalization was partly political—the rejection of an "era of confinement" and the promotion of the human rights of persons with mental illness—and partly economic. In countries of the Global South, psychiatric institutions were few and institutionalization was less of a concern. Still, the WHO promotes the policy of care in the community and the delivery of mental healthcare through primary care systems (World Health Organization 1975; World Health Organization and World Family Doctors Caring for People 2008). The call for deinstitutionalization has been a feature of global mental health, gaining additional moral force from the expansion of rights-based approaches to mental health, but its implementation has been uneven (World Health Organization and World Family Doctors Caring for

People 2008). A widely promoted method of strengthening the health system, endorsed by global mental health actors, concerns what is known as "task shifting." Task shifting involves the delegation of less specialized clinical and administrative tasks to lower-level workers (World Health Organization and World Family Doctors Caring for People 2008; Maes 2015). These workers might be new cadres of personnel employed directly by the health service, but they might also be community volunteers, nongovernmental organization (NGO) staff, traditional and faith healers, and, through forms of "self-management," patients and families themselves (Brodwin 2017; Davis 2018). Both clinicians and task shifters are engaged in various tasks that move beyond the clinic walls and into the community, in the form of community engagement, "sensitization," "education" and "awareness raising," distribution of pharmaceuticals, home visits, and various forms of screening and surveillance bringing coercion to the doorstep (Lang 2019).

In medical genetics, the place of hospitals in the Global South is slightly different. The highly technical environment necessary for the implementation of genetic testing and screening, combined with the tertiary-care status of genetic expertise related to rare disorders, led to large hospitals playing a crucial role in the evolution of the discipline. Nevertheless, the WHO did attempt to open a path outside the hospital for genetic medicine through its promotion of community genetics in the 1980s and 1990s (see chapter 1, Localization in the Global).

Answering the 1978 Alma-Ata call for comprehensive primary health care and aiming to implement a population-level approach for the prevention of the genetic disorders that are most frequently inherited worldwide (namely, inherited blood disorders and cystic fibrosis), clinical geneticists and pediatricians gathered in several committees in the early 1980s (Modell and Kuliev 1998). These groups participated in the definition of guidelines and in the creation and conduct of large-scale experimental programs such as the management of beta-thalassemia in Cyprus (Angastiniotis, Kyriakidou et al. 1986; Ruault, Beaudevin et al. 2020). While the treatment of targeted disorders was mostly hospital-based (including in the Global North), these programs aimed to extend the availability of genetic counseling and screening to primary health care facilities for a small number of inherited diseases (World Health Organization 1999). However, besides Cyprus and countries like Iran, Cuba, and Oman, few countries of the Global South implemented this approach for many reasons, including politics and logistics and, of course, cost. In countries where clinical medical genetics (i.e., diagnostic expertise beyond access to screening tests) is nowadays available, it largely remains a hospital-based enterprise.

Our dual historical and anthropological investigations into the domains of TB, mental health, and genetics left us facing the ambiguous status of hospitals in our fields. Hospitals are continuously targeted by critics within public health and health systems science. As such, they are not explicit targets of global health interventions and hence are not part of what we define in the introduction as the specific field of global health. We contend, however, that the hospital, as an infrastructure and site of care, is centrally located within the larger processes of health globalization. In order to explore this centrality, we bring materialities to the fore. In contrast to the desire on the part of global health players to simply see through hospitals to the challenges and interventions beneath, we approach hospitals as infrastructures. On a first analytical level, hospitals represent major targets of referral within healthcare systems; on another level, we contend they are material, spatial, and relational infrastructures, defined and built by the people who staff, use, and need them.

The three cases stemming from our inquiries in East Africa, Asia, and the Middle East instantiate some of the manifold ways in which novel global health diseases and technologies use, affect, reconfigure, and expand the hospital and its infrastructure—notably by creating new priorities. Our first case focuses on how medical genetics as a new and globalized specialty enters the public hospital in Oman, and how it mobilizes and changes its infrastructure, with the genetic clinic becoming an important node in the training, research, and care infrastructure of the country. The case also shows the relevance of digital infrastructure as a crucial component of processes of health globalization, even as these processes are adapted to local needs. In the second case, we show how the treatment of multidrug-resistant tuberculosis (MDR-TB) builds on, as much as reconfigures, the infrastructure of a prominent TB hospital in Tanzania. Our final case shows the centrality of a state mental hospital in India in the mental health infrastructure of the country. It explores how this hospital has expanded its treatment, teaching, and research infrastructure beyond the clinic's walls to pilot and implement community mental health through shifting tides of mental healthcare in India. The advent of digital technologies has further expanded the reach of its training and care, as have novel mental health priorities such as depression as well as reconceptualization of the community as a middle-class neighborhood. These developments have taken place despite the neglect of the hospital in global mental health policies and publications. Taken together, our cases demonstrate the strong presence and "nodality" (i.e., both centrality and connectivity to other health facilities) of the hospital in states' care, training, research, and referral infrastructures. The cases also show that hospitals are open to change and that their infrastructure expands and is reconfigured as novel diseases and tools flow through them.

CRAFTING MEDICAL GENETICS IN AN OMANI HOSPITAL

The globalization of health processes we followed include growing medical genetics activities, which mostly result from the increased visibility of the millions of people affected by myriad inherited disorders. As such, this clinical practice (and its commensurate research activities) is a new feature of many healthcare systems outside of Europe and North America. In the Arabian Peninsula, the Sultanate of Oman is no exception. The following section explores how medical genetics as a recently practiced specialty enters contemporary Omani hospitals, modifies their infrastructure, initiates relations with other health facilities and the world, and participates in shaping their position in the national referral system.

There are some fifty state-funded hospitals in Oman (Ministry of Health Oman 2020). The Ministry of Higher Education administers one of them, Sultan Qaboos University Hospital (SQUH). Located in the capital area and inaugurated in 1990, it is the oldest and largest of Oman's two teaching hospitals. SQUH lies at the foot of the Western Hajar Mountains, approximately six miles from Indian Ocean beaches, on the coastal plain that runs from the mountains next to the Strait of Hormuz to Muscat. Once remote, this area is now central, following the massive urbanization of the coast in the 2000s. SQUH's main building sits on the edge of the national university campus, adjacent to the Colleges of Medicine and Nursing. With about 650 beds and 3,000 staff members (including 450 physicians), SQUH provides the population of the capital area with secondary care and is a tertiary-care referral center for the whole country (College of Medicine and Health Sciences 2016; Ministry of Health Oman 2017). This hospital is both a massive material complex and a crucial node of Oman's healthcare system. Here we present the case of one of SQUH's newest departments, the Clinical Genetics and Developmental Medicine Clinic (hereafter, "the genetic medicine clinic," as the chapter focuses on its medical genetics activities).

A recent addition to the panel of specialized care offered by SQUH, this clinic is the university hospital's answer to the growing need for genetic diagnosis and treatment of rare as well as more common inherited disorders in a sultanate that has been undergoing a massive epidemiological transition. This unfolding of medical genetics in Oman occurred after the Ministry of Health acknowledged the need for genetic medicine in primary health care facilities targeting specific disorders. The original governmental objective dealt with screening engaged couples for common inherited blood disorders (thalassemia and sickle cell anemia). During the late 2000s, the Ministry of Health bought high-performance liquid chromatography (HPLC) machines that would allow for on-site hemoglobin analysis in many primary health care centers and governorate hospitals.[1] In line with the original aims of the 1980s WHO Human Genetics Program (see chapter 7, Provincializing the WHO) and after the 2002 visit of WHO consultant and geneticist Bernadette Modell (see chapter 7 and chapter 1, Localization in the Global) to Oman, the goal was to target the most common inherited disorders with a decentralized screening and counseling preventive program—namely, community genetics. In the decade that followed, the difficulties of implementing such a program and the need to expand clinical genetics expertise beyond commonly inherited blood disorders shaped the further unfolding of medical genetics in Oman. On the one hand, the community genetics program remained centralized until the 2016 training of several regional hospital nurses in basic genetic counseling (see chapter 3, Triage beyond the Clinic). The courses mostly deal with hemoglobinopathies and how to care for existing cases of other relatively common genetic disorders such as Down syndrome. On the other hand, since the early 2010s, young Omani doctors and biologists have come back home after having specialized in genetics abroad, thus expanding the scope of the available medical genetics expertise in the country.

The multidisciplinary expertise necessary to diagnose and manage genetic disorders, as well as the multiplicity of diagnosis tools involved, make medical genetics a mainly hospital-based specialty. In Oman, except for the community genetics approach toward hemoglobinopathies, medical genetics is centralized in SQUH and in the Royal Hospital, the country's two main public referral hospitals located in the capital. The returning doctors took positions in these two institutions. Both sites provide the necessary infrastructure for a tertiary-level combination of clinical and laboratory genetic expertise, diagnostic technologies, and genetic counseling. Their routine activities mainly pertain to rare disorders, and especially dysmorphologies and metabolic diseases—in other words, confirming diagnoses in newborns and diagnosing and genetically confirming various congenital diseases including Down syndrome, Huntington disease, and cystic fibrosis. Patients affected by potentially inherited forms of cancer attend the clinic, as do young patients of rare metabolic disorders, for follow-up. The clinic's activity is thus a combination of highly specialized diagnosis, regular treatment for chronic genetic disorders, and specific research activities related to the College of Medicine. Such activities involve complex referral trajectories and the circulation of genetic information across the country, which both necessitate specific material arrangements and the involvement of numerous individuals—staff and patients.

Opened in the summer of 2011 as a new department offering novel medical services, the genetic clinic deals with all sorts of genetic disorders, but not with the ones that community genetics is tasked with targeting throughout the country. Treatment of inherited blood disorders—the initial target of community genetics—occurs in the hematology department. The genetics clinic's medical and paramedical team gathers geneticists, pediatricians, genetic counselors, dieticians, nurses, a social worker, a psychologist, and two administrative officers. They all provide outpatient consultations, as well as some visits to patients in hospital wards, and work in close collaboration with the genetic laboratory of the College of Medicine, where all in-house tests are performed.

The clinic is located outside SQUH's main building, on the ground floor of a 4,200-square-foot structure that once housed the laundry. Reorganized to accommodate the clinic, the premises now feature a checkered layout, with a peripheral zone for offices and consultation rooms and a central windowless area with three tiny, shared physicians' offices and two counseling rooms. The site feels undersized for its intense clinical activity: about twenty consultations per day, often involving several family members of the patient and lasting for more than thirty minutes.

The backdrop to this situation partly explains this scarcity of space: The aftermath of the 2008 global financial crisis, combined with successive drops in oil prices, has led the Omani government into unfamiliar austerities. In the past, state finances usually absorbed deficits without disclosing them. In 2016, for the first time, these shortfalls were partially offset by officially acknowledged public budget cuts, and the resulting shortages have begun to affect health-related expenditures in the public sector (Oman News Agency 2015, 2016; Reuters 2016; Valeri

2018).[2] For instance, the planned neighboring hematologic center at SQUH stands as a warning to any expansionist ambitions: an empty five-floor vessel in bare concrete, trapped in scaffoldings, without an official date of inauguration. As a reminder of the budget constraints, there are recurrent administrative requests from hospital management that the clinic does not increase its consultation activity. No larger building is planned, despite attendance doubling since 2012. And referrals continue to grow, with approximately twenty new referrals every week that could also trigger consultations for these patients' relatives.

Room management in the genetic clinic is a quotidian challenge that embodies these tensions. Counseling occurs in a windowless thirty-square-foot room that nevertheless contains two large faux-leather sofas, a coffee table, a small computer desk and a fridge for medications. When the schedule shows two simultaneous sessions, one of the counselors sits with her patients in the department's meeting room. The scarcity of space also has a direct impact on patients' lives, since SQUH has a limited storage capacity for medication. Thus, parents of infants affected by inherited metabolic disorders requiring specific milk can only get a few weeks' supply of it at each visit. Besides these logistic adaptations and the relative plasticity of the hospital infrastructure, improvisation skills among health professionals also emerge when dealing with the information technology (IT) elements of their daily activities.

The materialities necessary for clinical genetics go beyond cutting-edge DNA sequencing machines. They involve sufficient working space, furniture, package deliveries, machines, tools, and roads for patient transportation. Moreover, digital infrastructures matter. These can take the form of computers, software, servers, broadband Internet, smartphones and their apps, online interfaces, online databases, email clients, patient file software, backups, and storage space—of unprecedented size for hospitals' IT departments. All these tools are, of course, required for the operation of the genetics laboratory (located in the nearby College of Medicine), but they are also indispensable in the clinical area for storing and organizing personal health data, consultation schedules, and referrals; interconnecting health facilities; and exchanging results between practitioners and institutions, as well as analyzing clinical data for research purposes.

Operating under a different ministerial umbrella (the Ministry of Higher Education) than the Royal Hospital and other Ministry of Health facilities, SQUH's genetic medicine clinic also uses a different hospital information system. The lack of interoperability sheds light on the relational way in which genetic medicine operates despite such disconnectivity within official digital infrastructures. This hospital's infrastructure is the instantiation of the regulatory framework, as well as the condition of possibility of the professional practice of medical genetics. The novelty of the profession of genetic counseling in the country and the very small number of formally trained practitioners deprive this activity of a clear status in the medical hierarchy. Genetic counselors typically train locally as nurses or biologists before traveling abroad for specialized training in countries where genetic counseling is an established profession. These health workers study in places such as the United Kingdom, the United States, and South Africa, depending on their personal networks and Oman's historical connections. In their everyday practice of counseling in Oman, however, the status of their original education largely defines their professional autonomy.

The various hospital information systems mirror the fuzzy status and daily negotiations of the genetic counselors. The systems allow data access and input based on professional status. Nurses may thus not hold the necessary credentials to request further genetic tests—or, rather, the software technically prevents them from doing so. Similarly, biologists may not be granted access to add remarks in the "medical" fields of a patient's file, even if their genetics-related activities require them to do so. For all of the genetic counselors, negotiating their new status in the healthcare system directly relates to bridging infrastructural discontinuity between various parts of the system. The medical results they can access on-screen, the selected referrals they are allowed to arrange, and the field dedicated to their remarks in the patient file are all crucial matters for them to control, since they determine the precision of a patient's therapeutic itinerary.

In addition to these discontinuities, a striking, institutional disconnect takes place between SQUH and public healthcare facilities under the umbrella of the Ministry of Health. Numerous professionals try to collaborate despite this situation, which triggers improvisation, especially when dealing with intractable information systems. Interestingly, WhatsApp, a Facebook-owned smartphone messaging app, is the main tool used to bypass these obstacles. WhatsApp is the quickest way to share information between SQUH hospital doctors and their counterparts outside—especially useful in advance of the weekly seminar where cases might be discussed. One can thus observe WhatsApp discussions about pedigrees and medical images moving from SQUH to medical professionals in other hospitals via servers in California.[3] In addition to the circulation of medical data between institutions, WhatsApp also serves as a crucial link between SQUH and its patients. It can stand in for a home visit when dieticians deliver advice and follow-up instructions over the app to those patients who live too far away from Muscat to attend the clinic in person. Staff members then transcribe the contents of those online exchanges into the patient record, using vague language such as "patient contacted us." Many nurses and administrators also find the application useful, since it allows for leaving voice messages for nonliterate patients, whereas Omani mobile phone packages do not include this service.

Other nonexplicit Oman-California connections occur on an everyday basis when it comes to ordering molecular genetic tests outside Oman. If a prescribed test is not available or is too costly to do in-house, the DNA sample travels abroad. In SQUH, genetic counselors (trained in human genetics) deal with this aspect of their work, and they have built an ad hoc digital procedure around it. The first step is exploration of the online market for medical genetic tests, a process that starts with a Google search for the online prices of the specific test needed. Out of the usual five to seven test providers (based in the United States, Germany, or France, usually), genetic counselors then select the one they deem appropriate, in terms of the current price, potential pre-negotiated discounts, and the proposed turnaround time. Then, in an Excel spreadsheet of the clinic's patients, the counselor fills in the type of test and the chosen testing company. The next step takes place in another Google service: Gmail. Because of the unreliability of hospital email—notably in the aftermath of the massive 2017 hacking campaigns against hospitals worldwide—the clinic mostly uses Gmail accounts, which allow genetic counselors to upload patient consent forms, the companies to send results and invoices, and the accountancy manager of the clinic to launch the payments. Shipping companies such as UPS or DHL then transport the DNA, collecting samples every week from the clinic.

Once the test results arrive, in a PDF file, the improvised process continues. European and North American companies' test results determine the potential pathogenicity of genetic sequences based on international databases,[4] which often do not account for local variations. In several cases, Omani patients carrying a supposedly nonpathogenic mutation showed symptoms. The team is aware of these epistemic gaps and pays attention to the necessary negotiation between their own database, the test reports, and clinical information.

The noninteroperable information systems and databases strongly affect referral pathways in Oman. Looking at the Ministry of Health's network of health facilities, one notices that its information system allows every public healthcare facility to connect to the others over a dedicated network—distinct from the Internet, for security reasons. Thus, with the proper credentials, professionals can access the medical history of any of their patients, whichever facility stores the information. As a corollary, referrals are supposed to occur exclusively through this network. A practitioner, when organizing a referral, should only need to select the right name in the facilities list on their screen and send a short message along with the referral. Once these steps are performed, the referral process automatically starts and patients get a text message on their mobile phone with an appointment date. Problems occur, however, when the referral target is wrongly coded or not listed. As one geneticist explained in 2017, "We are listed 'Muscat Genetics' in [another tertiary hospital system], which isn't the official name of anything. As a result, nobody is actually referred if they don't double ask by fax: the referral does not pop up into our appointment list." This example shows how a digital infrastructure meant to connect providers actually blurs referral trajectories and ends up increasing the relative isolation of the newly created genetic centers.

As an outsider to the Ministry of Health's facilities network, SQUH uses its own guidelines. One of them is theoretically iconoclastic in a system that fosters professionally oriented referral paths: The clinic accepts "self-referrals." The clinical team knows that this policy tends to increase the patient load, even more so since many patients consider SQUH as a logical self-referral place, even after they have consulted specialists in the Ministry of Health facilities. However, it is considered a necessary workaround given the rigidity of the national referral system. The numerous trainees (medical residents, student nurses, nurses and doctors on continuing education programs), once back in their home-institutions or appointed

to their first job, use their personal network to organize referrals and thus also contribute to the bypass of the official referral system.

This exploration of the everyday processes that allow a medical specialty to
perform care on a national level shows the crucial role of hospitals and, more specifically, hospital staff, hospital infrastructure, and hospital expertise. It also
sheds light on the interstices within governmental systems and the long-living
institutional traditions left open to professional tinkering.

Providing Multidrug-Resistant Treatment
in a Tuberculosis Hospital in Tanzania

> It is not by chance that we work in this hospital. It was a plan, a strategy by the
> government to send us to Kibong'oto so that they can build skills to be able to
> manage MDR-TB in the country, because the country has dedicated to trans-
> form the hospital from a mere hospital to become a center for managing MDR-
> TB. First, [the government] strengthened its infrastructure in terms of wards,
> laboratory, and staff, capacitate with knowledge, and [second] they tried to link
> it with other partners and stakeholders, Ministry of Health, USAID, and others
> who support these efforts by the government.[5]

This quote from Kibong'oto hospital director introduces key issues in relation to
the adaptation strategies of hospitals when confronted with a novel global health
problem. In 2009, the Tanzanian Ministry of Health decided to select this long-
existing hospital to be at the forefront of treating multidrug-resistant tuberculosis. The government's revitalization of Kibong'oto included training human
resources, developing research skills, and expanding infrastructure. We argue that
this reassignment of Kibong'oto played a key role in MDR-TB care in Tanzania
because of the hospital's capacity to provide reliable infrastructure and attract
international actors to support the government's goal. However, as we will show,
hospital staff struggle to cope with the difficulties of long hospitalization and TB
treatments, most notably with the side effects of drugs, stress, homesickness, and
the inadequacy of food provision. In this hospital, we see the infrastructures,
people, surveillance, and care. The multiple risks the disease poses both to life, to
the senses, and the hospitals' long-standing ability to bring multiple forms of expertise in a centralized location are indeed key. Just as drug resistance is stretching
the limits of global health, the hospital's overarching role as a consolidator of services becomes central.

The term MDR-TB refers to TB bacilli that have evolved to tolerate the standard pharmaceutical regimens used to treat the disease. MDR-TB treatment has
been a motor of global health innovation since it entered the field as a crisis of pharmaceuticals and disease control. Worries about drug resistance have led to new
funding mechanisms, new diagnostic technologies like GeneXpert (see chapter 5,
Tech for All), new drugs like bedaquiline and delamanid, new forms of support,
and unfortunately, new forms of resistance—extremely resistant tuberculosis, or

XDR-TB, is a bacteria resistant to at least four anti-TB drugs. TB's resistance runs ahead of global health, and global health institutions that give care and work to produce knowledge have been pushed to keep up with the disease and its constant challenges to biomedicine. In short, MDR-TB as an evolving disease has caused global health, too, to be dynamic and begin to address those less cost-effective areas of disease control.

At the end of the 2000s, MDR-TB as a novel global health concern had the potential, through negotiations with international partners and decisions at a governmental level, to transform Kibong'oto hospital, a TB hospital at that time on the decline. The hospital was on the decline precisely because tuberculosis was mostly treated at home with the support of a network of health centers providing drugs in line with the DOTS strategy. When national TB experts in Tanzania decided to rehabilitate Kibong'oto for MDR-TB research and treatment, they were also deciding in favor of hospital-based TB care, despite a global trend supporting the treatment of TB "outside" the hospital. The WHO, through the 2011 guidelines on the management of multidrug-resistant tuberculosis and until the most recent 2019 consolidated guidelines, has consistently advocated for decentralized models of care stating that "patients with MDR-TB should be treated using mainly ambulatory care rather than models of care based principally on hospitalization" (World Health Organization 2014). However, for Tanzanian health officials and their partners, it was important to be able to isolate multidrug-resistant patients in a closed and secured health infrastructure where they could be treated and closely monitored. Globally, isolation and hospitalization of TB patients remains questionable, and most organizations advocate for applying DOTS or DOTS-plus, in the case of MDR-TB, because hospitalization is considered too costly and disempowering for patients. More than direct hospital expenditures, indirect economic and social costs such as loss of work and income, discrimination, and stigmatization matter (Bieh, Weigel et al. 2017). Besides, hospitalization of MDR-TB patients also increases the risk of re-infection for other patients.

The question of whether or not to hospitalize tuberculosis patients has a long history in international and global health. Hospitalization was for a long time the only treatment for TB, associated with the sanatorium infrastructure and architecture. The sanatorium provided for long (often palliative) stays in environments with fresh air and light. With the discovery of antibiotics, interventions changed and sanatoriums were either abandoned or transformed into something else. Kibong'oto in Tanzania was such a hospital. It was founded in 1926 by a British colonial doctor, on the hills of Kilimanjaro, to serve as a sanatorium and provide fresh air to patients. In 1956, Kibong'oto became the national TB hospital, and today it is Tanzania's national referral hospital for tuberculosis. The hospital was almost abandoned in the 1980s and again the 1990s, however, after the country adopted a policy of shortening and decentralizing TB treatment. In this section, we argue that MDR-TB has provided new life to this old TB hospital by enacting a substantial rehospitalization of tuberculosis patients in Tanzania. Ultimately, the long history of a specialized TB hospital in Tanzania provided dependable infrastructure that mattered for MDR-TB care and control, such as functional and adaptable buildings with good air circulation (for isolation wards) and a team of experienced healthcare workers.

The rehabilitation of Kibong'oto actually started during the HIV epidemic. When HIV combined with TB in a co-epidemic, the government opened new HIV services in this hospital, renovated buildings, employed more staff, and garnered logistical support and drug supplies from the Global Fund against HIV, TB, and malaria. Other partners such as LHL International (a Norwegian NGO) and KNCV[6] (a Dutch NGO) provided support for patient welfare, prevention, and diagnostic activities in the villages around the hospital. In order to start the MDR-TB program, the Global Fund provided free drugs and the University of California, San Francisco (UCSF) provided clinical expertise and training for Tanzanian experts. The Curry International TB Center at UCSF also helped to design the MDR-TB program, contributing to the development of the national drug-resistant guidelines as well as tools, policies, and programmatic quality-improvement initiatives that benefited the hospital.

During fieldwork at Kibong'oto in 2017 and 2018, prolonged hospitalization for MDR-TB patients was the norm, lasting for a period ranging from twelve to eighteen months, usually in the initial phase of treatment. From 2017, the Ministry of Health developed a decentralized approach in which patients would be transferred to health centers near their home, and several regional or district hospitals were also able to start MDR-TB treatment. Whether it is possible to treat MDR-TB without hospitalizing patients for a long period was not a question asked in Kibong'oto during our fieldwork. MDR-TB patients were generally considered to be very sick and very infectious. This dissent with global health guidelines for community-based MDR-TB treatment explains why global health actors' presence was hardly felt. The state's almost invisible support to the hospital stood in stark contrast with the highly visible, and often destabilizing, presence of global health actors in other public hospitals in the Northern Tanzania region of Arusha, hospitals that created enclaves of HIV care (Sullivan 2011). At the same time, prolonged hospitalization is problematic, and it is questioned even by the staff at Kibong'oto. Most of our interlocutors in the hospital pointed to the pitfalls of long hospitalization away from home. They worked daily to improve material and emotional conditions for their patients, for example, by trying to find ways to shorten the duration of treatment. In the meantime, however, the hospital remains a highly symbolic place for Tanzanians and a national hospital infrastructure capable of both adaptation and resilience.

When national health authorities chose Kibong'oto hospital to start MDR-TB treatment, both the long history of the site in dealing with TB and its remote location mattered. International partners and experts from the U.S. Centers for Disease Control (CDC) supported the Tanzanian government's assessment: "Their recommendation was that the place is very nice. [We] don't need mechanical mechanism[7] of infection control—what [we] have is a natural intervention [that] we were asked to maximize in terms of opening the windows."[8] Thus, the facility was deemed conducive, and staff simply kept all windows open to allow for the maximization of air circulation and natural light. Of course, the infectious nature of patients' disease, and by extension of the place, was a constant concern for the staff. Healthcare workers thus embodied a paradoxical relationship to the environment. Environments could be perceived as threatening if, for example, patients did not follow the rules or windows were closed, but at the same time, they were considered pivotal for the treatment of TB:

> We believe that a pleasant environment can be a therapy in itself. . . . We try to ensure the environment is very clean and supportive, we target what can quickly contribute to recovery of patients: the availability of water, toilets, bathroom . . . if we notice a problem we report: the availability of trees, shade down there, if there's no trees we try to advise.[9]

Every morning before nurses make their rounds to distribute medication, several medical attendants perform a thorough cleaning of the wards, with most patients staying outside while this is being done. Then nurses distribute pills, observe patients, and document this visit with a cross in each patient's file. But doing rounds is only one of the ingredients of the daily care of MDR-TB patients. Much of the job of hospital staff revolves around maintaining the facility and fostering pleasant relationships with patients. For most of the nurses we talked to, however, securing a hygienic environment was a prerequisite for the real work of offering "standardized care for patients" or "DOTS," which was about observing and documenting: "We observe the patient while taking the drug . . . [we] check if he has swallowed and no vomiting."[10]

Kibong'oto hospital is characterized both by its remoteness and its exceptional status in the healthcare system, in particular its role in the management of MDR-TB. Health staff members were especially concerned about several challenges related to hospitalization of MDR-TB: the extended stay of patients with extremely limited family visits (once a month); the toxicity of drugs; and the absence of recreational activities. This necessity for MDR-TB hospital to be a closed infrastructure can at any moment turn it into a threatening place, a situation that makes its inevitable loopholes and shortcomings fearsome.

In TB treatment, food has often been considered crucial to treatment success and to the ability to withstand long, antibiotic chemotherapy, and yet global health programs often fail to secure the provision of a good and balanced diet. In Kibong'oto, patients mostly eat *ugali* (maize porridge) and beans, and this was considered grossly insufficient. There was never enough food, and it was always the same and not appropriate for some patients—most notably Masai patients accustomed to meat and milk. It is common knowledge at the hospital that food is crucial for TB treatment (the hospital director notes it is in the literature), and many others know the importance of a good, balanced diet for patients to recover and for staff to avoid illness—especially in cases of MDR-TB. One nurse at Kibong'oto goes as far as to say, "People contracted this infection because of poor nutritional status."[11]

Staff views the provision of sufficient and diversified food as one of the most important reasons for the hospital's centrality in patients' recovery. As one medical attendant states:

> It was . . . like three to four years now, many patients were cured. I have gone to Dar-es-Salaam two times to pick the patients. You find a patient is very weak, helpless from the health center, but when they reach here they got cured, good food was available. Nowadays patients are given porridge only. . . . That's why there are many deaths. A patient cannot withstand the medicines with low immunity.[12]

Another concern at the hospital is the toxicity of the MDR-TB drugs and the extended hospital stay for patients away from home. One nurse reports:

> I [remember] a patient who developed psychosis, mental illness disturbance due to cycloserine. The patient was violent and very aggressive. He came from the ward and he wanted to go around the hospital and couldn't be stopped. We thought he might even take a stone and throw it to us.[13]

Hospitalizing MDR-TB patients allows clinicians and nurses to closely monitor side effects, especially the side effects of injectables, such as cycloserine, that often bring hearing loss and psychosis. Mental disturbance, according to nurses, can also result from being alone in a hospital far away from home for extended periods of time. Generally, a patient will stay until the sputum is converted to negative, which, in the case of MDR-TB treatment, can take up to eighteen or twenty-four months.

Thus, not only is infectious bacteria everywhere and always a threat for health workers, but patients themselves can become dangerous because of the side effects of certain drugs. This has led to some infrastructural changes, such as building a fence around the facility. According to a local resident who worked in the hospital from 1958 to 1998:

> The fence has just been introduced recently, after finding out the patient[s] escape from the hospital and they go out to the village to drink alcohol and they can infect other people. They thought it was better to build fence and employ security guards to make sure patients stay inside.[14]

MDR-TB has also changed the infrastructure at Kibong'oto. In 2018, in response to the concerns over diet, the hospital launched a nutritional program. Staff screened all patients for their nutritional status and provided those suffering from mild or severe malnutrition with nutritional supplements. Similarly, management addressed hearing loss as a side effect of MDR-TB medication by procuring an audiometry machine and training staff to assess hearing loss among patients. The hospital also constructed an isolation room for patients who demonstrate aggressive and dangerous behaviors, as part of a new ward for MDR-TB. Finally, the head of the hospital's Community Medicine Department, with funding from a South African organization (TB in the Mining Sector in Southern Africa), opened an outpatient occupational health clinic within the hospital premises to help miners and their families who were heavily affected by TB, HIV, and other diseases. This expansion of the hospital toward the treatment of other diseases is a clear indication that despite persisting as a hospital behind closed walls, the hospital has a capacity to work on its environment, through outreach, case-finding activities, and treatment of diseases beyond TB.

Kibong'oto hospital is a key node of infrastructure for MDR-TB in Tanzania. The presence of this TB hospital infrastructure matters heavily and has influenced a national policy in Tanzania that favors hospitalization of patients as the place gathers expertise and experience about everyday, long-term management of the disease and the drugs' side effects. At the same time, we can notice the relative invisibility of this hospital in the global health field. Global health actors, such as European TB NGOs or clinicians from UCSF, provide technical or financial support, but there is no global health program installed in the hospital or clinical trials promoted there by global actors. It is mainly the Tanzanian state that deems relevant this hospital and its MDR-TB related activities; as such, the hospital also bears the promise of the state's state-of-the-art research, geared toward global science. In Tanzania as elsewhere, the (public) hospital *is* the state, its power as well as its shortages (Kehr and Chabrol 2018).

The Mental Hospital and Community Mental Health in India

Global mental health largely neglects psychiatric hospitals (Thornicroft and Tansella 2004; Cohen, Chatterjee et al. 2016; Cohen and Minas 2017). This is particularly relevant not only since they are often the sole sites of care for the mentally ill in many low- and middle-income countries but also, as Alex Cohen and Harry Minas (2017) have discussed, because they are often sites of neglect and abuse. As we suggest in the case of the National Institute of Mental Health and Neuroscience (NIMHANS) in the South Indian metropolis of Bengaluru, however, the psychiatric hospital can be a site of progress and innovation, albeit largely outside the interventions of global mental health. Our discussion poses questions about global mental health's ethics of action—an ethics that is based on the assumption that mental healthcare is somehow absent in places where psychiatric hospitals, mental health infrastructure, and expertise are present. In other words, the case of NIMHANS challenges the idea in global mental health of a blank space—a therapeutic gap—into which global mental health interventions are rolled out.

In India, deinstitutionalization of mental healthcare did not mean dismantling large mental hospitals. Rather, efforts at modernizing the mental health infrastructure have aimed at transforming the mental hospital from a site of care to a site of specialist training and research, while promoting psychiatric care in general hospitals and primary health centers. By focusing on shortened stays and outpatient treatment, former mental hospitals have become vibrant sites of treatment, research, and training. Despite an overt commitment to community care, however, confinement of severely and chronically ill long-term patients continues, though in the less visible spaces of public and private institutions (Pinto 2014; Varma 2016).

NIMHANS is a prominent site of specialist care, training, and research that has been emblematic and formative of India's mental health infrastructure and the transformation of mental health in India in collaboration with the WHO. The twenty-five-acre campus, with its extensive gardens, exists as a calm and cool oasis in the middle of bustling and smoggy Bengaluru. Located on a congested arterial road, NIMHANS is a prominent center of care for the mentally ill, with patients hailing from all parts of India and families queuing for hours in the crowded outpatient department, waiting for a short consultation for one or more suffering family members before heading back to their homes hours and sometimes days away. Although designated as a tertiary-care hospital, its reputation and the long-term bonds between doctors and families have made it a site of primary and secondary healthcare for many. As compared to images of the asylum as a total institution—a site "where a large number of like-situated individuals, cut off from the wider society for an appreciable period of time, together lead an enclosed, formally administered round of life" (Goffman 1961, xiii)—NIMHANS is a permeable space. Its open walls have enabled flows of ideas, knowledge, experts, policies, and patients, and it has also been a nodal point in India's community mental health infrastructure, as it has expanded and shifted in the moving seas of mental health modernization. Moreover, NIMHANS has been deeply involved in the national and global production and dissemination of knowledge. While the clinic's walls came down, this hospital has remained a monument in the shifting tides of knowing and treating mental illness in India. By focusing on this institution as a key node in the infrastructure of mental health knowledge, training, care, and policy in India, we show how global mental health's priorities and targets have affected and reconfigured the infrastructure of both the mental hospital and wider mental healthcare in India.

While actors, targets, tools, and priorities have shifted, NIMHANS has adapted and continues to be an iconic site and a lived and acting infrastructure of mental healthcare in India (Murthy, Isaac et al. 2017). A strong symbol of progress, development, and modernity, NIMHANS makes material the state that supports it (Amin 2014). The history of NIMHANS as a successful hospital differs from other accounts of "failed hospitals," "unstable places" (Street 2014), and sites of "improvising medicine" (Livingston 2012) that in other places represent fragile postcolonial states. Contrary to a global health depiction of the hospital as decaying, in crisis, ruined, or inefficient, NIMHANS is a case of fulfilled promises in the Indian postcolonial state. As a node in the mental health infrastructure that connects Bengaluru with Delhi and Geneva, on the one hand, and that enables South-South circulation of experts and expertise on the other, NIMHANS has been key in developing and implementing community mental health in India and beyond. At a time when the Indian state is working to reorient asylums as centers of excellence, with a focus on research, training, and outpatient or short-term treatment, NIMHANS has long been the emblematic institution that unites this double movement of decentralization of treatment and centralization of expertise, training, and research (Varma 2016).

Although innovation routinely occurs at NIMHANS, and the center has closely collaborated with the WHO in building community mental health in India, the hospital is largely invisible in global mental health publications and programs, as a result of the shifting epistemes and networks that have guided mental health innovations in the twentieth and twenty-first century. By ignoring India's infrastructure of community mental health, in which NIMHANS has been centrally involved, global mental health activists portray novel, foreign-financed research and intervention projects that create enclaves of community mental healthcare as populating a wasteland of mental healthcare in India (Ecks 2016; Lang 2019; Lovell, Read et al. 2019).[15] We will further use the emergence and transformation of NIMHANS in producing, disseminating, advocating, and researching community mental healthcare as a lens on the transition from international public health to global health. In doing so, we will demonstrate the shifting mental health infrastructure and assemblage of actors, targets, and tools as they manifest in India. While NIMHANS is not a "global mental health site," it has always been and continues to be affected by processes of mental health globalization.

Historians date the origins of NIMHANS to 1838, when Charles Smith, colonial doctor at the Hospital for Soldiers, Peons, and Paupers, established a separate ward for the insane (Radhika, Murthy, Jain 2015; Radhika, Murthy, Sarin et al. 2015). The clientele was largely poor; the affluent preferred traditional Indian medicine (Radhika, Murthy et al. 2015a). Twelve years later, the Lunatic Asylum, a separate large and airy hospital, was built with extensive gardens on the banks of a lake, in the vicinity of a jail, a TB hospital, and a leper's asylum. Treatment was largely "moral"—that is, aiming at strengthening reason and character, it focused on regimenting daily life but also the administration of sedatives and baths, and patients were engaged in occupations such as gardening or tailoring (Mills 2001). Diagnoses and care corresponded to practices in Britain, and changes in one location quickly followed suit into the other (Ernst 2007; Radhika, Murthy, Sarin et al. 2015).

In 1936, when the city of Bengaluru began to overrun the asylum, the renamed Mysore Government Mental Hospital moved to a quiet and salubrious environment at its present location on a hillock at what was then the outskirts of the city. While segregation between British and Indian elite patients, on the one hand, and "native" patients, on the other, was protocol at other mental hospitals, at NIMHANS social distinction in the wards was rare (Jain and Murthy 2006). Inspired by the architecture of Bethlem hospital in London, architects and horticulturalists planned the new hospital grounds as a therapeutic environment, with several pavilions in the midst of vibrant gardens. The often-told story that Bangaloreans once used the hospital gardens as a picnic spot testifies to the absence of hospital walls and the permeability of hospital space for patients and nonpatients, even in its early years. Like most hospitals, the institution kept pace with medical innovations over the decades, watching state-of-the-art treatments, like cardiazol shocks or leucotomies, become failures and barbarisms as new tools and methods were developed.

WHO involvement in the hospital began in the mid-1950s, with a program of postgraduate, psychiatric training at the newly founded All India Institute of

Mental Health (AIIMH)—which later became NIMHANS. Under its director M. V. Govindaswamy, the institute set up the first psychiatry degree in postindependence India. The program was broadly modeled after the Institute of Psychiatry in London, where many Indian psychiatrists had themselves been trained. The WHO supported the establishment of AIIMH as a training institution by bringing in consultants. From the start, psychiatric training at AIIMH included psychiatry, psychology, Western and Indian philosophy, and literature, as well as the basic sciences, and research included religious and anthropological aspects of mental health along with classical science fields, at least until the mid-1980s, when the focus was redirected toward biological psychiatry. NIMHANS currently has a number of departments, including psychiatry, neuroscience, epidemiology, psychology, nursing, social work, and others.

From the 1960s onward, psychiatrists who were trained at NIMHANS, and shaped by emerging discourses of deinstitutionalization, staffed the new psychiatric units in general hospitals, leading to an expansion of services in India. With the advent and growing availability of psychopharmaceuticals, outpatient and short-term hospital stays became more possible. Reform experiments in India since the 1950s have not questioned the hospital, as such, as a locus of care, but rather the exclusion of families and the focus on custodial rather than recovery-oriented care. In response, NIMHANS opened family wards to involve kin in the care of their hospitalized relatives. The first wave of deinstitutionalization in India in the 1960s did not yet aim at moving mental health out of the hospital, but rather at shifting care out of the asylums and into general hospitals. Throughout all of these changes, NIMHANS has not only been on the forefront of psychiatry, neuroscience and psychological treatment, training and research, but it has also housed and shaped a series of debates on and experiments with yoga, Ayurveda, and what is called "Indian psychiatry and psychology" in the hospital and the community.

The NIMHANS Community Psychiatry Unit, established in 1975, continued moving mental healthcare beyond the hospital walls. Around the same time, the community mental health movement was beginning to gain steam. Psychiatrists at NIMHANS felt that they wanted to take advantage of the moment, Dr. Srinivasa Murthy, one of the pioneering figures of community psychiatry at NIMHANS, explained.[16] According to Murthy, NIMHANS started the Community Psychiatry Unit to operationalize the recommendations of a WHO report (World Health Organization 1975) that urged member states to carry out pilot programs testing the feasibility of community mental health (Isaac 1986). NIMHANS set up a Rural Mental Health Center to train general physicians and community health workers in rural areas and develop models of mental healthcare delivery outside the hospital. The psychiatry unit soon became a nodal point of community mental healthcare in the country. It was key in initiating and implementing the National Mental Health Program in 1982 in collaboration with the WHO, a program that envisioned extending mental health infrastructure and integrating mental health into primary health care. From 1985 to 1990, the unit piloted a district-level community mental health project in the Bellary district and trained primary health care general physicians, community health workers, and mental health professionals from several Indian states to organize and deliver mental health services within the primary health infrastructure. The Bellary pilot project later became well known as the prototype of the District Mental Health Program, which India launched in 1996 in order to shift the identification and treatment of mental health problems from the hospital to primary health centers in all districts in India (Sarin and Jain 2013; van Ginneken, Jain et al. 2014).

In 1986, NIMHANS became a WHO-collaborating center for research and training in mental health, and the development of community mental health programs and services was a shared priority. As the designation document states: "During the past ... decade, the broad policies, aims and objectives and commitment of the Institute [NIMHANS] have been fairly similar to the objectives of the WHO's global medium term programme in mental health."[17] The document also includes plans to develop NIMHANS as a node in the mental health infrastructure of Southeast Asia and other WHO regions, to be implemented in the following years.

This original state-based, NIMHANS-centered community mental health infrastructure has connected community mental health pioneers, the Ministry of Health in Delhi, India's primary health infrastructure, the WHO in Geneva, and mental health professionals in other South and Southeast Asian countries and beyond. The main collaboration between NIMHANS and the WHO in mental health until the early 1990s involved training mental health professionals in organizing services using the primary health care infrastructure, but also in social psychiatry and epidemiology. This infrastructure allows for the production and circulation of knowledge, experts, and policies and reaches hundreds of thousands of patients, mainly with severe mental disabilities. As a WHO-collaborating center, NIMHANS has frequently followed WHO guidance for the modernization of mental health systems.

More recently, NIMHANS has further expanded the community mental health infrastructure in India through the creation of a digital infrastructure in collaboration with the Indian Space Organization. Using technologies like e-learning and tele-clinics to expand India's community mental health infrastructure, the renamed Telemedicine and Community Psychiatry Unit has created a digital academy to conduct courses in community mental health and counseling and grant degrees. This academy connects general physicians, psychologists, nurses, social workers, and volunteers to mental health professionals at NIMHANS. Digital training and care expands community psychiatry to areas barely covered by India's District Mental Health Program. Moreover, recently piloted "tele after-care services," which follow one-month inpatient treatments, save patients the long and expensive journey for an outpatient follow-up at NIMHANS. Tele-trainings and tele-assisted consultations significantly expand the NIMHANS training and clinical infrastructure and move the psychiatric gaze further out of the hospital space.

A more recent, parallel community mental health research and intervention infrastructure has emerged in India since the 2010s as part of the Movement for Global Mental Health. This movement assembles agencies, research funding bodies, philanthropies, NGOs, advocacy groups and prominent academic journals engaged in the production and circulation of technologies, principles, and practices. In India, as elsewhere, research trials of mental health interventions that are based on "task shifting" and "task sharing" provide mental health services, with a focus on counseling and common mental disorders, as part of randomized and controlled intervention trials. The results appear in high-profile global health journals, notably in *The Lancet*.[18] These trials are built into the existing primary health infrastructure, even while the provision of care largely resembles enclaves or islands of global health interventions. Nonetheless, both NIMHANS as a nodal site for the production and dissemination of knowledge and training in community psychiatry and the state-based community mental health infrastructure it helped to build remain largely invisible in the Movement for Global Mental Health and its publications. It is no surprise, then, that some of the psychiatrists who have built India's community mental health infrastructure, while sympathetic and supportive of the aims of the Movement for Global Mental Health, are skeptical of short-term and highly transient global mental health interventions and their capacity to strengthen health systems.

In the 2010s, NIMHANS has expanded its infrastructure to target novel forms of suffering in urban and middle-class contexts by establishing the NIMHANS Centre for Wellbeing. According to the website, NIMHANS launched this "innovative mental health promotion initiative by stepping out of the institution and locating itself within the community."[19] While India's community mental health infrastructure, with its roots in pre-Alma-Ata WHO imperatives to integrate mental health within rural primary health care, has targeted severe forms of mental disorder, this new form of community mental health targets the more common mental health challenges of urbanized middle-class youth and expands community mental health to include urban middle-class neighborhoods. The center is located a few miles away from the hospital in a double-story house with a quiet garden in a middle-class residential area, and NIMHANS psychiatrists and psychologists emphasize that in this "youth-friendly" mental health space anyone can just drop in and talk to a practitioner without waiting in long lines as at the NIMHANS outpatient department. The center offers counseling and psychiatric services mainly for teenagers and young adults and focuses on well-being and positive psychology, stress management, marital problems, and the use of technology. Doctors hope the idea will be replicated in other parts of Bengaluru, as well as in other states. This shift toward "common mental disorders" is indicative of how global mental health's novel targets and techniques enter the expanded hospital and reconfigure hospital spaces, practices, targets, and tools. At the same time, it speaks to the issues that concern India's growing urban middle class. With a shift of target came a shift in clinical actors and techniques. A majority of the staff of the Centre for Well Being are psychologists (along with some psychiatrists and social workers) and treatment is largely based on psychotherapy and counseling—as compared to NIMHANS outpatient clinic, where treatment focuses on psychiatrists prescribing psychopharmaceuticals.

The center is a friendly and informal space that people experience as pleasant rather than stigmatizing and threatening—a frequent complaint about NIMHANS. Instead of talking about mental disorders, staff and promotion material talk about "mental health challenges" and "difficult life situations." Rather than bringing together mental disorders and physical diseases in the realm of primary health care, with the Centre for Well Being, NIMHANS expands its infrastructure toward everyday challenges—tension and stress in modern metropolitan life. This change is illustrative of a larger turn from severe mental disorders toward well-being and the common stresses and tensions of daily life, especially in cities (Fitzgerald, Rose et al. 2016), and an increased demand for preventive mental health services among India's middle class. This integral yet outsourced turn toward well-being by NIMHANS thus illustrates the impact of larger health globalization forces on the Indian mental health infrastructure.

Combining innovative targets and tools, NIMHANS has further expanded its infrastructure to reach young, tech-savvy individuals with novel apps. The "Push-D" (Practice and Use Self-Help for Depression) app is a digital tool that offers information, psychological self-management based on evidence-based psychotherapeutic techniques, and monitoring by NIMHANS experts for users dealing with symptoms of mild depression. The "Digital Detox" app tracks smartphone usage and offers advice for unplugging. With these new mental health tools, the NIMHANS digital psychiatric and psychological infrastructure merges novel ideas of self-care and self-responsibility with state-based forms of care, thus expanding its reach.

Clearly, NIMHANS has shaped India's mental health infrastructure through training, treatment, and research innovations. At the same time, the new targets and tools of global health—some of them are part of global mental health yet overflow the field in that they are part of larger processes of the globalization of health and sciences targeting the psyche—have also impacted the NIMHANS infrastructure of knowledge production and distribution and of care. NIMHANS has not only been a node in mental health infrastructure in India, but it has also incorporated—and partly shaped—larger trends in international and, later, global health, such as community mental health, human rights, the turn toward common mental disorders and well-being, and the use of digital mental health technologies. While these changes have further strengthened the relevance of NIMHANS as a site of care and knowledge in India, its expanded infrastructure and its key position in the mental health infrastructure of India has largely been invisible in global mental health publications and debates. Similar to Kibong'oto TB hospital and Sultan Qaboos University Hospital, NIMHANS is not an avowed target of global health interventions, and yet new global health targets and larger health globalization processes affect and change it.

Conclusion

This chapter explored the ways in which state-run hospitals, in spite of their apparent invisibility to global health, remain central to global health interventions by focusing on their daily operational presence in national healthcare systems. The cases show how global health does not target hospitals as sites of intervention and yet works through them as loci of care, training, and research.

These hospitals are complex infrastructures, both in the sense that they remain crucial nodes in the health system and material organizations whose activity implies multiple layers of logistics. Buildings and their environments, personnel, equipment, and digital infrastructures are key to both hospitalized and de-hospitalized care. The three hospitals we discussed are tightly woven into their local social environments and respond to specific national health needs. As specialized hospitals, they persist in the era of global health, echoing both global health's vertical approach and states' investments in prestigious hospitals that are imbued with symbolic power.

Hospitals thus figure prominently in arenas of health globalization and are strongly impacted by these processes. They incorporate novel targets, techniques, and tools originating in, or associated with, global health, and these incorporations mobilize and change their infrastructures. In Oman, the field of medical genetics builds on and expands the infrastructure of two specialized state hospitals through new spaces of diagnostics and care, equipment, expertise, and digital infrastructures. In Tanzania, MDR-TB triggered the transformation of a historic hospital from a declining facility to a center of treatment, care, training, and research. It was precisely the hospital's material and relational infrastructure that enabled the rehospitalization of MDR-TB, following decades of TB deinstitutionalization. In India, policies of task shifting and care in the community in the realm of mental health have built on and expanded the infrastructure of a prestigious mental hospital. More recently, increased attention to common mental disorders, urban and middle-class youth, and digital, therapeutic technologies have further expanded its material and relational infrastructure. Indeed diagnosis, treatment, and training increasingly incorporate private, globalized digital infrastructures and applications for the circulation of knowledge and information and therapeutic techniques of self-care that build on and expand the hospital infrastructure. The Omani case shows, for instance, how Gmail can sometimes help bridge the gaps in state-run digital infrastructures, as well as the importance of WhatsApp and UPS for the (trans)national circulation of genetic information and the building of genetic knowledge.

In other words, global health as we know it would not exist without hospitals as nodes of dissemination and adaptation. What has, however, not radically changed in the three decades of health globalization is that public hospitals—plugged into global health or not—face multiple forms of scarcity and must constantly engage in local, clinical triage in order to manage their outcomes, often by filling in the gaps of global health standards.

CHAPTER 7

Provincializing the WHO

Christoph Gradmann, Olivia Fiorilli, Jean-Paul Gaudillière,
Caroline Meier zu Biesen, Lucile Ruault, and Simeng Wang

How did the World Health Organization (WHO), arguably the center of international health in the period after World War II, come to be a backwater of global health? Historians who have written about the WHO agree that it enjoyed a more hegemonic position in international health until it entered a crisis in the 1980s (Birn 2009; Packard 2016; Cueto, Brown et al. 2019) that was a decade of political and economic turmoil. Most visibly it was a financial crisis, triggered by the decision of the United States to suspend budgetary contributions. Underneath, however, it was the crisis of an institution that struggled to define its role in the rapidly changing landscape of the 1990s after getting used to dealing with state actors during the Cold War and giving a decisive voice to the self-identified Third World (Chorev 2012; Cueto, Brown et al. 2019). During the 1990s, the WHO's position was financially, politically, and morally challenged by the rise of new actors like the World Bank and a plethora of new global health nongovernmental organizations (NGOs) deeply involved in the transition toward economic triage and a neoliberal model of international governance. The weakening of the WHO was also a result of it being a political body in a sea of institutions organized as corporations or foundations such as the Rockefeller Foundation.[1]

How can we write this history and understand its significance for global health? A consideration of available sources is helpful. History, while concerned with what has happened, is written from what has remained. This may seem a trivial piece of insight when we look at histories that can be assembled from numerous and well-furnished archives, but it is a critical consideration when documentation is scarce and uneven. In medical history, to give an example, the accounts of doctors tend to dominate what is written because their lives and work are usually documented in more depth than those of patients (Condrau 2007). In the historiography of international and global health, we see an uneven availability of archival sources, which can help us to understand why institutions like the Rockefeller Foundation or the World Health Organization receive more attention than they might merit in the larger picture (Löwy 2001; Birn 2006; Cueto 2007).

Thinking about the popularity of the WHO in the historiography of health glo-balization and global health and the air of nostalgia for the WHO's past grandeur, it seems reasonable to assume that such discourse originates in two places: first, from political critique of global health as a neoliberal enterprise and, second, from the convenience of documentation through the existence of a rich and accessible WHO archive. Indeed, many other players in global health lack one or the other or both: Postcolonial states and their institutions often have poorly maintained archives, and the efforts of local scholars to amend this receive little recognition (Feierman 2019). The NGOs that dominate in global health might have archives, but they lack a culture of political accountability and access, which a political organization such as the WHO is required to have. Of course, every group com-municates with the public in some way, but there is a difference in the strategies of accountability. Private corporations and foundations are accountable to their owners or members but do not necessarily answer to the political sphere (Maha-jan 2018; Reubi 2018). They may grant access to archival materials or deny it, and they may even, as it has happened to one of the authors of this chapter, flatly (and falsely) deny they ever had an archive in the first place. For the WHO as a political body, on the other hand, much of its still-existing prestige rests on public appear-ance, which takes the form of publication series, international commissions, a parliament-like assembly, and finally, an accessible archive. Thus, it is no contra-diction that recent histories of global health emphasize the declining and limited influence that the WHO possesses while at the same time continuing to give it rela-tively more attention than other big players.

Interestingly, the WHO complex in Geneva, which houses its archive, can be seen as an architectonic exemplification of the organization's obsolescence. The stylish, late-1960s buildings embody the glory days of the organization, and it is equally evident that the complex has not seen much renovation since.[2] Those who visit the archives it houses, and who care to look at the period from 1960 to 2000, get an almost visceral experience of the bleeding of resources that shook the insti-tution in the late 1980s. For instance, in the field of tuberculosis control, files that begin in a comprehensive and well-maintained way become shorter and more frag-mented. In some cases, they seem to physically disintegrate, missing copies of outgoing mail, for instance. The dynamics of the WHO after World War II have been described as the successful building of a bureaucratic apparatus (Birn 2009). Judging from the state of its archive, this apparatus was beginning to fail in the 1980s. While this conclusion is fairly unanimous in histories of the WHO, we need to think more closely about what it means for global health.

In order to explore the crisis of organizations identified with an international order, which saw the end of European colonial empires and the rise of the Third World, we draw inspiration from postcolonial thought, particularly Dipesh Chakrabarty's critique of European historical thought put forward in his *Provin-cializing Europe* (Chakrabarty 2008). Throughout the 1990s, the WHO had to say goodbye to the aspirations to hegemony that it may have held in its heyday and instead had to learn to adapt to an environment of powerful new players, the economization of health, and emerging narratives that evolve around Indian and Chinese histories, which do not point to Europe as the origin of modernity. Just as European grand narratives become fodder for subaltern critique, we argue the WHO has become "at once both indispensable and inadequate" (Chakrabarty 2008, 16)—inadequate because it embodies a narrative of Western progress that remains a reference although quite out of date; indispensable since its present forms of action carry decisive continuities concerning the political dimensions of inter-national and global health beyond its proclaimed economization. Understanding the demotion of the WHO, as well as its peculiarity and retained influence, helps us to understand why historians of the WHO, when writing about its fate after the "health for all" days, tend to employ a nostalgic tone that obstructs the view of some fundamental changes that have occurred beyond the perpetuation of the North-South divide. Following the inspiration drawn from Chakrabarty, this chapter shows how the marginalization of the WHO happened and how other networks created their own forms of knowledge.

Our journey from within the archives of the WHO and other institutions will take place in five steps, drafting a complex picture that stretches over several decades. First, we will show how pressure worked and look at developments around the global control of tuberculosis (TB) in the 1980s and 1990s. In this case the World Bank engaged massively in support of creating the directly observed treatment short-course (DOTS) strategy to control TB. The strategy was invented against the WHO's own policy of control for that condition and met stiff resistance from Geneva originally. Next, we will look at a rather different image of collaboration, reconsidering what is a key element in the current historiography—namely, that the WHO was pressured into a form of alignment with neoliberalism by new actors in the emerging global health field, with an exploration of the ways in which the WHO already collaborated with the World Bank at the peak of the primary health care and "Health for All by the Year 2000" strategy in the 1980s. The third scene shows a promising agenda to diversify programs beyond infectious diseases. It delineates how WHO experts gave visibility to the paradigm of community gene-tics in the 1980s and 1990s, which they dropped when global health and genomics came to the fore during the next decade. The fourth moment reveals similar ambiv-alence, as it illustrates the continuity of the WHO's normative role but limited practical consequences in the context of trade and drugs circulation of Ayurvedic pharmaceuticals crossing the Indian Ocean. Finally, we look at China's health interventions in Africa, showing how a country whose experience was pivotal in discussions about primary health care with the WHO and the United Nations Children's Fund (UNICEF) has become the dominant player in South-South devel-opment aid, no longer paying much attention to the WHO.

In doing so, the chapter will argue for three historiographical considerations: First, the WHO's former glory was bound to a world of North-South dependen-cies typical of international health in the era of the Cold War. Second, South-South cooperation and exchange, in contrast, structure the current processes of health globalization, if not the entire global health field. And third, the WHO's remaining power is in large part an echo of what that organization's historical roots in interwar international health entailed—namely, soft power that rests on documentation, epidemiological data, and its function as a platform for normative activities, mastering politics and diplomacy rather than practice.

TUBERCULOSIS, THE MAKING OF DOTS, AND THE DECLINE OF PRIMARY HEALTH CARE

International TB control strategies provide an instructive example of the WHO's influence in the days of international health; they also help us understand the forces that grew to challenge the WHO's influence in the transition to global health. The WHO's involvement with tuberculosis started right from its foundation after World War II. Indeed, the late 1940s were a unique historical period that placed tuberculosis at the center of international health. Over the course of the first half of the twentieth century, TB had already been much reduced in industrialized countries. It is likely that improved living conditions and preventive medicines were the cause of its reduced prevalence (Mercer 2014, 118–130). During this period, vaccines, antibiotics, and chemotherapies became widely available. The Bacillus Calmette-Guérin (BCG) vaccination for TB, though developed in the interwar years, now came into widespread use, while antibiotics and other pharmaceutical treatments for TB were introduced at the end of the war (Brimnes 2008; Greenwood 2008, 141–207). Low-income countries were the main field of application for vaccines and modern therapies after WWII, and tuberculosis control changed character. What had essentially been framed as a social disease in the interwar period—where no progress could be expected without looking at housing or food—became a malady that could be controlled independently of such conditions by using technologies such as BCG or chemotherapies (Amrith 2004). The WHO did not initially predominate in developing or implementing such control strategies, but as the influence of researchers associated with (former) colonial powers such as the British Medical Research Council (MRC) declined over the years, its influence grew.[3]

By the 1970s, the WHO was working with local authorities to create TB control plans for newly independent countries seeking to improve on the weaknesses of the control trials run by the MRC in the previous decades. Such trials had produced a host of treatment regimens mostly designed to either cut costs, improve outcomes, shorten treatment, or, most notably, facilitate outpatient treatment.[4] These strategies, however, had by and large, remained confined to clinical trials and had not translated into comprehensive national control programs. As an MRC bureaucrat commented in 1962, advanced trials were in danger of becoming a surrogate for comprehensive control: "We must not delude ourselves into thinking that the trials by themselves will solve the numerous problems of tuberculosis in East Africa. The trials are essentially confined to treating advanced cases. . . ."[5] It was against this backdrop that the WHO promoted integrating TB control into primary health services and prioritizing prevention over treatment. For countries struggling with a lack of effective treatment infrastructure, these policies were enticing. Moreover, the efficacy of the BCG vaccine was favorably evaluated in those days, and thus it made sense to imagine a control strategy that rested on vaccination and to assume that clinical cases of TB were a residual problem that would decline in numbers as more and more people were vaccinated (McMillen 2015; Brimnes 2016).

It is no coincidence that this reminds of primary health care policies promoted in the 1970s by the WHO (Cueto 2004). In fact, these WHO policies were inspired by TB control programs in low-income countries, most notably India (Brimnes 2016). Halfdan Mahler, before becoming director general of the WHO in 1973, had been the WHO official responsible during the creation of the Indian national tuberculosis program. Although it was not absolutely certain that a combination of affordable technology, prevention, and treatment by primary care providers would be successful in all cases, tuberculosis control programs had become part of primary healthcare policy and the available data did not contradict the notion that this worked. In East Africa, for instance, there seemed to be slow but steady decline in rates of TB (Kent 1976; Second East African/British Medical Research Council Kenya Tuberculosis Survey 1978; Swai, Edwards et al. 1989).

Those who wished to challenge such approaches could do so in two different ways, and both were practiced in the 1970s. First, they could challenge BCG vaccine efficacy. Second, they could argue that more specialized, technological approaches in treatment were superior to the simple treatment delivered through the general health service. In the case of BCG, consensus slowly turned against it after long-term trials in 1979 showed that the vaccine offered much less protection than previously claimed (McMillen 2015, 117–119). Concerned about specialized versus simple treatment, the International Union Against TB and Lung Disease (IUATLD) started trials in three East African countries in the late 1970s to show that using more expensive "short course" treatments, which had previously been developed by the MRC, delivered substantially better treatment outcomes than simple regimens.

The IUATLD became involved with several national control programs through its Mutual Assistance Program. This program had begun by providing assistance to smaller projects, but from the late 1970s on, it aimed at building national control programs (Rouillon 1991). The WHO refused to participate in the IUATLD project, which, funded by the Swiss and Dutch governments, started in Tanzania in 1977. Interestingly, the project began by testing the efficacy of the WHO-recommended simple treatment regimens while creating thinly disguised, vertical, specialized TB services, which also produced a wealth of data. Evidence was quickly gathered that indicated a low efficacy for WHO-compliant regimens reliant on cheap drugs, outpatient self-monitoring, and a long course of treatment (twelve to eighteen months). In a second step from 1982, the IUATLD went on to test rather advanced MRC short-course regimens and combined this more expensive treatment with a period of initial hospitalization lasting two months. Treatment now took only eight months. Quite accurately, this was seen as an all-out violation of primary health care (PHC) principles, and open conflict between the

IUATLD and the WHO erupted. In an April 1983 letter to Annick Rouillon, the IUATLD's executive director, Halfdan Mahler portrayed the Tanzanian trials as an attack on WHO policy:

> We know, however, that when healthcare delivery is excellent the actual treatment regimen is of little importance. National tuberculosis programs have not failed because of faulty technology, but because of a lack of productive interaction between the health system and the people. . . . The question is not whether primary healthcare can improve the delivery of tuberculosis programs, but how the tuberculosis program should contribute to primary healthcare.[6]

In fact, the WHO was so incensed that it attempted to stop the whole endeavor by going after its financiers and reminding them that they were funding a violation of WHO policy (Gradmann 2019). However, the trials that the WHO would have loved to nip in the bud succeeded—the National Tuberculosis and Leprosy Control Program was completed in 1987—and were embraced by the WHO's critics. These programs provided a comprehensive antithesis to PHC: a specialized, technology-driven, vertical-control program deemed both effective and efficient. When the World Bank assigned a postdoctoral researcher in the late 1980s as consultant to identify cost-effective, specialized treatment programs for major health challenges, the IUATLD trials came to be seen as the blueprint. Producing a rich harvest of epidemiological data (the responsible consultant being an epidemiologist), the trials provided a basis for the World Bank's preferred mode of analysis, employing health systems research tools. These were added to the classical public health science that IUATLD's program had employed, and they appear in joint publications in the early 1990s (Murray, Styblo et al. 1990; Murray, Dejonghe et al. 1991). The IUATLD had considered cost an immediate practical concern and calculated a cost-of-treatment-per-patient, aiming to deliver an effective service at a reasonable price; for the World Bank, cost became a matter of economic analysis of entire societies and of projection into the future.

Treatment was now seen as an investment, which would produce a downward trend of tuberculosis infection in the years to come. With fewer patients to treat (or "deaths averted," as they were called in the analysis), the costs of the condition's control were projected to decline. Without yet using the disability-adjusted life years (DALY) metric, which was to be introduced shortly after in the 1993 *World Development Report*, the World Bank began to describe the Tanzanian TB control program as cost-efficient rather than low-cost, because it was an investment that promised returns (i.e., fewer cases to treat in the future). When the trials were applauded in the *World Development Report* and the responsible consultant—Christopher Murray, today's director of the Institute for Health Metrics and Evaluation (IHME)—experienced a meteoric rise in global health epidemiology, the WHO had to concede. Thus, by about 1990, primary health care policies were abandoned by the WHO because of changes in the very field that had been one of its inspirations, tuberculosis control (Ogden, Walt et al. 2003). Instead, a set of principles derived from the IUATLD trials became the standard with which a national

TB control program had to comply if it wanted to access donor money. The control strategy, which came to be called DOTS, was implemented beginning in 1994. Slightly earlier, the WHO, having given up on its own control strategy, now had to be content with the role of door opener for the World Bank in China, where the East African trials were tested on a large scale in 1991 (Dirlikov 2015).[7] What was initially called DOTS changed form over the years, taking into account, for instance, the importance of HIV complications or drug resistance. It has also changed names and is currently called StopTB. Arguably, the role of the WHO in the creation and management of DOTS illustrates that it is an organization that garners quite a bit of publicity but whose policies have become memories or are of a more normative character, such as connecting drug access, policies, and treatment standards in the field of drug-resistant tuberculosis through its "Green Light Committee."

The WHO and the World Bank: Revisiting the "Takeover"

On February 24 and 25, 1975, Dr. Thomas Lambo, then deputy director general of the WHO, and several heads of WHO departments hosted a delegation of the International Bank for Reconstruction and Development (IBRD) in Geneva for a consultation. The meeting explored issues as diverse as environmental health, rural development, healthcare delivery systems, and workforce and health sector reviewing. On the World Bank side, the archival documents associated with the preparation for this meeting include a sheet with a series of general questions. Question 4 asked, "Should the Bank enter any cooperative arrangements with WHO at this time? What about a broad memorandum of understanding?" An unspecified reader, presumably Dr. Michael Hoffman, the World Bank's director of international relations, responded in handwriting to these questions "no" and "yes respectively."[8]

The internal memo written by Dr. Shirley Boskey from the World Bank's Population, Health, and Nutrition (PHN) division on her return from Geneva helps us make sense of these responses. She suggests that WHO officials were disappointed when the World Bank made clear that it did "not [want] to become a health organization" and that it was cautious about financing "health sector projects," which in World Bank parlance meant "conventional health services delivery and services." She adds in her memo, "When we had the opportunity (unfortunately after we had left Geneva) to read a WHO/UNICEF study on health needs handed to us while we were there, we came to see the reason for the WHO reaction."[9] In other words, WHO officials had misunderstood caution in respect to health services as an absence of interest in health. Boskey then insists that "the trend of our rural development projects is entirely in line with the trend in WHO." In other words:

> Unless the health sector and those responsible for it are consulted—which is usually not the case—it is not possible to realize the full developmental potential of activities in other sectors, such as nutrition, family planning and education of

women. Thus through association with the Bank, WHO would hope to achieve greater leverage and scope for its own immediate concerns in the health sector.[10]

She notes that at the end of the meeting, WHO officials described two initiatives the organization had taken to develop primary health care: first, to define the tasks and necessary training of village health workers; and second, to initiate health programming in a dozen nation-states. Ultimately, she concludes, "The Bank attaches great importance to the fact that it is possible to expand coverage within existing means or at least to provide minimum inputs acceptable to the governments under present constraints."[11]

The idea of the WHO and the World Bank coming together under the common umbrella of the primary health care strategy is surprising. Such development is at odds with the tensions between the two organizations, which historians usually associate with the World Bank's role in the emergence of global health and its insistence on redefining the PHC strategy along more "selective" lines (see chapter 3, Triage beyond the Clinic). However, the 1975 visit and the various memorandums of understanding it initiated actually point to a period of intense collaboration between the World Bank and the WHO that preceded the former institution's "health turn" and official endorsement of health investments as a priority for development. The collaboration between the two organizations in the 1980s neither implied total alignment nor an absence of tensions. If PHC was a strategy of mutual interest, it was approached and understood along different lines and led to different hierarchies of initiatives and programs. Convergence, mismatches, and open tensions thus plagued a decade critical for the strategy's implementation, economization, and "verticalization."

In the early 1980s, the list of projected World Bank loans that fell under the category of "health" expanded radically. Kandiah Kanagaratnam, the senior adviser in PHN, bluntly explained the motivation for this change to Petros Barvezian, the head of WHO Family Health, in January 1981, in a letter pleading for greater collaboration: "As you know we consider Maternal and Child Health [MCH] as a significant vehicle for both PHC and for Family Planning delivery; the attention given to MCH will be significant for both our population as well as our health efforts. In addition health education provides one useful communication strategy in demand creation [sic] in family planning."[12] That the World Bank would seek a more active engagement by the WHO in the domain of "population control" is not surprising, given the latter's cautious moves in a field whose Malthusian logic and suspicion of health as an aggravating factor was notorious (Connelly 2008).

This perspective was to turn family planning into an ingredient of primary health care, and the World Bank would invest in health infrastructures when they included such a component, rather than stressing the indirect health impact of family planning projects. This transition had deep roots in the contestation of population programs, which became more and more politically controversial as illustrated by the situation in India during Indira Gandhi's 1975 state of emergency (Rao 2004; Connelly 2008). Even pursuing population control programs in a less coercive way—within the framework of rural and community health—required some caution. The WHO's regional and national bureaus were always adamant that they be involved in the implementation of such programs. In April 1978, apprised of a forthcoming World Bank mission to prepare a second population initiative for the Philippines with a strong focus on PHC, the West Pacific Regional Office (WPRO) asked Geneva headquarters to request a postponement to let the WHO conduct its own assessment of the situation. WHO regional offices worried that the Bank initiative might undermine the local acceptance and development of health services because of the perception that priorities were being imposed on local communities without their input. As the request states:

> This suggestion is based on the concern that future Bank assistance in the area of rural health should be in line with the PHC policy. As you are aware, the promotion and implementation of the first population program, dealing with the construction of rural health units and training of midwives was designed according to predetermined facilities and manpower rather than through consultation with the community, which is one of the essential elements of PHC.[13]

The World Bank refused to delay the mission, citing time constraints in completing the loan, but agreed to conduct it in closer consultation with the WPRO.

There is little doubt that this convergence contributed to the late 1980s realignment of primary health care policies along more selective lines oriented toward maternal and child health. The same pattern significantly altered World Bank policies, legitimizing projects aiming at strengthening PHC facilities. Assessing the loans issued from 1986 to 1989, the PHN division thus singled out thirty-four loans with "maternal healthcare" emphasis—half of them located in Africa—whose core objectives were prenatal and postnatal care, drug supply, improved referral system, health education, and unsurprisingly, integrated family planning. The Bank thus spent $300 million to $400 million on a combination of facility building, personnel training, transportation, and therapeutic kits.

While self-reliance was central to the primary health care approach, the WHO recognized that external aid was an inevitable ingredient for the development of a country-level PHC system, at least in the implementation phase.[14] For this reason, it had been calling for new mechanisms to attract bilateral and multilateral aid since 1978. Between November 1978 and December 1979, the WHO held two informal consultations with multilateral and bilateral donors, as well as selected recipient countries, to determine how the organization could secure increased extra-budgetary support for the implementation of Health for All by the Year 2000.[15] The meetings endorsed the creation of a consultative group representing "developing countries and donors," including the World Bank. The avowed aim of the newly established Health Resources Group (HRG) was to promote the mobilization and "rationalization of health resources" toward PHC activities "in accordance with priorities recognized by WHO member states."[16]

The motivations of the WHO, and its director, in the creation of the HRG were three. First, the WHO was conscious of the growing role of extra-budgetary funding in its activities[17] and wanted to make sure that "all funds channeled through it are devoted to activities that conform to its policies."[18] Second, the WHO wanted to make sure that countries were engaged on a policymaking level with PHC strategy. Creating a mechanism to link an increase in external funding to PHC implementation could be read as a way to secure countries' "compliance" with the strategy. Third, the WHO wanted not only to increase donor funding for health but also to make sure that resources were actually directed toward PHC.

Though some WHO and World Bank interests converged, the encounter between the two organizations in the Health Resources Group proved complicated. Tensions coalesced around two issues: the governance of the new body and the nature of its functions. These tensions were grounded in donors' concerns that the new body might interfere with their freedom to make funding decisions based on their own priorities. Indeed, since the inception of the meetings, donors had made it very clear that they did not want the HRG—or the WHO—to exercise any form of control over resources.[19]

The equivocation on the part of donors—primarily the World Bank—resulted in repeated attempts to undermine the WHO's control over the HRG. The strongest challenge to the WHO's leadership came during the early phase of negotiations. Even before the creation of the body, some donor countries had proposed that the group should be located outside the WHO (World Health Organization 1980, 153). In response, the director general stressed that "no group concerned with the international transfer of resources could exist in [the WHO] without the presence of recipient countries."[20] Indeed, the WHO repeatedly insisted that the HRG was not meant to be a "donor club."[21] Nevertheless, in September 1980, an interim planning group was created to prepare the second HRG meeting in December 1980. Its membership included the World Bank, the Swedish International Development Agency (SIDA), and the U.N. Development Program (UNDP), among other donors.[22] The group proposed to change the HRG's governance in a way that actually undermined WHO authority. Although a simple change, the proposed governance reform wrested control away from the WHO by submitting the HRG (renamed the Health Resources Consortium) to the control of an independent secretariat and steering committee elected by HRG members. In addition, membership in the refashioned Health Resources Consortium had to be voluntary rather than populated by the WHO. The new architecture proposed by the interim planning group was approved in the second meeting in December 1980, but it did not take long for the WHO to react to what it viewed as a coup. In January 1981, its executive board, sitting in its sixty-seventh session, reaffirmed that the HRG should be an advisory group to the director general and that the "WHO must participate in a coordinative role; that the secretariat cannot be freely standing."[23] Even though the planning group, which had now become the proposed steering committee, had to accept the executive board's decisions in order to avoid a crisis with the WHO, some of its members continued to voice their discontent. Unsurprisingly, the World Bank was particularly vocal in opposing WHO control of the HRG.

If the WHO was successful in imposing its formal authority on the HRG, ensuring that it functioned the way the organization had envisaged proved more complicated. Indeed, a second tension between the WHO and donors emerged around the nature of HRG activities and functions. As we saw, the WHO intended the HRG as a mechanism for raising resources for PHC, based on the needs expressed by Southern countries with the support of the WHO. The Country Resource Utilization (CRU) review was soon identified as the most suitable mechanism toward this end. A CRU was a country study of the resources available, and of those needed, for implementation of the PHC action plans elaborated by the country itself. Developed on the basis of HRG guidelines, the CRU provided information on the plan and its cost implications. It also detailed what proportion of this cost could be covered by country resources and what amount of foreign aid was required.[24] Once elaborated by the government, with or without the aid of the WHO, the CRU had to be presented at the HRG. In Mahler's vision, the CRUs were meant to present donors with "the specific needs . . . of countries having well-defined strategies for health for all based on primary health care and to present the material in the form of 'fundable packages.'"[25] Ideally, presenting a CRU to the HRG would lead to the "formation of 'consortia' of interested parties, who could then arrange their own meetings in the country concerned at the invitation of the government."[26] Ultimately, this process proved difficult to implement. Multilateral agencies and other donors had no intention of being pushed to fund projects developed by individual countries with WHO help. The UNDP and the World Bank were particularly vocal in protecting their autonomy as funders. They insisted that the CRU information was too imprecise to provide a reliable basis for investment and that donor agencies needed to perform their own reviews.[27] They also stressed the lack of managerial ability on the part of the countries presenting the CRUs, and suggested that this represented a major problem.[28] Finally, they insisted that the HRG was not meant to review and approve the CRUs but simply discuss them. Obviously, this skepticism meant that the CRU did not serve as an effective fundraising mechanism. In October 1983, the WHO progress report on the activities of the HRG lamented the fact that some donors "still prefer to commit resources to discrete projects in line with their own priorities"[29] and did not respond to national governments' invitations for consortia meetings.

Nevertheless, multilateral agencies did not reject CRUs altogether. Rather, they worked to turn them into something different from what the WHO had envisioned. Instead of providing a blueprint to which funders were supposed to stick, CRUs would better serve as "quality control exercises" that would assess if countries "possessed sufficient institutional strength and commitment to receive grant, loan or investment money."[30] A CRU could also be conceived as a tool for categorizing and leveraging internal resources for health for all. "[A] CRU might more usefully determine what the health authorities could do if there were no external resources," explained one representative of the World Bank during a December 1983 meeting.[31] CRUs would thus come to be exercises in rationalization—fundamental in times of growing budget restriction and scarcity—and a precondition for donor investment, given that the Bank was "unlikely to finance PHC in any country which had not recognized the need for proper management or for mobilization of internal resources."[32] These words are revealing if we consider that in the very same period, the World Bank was implementing structural adjustment programs in a number of countries, including some that had undergone or were undergoing CRU reviews.

Donors' ideas about how the HRG should function eventually overcame those expressed by the WHO. Indeed, as shown by the June 1984 progress report of the HRG, in the great majority of cases, CRUs did not give rise to the creation of donor consortia but were employed by governments in bilateral negotiation with donors.[33] Most often, they were used as background documentation on the health sector in UNDP roundtable discussions and World Bank consultative groups. In 1985, Mahler announced that meetings of the HRG were suspended indefinitely, as were those of the HRG committee, a more select group that since 1983 had de facto taken the HRG's place. None of these bodies, he argues, had been effective in matching needs and resources, as this could only be done through direct negotiations with the countries concerned. "Under these circumstances," writes Mahler, "I would not wish to continue raising false hopes about the potential capacity of a HRG or similar instrument at either the global or regional level for mobilizing additional resources for individual countries."[34]

In the end, the Health Resources Group did not provide the funding mechanism for PHC that the WHO had hoped for. Nevertheless, the experience produced important effects both on the WHO and the World Bank. Indeed, on the WHO's side, this experience paved the way for a different approach to funding PHC. After 1985, the WHO began to contend that provision of health for all could not be done through external aid and that more economically realistic plans had to be developed to deal with the fact of limited resources in general and the rise of fiscal austerity more specifically.[35] As for the Bank, collaboration with the WHO in the HRG contributed to pushing the agency into the international conversation about basic health needs and paved the way for its more direct engagement in "investing in health."

Another important collaborative project originating at the WHO in the 1970s was the tropical diseases research (TDR) program, which officially started in 1978 and lasted until the late 1990s (Weisz and Tousignant 2019). Another brainchild of Mahler, the TDR was thought to be a means of bringing the traditional targets of vertical initiatives—vector-borne epidemic diseases like malaria, for example—in line with PHC's broader understanding of health and social medicine. At the first meeting with potential donors, on October 1975 in Geneva, TDR was described as resting on three assumptions: (1) purely technological responses focusing on the eradication of vectors had failed; (2) no new means of intervention had emerged for decades, especially in the drug sector, since most pharmaceutical firms had deserted research in tropical medicine; and (3) previous research and development (R&D) initiatives had not helped countries in the Third World to build their own research capabilities and, worse, the technological gap had actually widened as a consequence of brain drain. Tropical diseases research should therefore be an initiative that took advantage of new innovations in fields, such as molecular and cellular biology, to rethink the development of therapeutic treatments and vaccines rather than focusing on vector-oriented control. As Mahler and Lambo explained in their introduction to the 1975 meeting, TDR was "to take over the role of the industry" by investing in chemotherapeutic and preventive research targeting six major diseases: malaria, trypanosomiasis, filariasis, leprosy, leishmaniasis, and onchocerciasis. What differentiated this program from previous initiatives, in their minds, was not only the globalized nature of the intervention but also the priority given to "capability" building. TDR was meant to support interdisciplinary research centers located in developing countries, and it was governed through "equal partnership" between the WHO and national governments. Such collaboration was not only deemed important to ensure the "social relevance" of the program but also—echoing the premise of Lambo's own research on psychiatric disorders in Africa—to adapt biomedicine to local needs, open new forms of knowledge beyond the classical screening of drugs, and give TDR a more holistic meaning.

World Bank officials had been invited to participate in the first meeting, but they arrived in Geneva after the event. What they then learned from WHO officials and other attending experts (UNDP and USAID representatives) confirmed their suspicions: The gathering had involved serious criticism of the proposal and little money had been pledged. Minutes of the meeting reveal a slightly less bleak assessment, with significant support coming from Northern European countries, but it is true that delegates from Canada, Australia, and the United States openly criticized the six diseases approach, the lack of interest in environmental control, the emphasis placed on Africa, and, even more decisively, the dominant role that the WHO hoped to play in program governance. Following the advice of the most supportive donors, the WHO decided that giving the World Bank a key position in TDR would ease the negotiations. Mahler thus asked the Bank's president, Robert McNamara, about the possibility of the Bank cosponsoring TDR in parallel with the WHO and the UNDP. Following further discussions between James Lee, the Bank's environment and health adviser, and the Geneva staff, the Population, Health, and Nutrition division of the Bank endorsed the main aims of TDR, even if it took the whole of 1977 to reach an agreement on the organizational and management structure. As McNamara recounts in his memo of October 1977, which urged the World Bank's Board of Directors to sanction participation in TDR, the fact that the TDR fund was to be administered by the Bank, as well as the establishment of a Joint Coordinating Board composed of sponsors, donors, and recipient countries, was enough to ensure autonomy from the WHO bureaucracy.

During its first years of existence, TDR became the pet program of the World Bank's PHN division. In 1979, its officials successfully argued that the Bank should finance 10 percent of TDR's yearly budget, at the time $25 million, thus fulfilling WHO hopes for a financial "safety net" that would favorably impress Northern state donors. Moreover, in 1983, as new financial concerns surfaced as donations leveled off, PHN leadership insisted that TDR was not only well managed—as an external audit conducted in 1980 certified—but it was fulfilling its mission, having identified innovative paths toward malaria vaccines and begun the development of two new malaria drugs: mefloquine and qinghaosu.

The latter is the Chinese name for artemisinin, a plant-based preparation against malaria that became the most celebrated symbol of TDR success. Qinghaosu originates in the Chinese and WHO drive to integrate traditional medicine into biomedical systems as a way to mobilize new, cheaper, and "more socially acceptable" technologies in developing countries. The 1978 WHO report on the topic provides a list of national initiatives thought to have potential, from the inclusion of traditional birth attendants in African healthcare systems to the standardization of Ayurvedic doctor training in India. These are combined with vague general statements regarding what "integration into primary health care" could look like. One way was to view traditional medical practices as a source of new treatments and, more specifically, new drugs. This move may be understood as reducing traditional medicine to its biological compounds, or "herbalization," as it (1) equated traditional remedies with medicinal plants, (2) defined problems in terms of access to safe and effective products, and (3) argued for national regulation (i.e., adopting the norms of evaluation and marketing authorization used for chemical drugs).

China played a critical role in the implementation of this integration strategy. In 1995, it was the only country in the world with seven research centers benefiting from WHO support as "collaborative centers" in traditional medicine; among these, two were involved in the professionalization of acupuncture and three were active in the development of artemisinin.

Qinghaosu development had been under way in China since the 1970s. So, what did the internationalization of artemisinin research under the TDR umbrella change? In 1981, the WHO set up a Steering Committee on the Chemotherapy of Malaria (CHEMAL) to evaluate research proposals. The projects CHEMAL supported during the next decade reveal two logics, pursued in China as well as in Europe and in the United States. The first logic was that of complete molecularization and total chemical synthesis. Pharmaceutical giant Roche defended this perspective and benefited from extensive CHEMAL funding. The second logic was to improve cultivation and extraction in order to avoid complete synthesis. Research in that direction included the selection of more productive varietals, the use of growth factors, and clinical tests of various herbal *Artemisia* extracts conducted in the Beijing and Shanghai institutes for Chinese medicine. By the early 1990s, the Roche pathway for complete synthesis was a research success, but the process was so complicated that its industrial application looked uncertain. In spite of this setback, at CHEMAL, all ambiguities regarding the "holistic" road had evaporated. The only thing that mattered was the production of purified artemisinin, and whether that was more easily achieved through extraction or syntheses was secondary.

As a successful framework for the development of antimalarials, TDR revealed a strong bias in favor of pharmaceuticalization. However, this was not a consequence of the tensions between the WHO and the World Bank, which were mainly about financial and managerial issues and did not threaten the Bank's continuous funding of the program until 1998. Rather, this bias was an effect of the precarious existence of the traditional medicine integration strategy within the WHO itself. In other words, it was a consequence of the WHO's own contradictions.

THE WHO AND THE MISSED OPPORTUNITY FOR A GLOBAL AGENDA ON HUMAN GENETICS, 1980S–2000S

An early articulation of the role of human genetics in international health manifested itself at the WHO as early as the mid-1950s, when concern over the effects of nuclear radiation on future generations led to a consideration of genetics broadly defined (Lindee 2014). During the following decade, in addition to the comparative study of birth in various countries through the collection of epidemiological data and the work on "vanishing" groups of "unusual" genetic interest, the WHO also supported collaborative research on the frequency of diseases with a genetic component. This research-oriented approach "relied on the initiative of single individuals or small interdisciplinary teams of scientists" located in industrialized countries (Chadarevian 2015). With regard to this, a significant shift occurred in the late 1970s.

Partially motivated by criticism of its emphasis on blood clotting disorders, a "substantial reorientation"[36] of the Human Genetics Unit at the WHO started with the hiring of Anver Kuliev, a young Soviet geneticist. Soon he was appointed as the head of the WHO Human Genetics Program (HGP). His goal was to establish a reformed hereditary diseases program. In June 1981, a "historical conference"[37] on a blood disorder, thalassemia, was organized in Sardinia by pediatrician Antonio Cao. This conference prefigured the composition and targets of the WHO working group on genetics in that key experts, such as the British biologist Robert Williamson, "[discussed] the desirability of a WHO program for the control of hemoglobinopathies."[38] The members of the working group started collaborating as soon as November 1981, after Kuliev managed to convince the six international experts reviewing the whole field of medical genetics[39] that "hemoglobin disorders were a priority." In fact, "he found it very difficult" to do so, recalls Bernadette Modell, a British clinical geneticist.[40] Ultimately, he relied on the argument that "in many developing countries . . . hereditary anemias [were] the commonest form of genetic disease."[41]

Given the ubiquity of hemoglobin disorders, the HGP advocated the WHO taking a leading role in the dissemination of genetic services and training in developing countries, as well as in the standardization of techniques for diagnosis and prevention of genetic disabilities. The various advisory groups and reports set up at the HGP took root in the general patterns that the WHO Working Group on the Community Control of Hereditary Anemia created. From 1981 to 1985, a dozen people who shared a "technical approach"[42] and a penchant for clinical knowledge gathered annually in areas where these conditions were endemic (e.g., in Sicily, Cyprus, Milan, Bangkok, and Crete).

To influence the WHO agenda, these geneticists pushed for a definitive recognition of the relevance of genetics to public health and preventive medicine. The broad concept of "community genetics" that emerged as such in 1990 (Modell and Kuliev 1998) marked the coming of age of their reoriented program, sanctioning orientations and methods they had been formulating for ten years. Key elements of their approach were technical improvements, empirical evidence, and prevailing WHO values and strategies.

The HGP members either encouraged or directly developed several technical evolutions: screening for a growing number of inherited conditions, new diagnostic techniques for the detection of gene carriers for fetal monitoring, and of course advances in the treatment of diseases. In particular, in the early 1980s, Modell contributed with the improvement of chorionic villus sampling (CVS), which entails removing a sample of tissue from the placenta and testing it for different genetic abnormalities, so that it could become a first trimester fetal diagnostic, which allowed potential earlier therapeutic abortions of an affected fetus. By increasing the general acceptability of prevention, CVS was instrumental in legitimizing the work of the HGP.

In addition, the inclusion of clinical genetics in public health relied on ongoing national policies formulated in the Mediterranean area (pilot studies occurred in Cyprus, Greece, and Italy), where hereditary anemia was widespread. Building on scattered interventions that demonstrated the feasibility of beta-thalassemia (the most severe form) management at the country level, the HGP members sought to standardize existing methods and promote the value of hemoglobinopathies control programs as serious public health initiatives elsewhere, such as in Southeast Asia. Large-scale Cypriot screening of at-risk couples, with the option of therapeutic abortion, was a "strong argument for providing population-based services" (Modell and Kuliev 1998) and inspired the core principles of the HGP approach for community control of hereditary diseases: an "integrated strategy" combining prevention and care,[43] thus targeting both genetic disorders and genetic reproductive risks.

Once formulated, such an approach was deemed relevant to the management of other hemoglobinopathies (mostly sickle cell disease) and, more broadly, other genetic disorders, leading to the creation in 1982 of the WHO Advisory Group on Community Control of Hereditary Diseases. This network sought, in Anver Kuliev's words, to "develop the principles of genetic counseling"[44] while tackling G6PD deficiency, cystic fibrosis, Tay-Sachs disease, and phenylketonuria (PKU), as well as lactose intolerance, mutational diseases, and a genetic risk approach to common diseases. In doing so, WHO experts used target diseases as paradigms of a community-based approach to genetics, at the expense of common congenital, genetic but not inherited diseases like Down syndrome. Indeed, with some exceptions, this network gave little attention to chromosomal disorders in the course of formulating a global program.[45]

A key principle of community genetics was the setting up of "comprehensive" control programs. The application of genetic knowledge at the community level included encouraging the formation of patient and parents support groups and collaborations between genetic services and lay associations that could promote a wider understanding of these issues and a shift in social attitudes. Lastly, training of general practitioners and other health workers in medical genetics would be a crucial component of health promotion.

The gradual unfolding of community genetics at the WHO showed a remarkable continuity, even under Victor Boulyjenkov, Kuliev's successor; more or less the same network of international experts worked together for twenty years, until the early 2000s. Although the group diversified over time, recruiting geneticists from Latin America or Africa, the roots of community genetics were found in Northern expertise and applied on a mass scale to countries then called "developing." As Robert Williamson puts it, "Thalassemia is a third-world country problem with a first-world solution."[46] The very idea of community genetics was therefore conceived by experts from Europe and North America who pioneered the mixing of strategies of medical genetics and "community medicine" (bearing the mark of British medicine).

Undertaking activities to centralize and spread information, these experts combined research and operational work. Indeed, as soon as 1981, the experts gathered in Cagliari, Sardinia, wanted the WHO to provide "authoritative information" in order "to raise the level of awareness and willingness to act of the governments concerned."[47] They regularly made recommendations on WHO priorities and where it "[could] play an important role in the dissemination of genetic services"— through quality control, standardization of laboratory techniques and nomenclatures, training courses, and conversations between scientists from "developing countries" and "developed ones."[48] In addition, over this period, a growing number of HGP reports promoted practical advances by providing educational materials and management guidelines for specific conditions.[49] They hoped, indeed, to directly affect policymaking. According to Kuliev, their main preoccupation was "how to formulate genetic tools for public health people," ideally in "a language that should be understood by the general physicians" and by "non-English-speaking people."

The group hoped to challenge the general perception of genetic disorders as secondary issues in developing countries by trying to tackle their epidemiology and calling for standardized data collection. Moreover, in the 1980s, HGP reports argued that medical genetics was worthy of investment, citing the relatively low cost of a hemoglobinopathy control program relative to the broad burden of these chronic diseases on health resources in the most affected countries.[50]

However, despite HGP hopes for WHO support to control genetic diseases across the globe, community genetics faced a rough and unstable trajectory. Disappointed by the relative disinterest of the WHO in their general framework for preventing the most common inherited diseases, some of the most active HGP expert working group members turned to other international health actors. The WHO Regional Office for Europe temporarily acted as an intermediary in the late

1980s to early 1990s through Marsden Wagner, regional officer for maternal and child health. They also continued to reflect on the organizational dimensions of community genetics services in a 1992 report (Modell, Kuliev et al. 1991).

Later, the WHO Eastern Mediterranean Regional Office (EMRO) warmly welcomed community genetics approaches to commonly encountered hereditary disorders in the region. The EMRO began to work to fight these disorders in the early 1990s, in dialogue with Iran's and Saudi Arabia's governments, to help establish WHO collaborating centers for prevention and control of thalassemia. It then distinguished itself in 1993 by creating a WHO task force in its headquarters in Alexandria, Egypt, to review the epidemiological situation and formulate a plan for the control of hereditary disorders in the entire region.[51] Ala Alwan, who joined the EMRO in 1992 as regional adviser for noncommunicable diseases, was a strong advocate of regional action. In its bid to control these hereditary disorders, the EMRO organized meetings promoting community genetics from 1993 to 1996, focusing on tailoring community genetics to the countries in the region,[52] identifying regional priorities (notably parental age distribution, consanguinity, and control of hemoglobin disorders), and putting forward policy recommendations for national programs.[53] Beyond these extensive efforts at the EMRO,[54] regional exchanges (especially those initiated by Greece and Cyprus regarding their successful programs) and national initiatives (like the Iranian program) were directly encouraged by some of the early HGP experts and developed over time. Even in the early 2000s, the development of the Omani prevention program for genetic blood disorders did not primarily rest on the regional or national WHO offices' influence per se. It was rather partly determined by the interpersonal relationship between the British geneticist Bernadette Modell and Anna Rajab, pediatrician, geneticist, and head of the Ministry of Health's central lab who pioneered community genetics in Oman (the former being a PhD examiner for the latter). This suggests a regionalization of the original HGP perspectives, in a way shifting the hub from Geneva to Alexandria. Furthermore, the scattered development of similar programs at a national level, especially as happened very early in Cuba, under geneticist Luis Heredero's initiative in the 1980s, and later in Oman, proves that a process of globalization occurred along the way.

This outline of the trajectory of "community genetics" as an international issue shows the relative failure of the HGP to guide WHO activities and urge the organization to drive global policy in that field. The vast number of reports the HGP members published over the period (more than a hundred) were granted advisory status and thus viewed as reflecting only the opinions of invited experts, rather than the organization as a whole.[55] The early HGP experts we interviewed reported that they did not have a strong voice within the WHO. All of them regretted the lack of enthusiasm the HGP's work faced at the Geneva headquarters. Williamson's written reply to a request from Boulyjenkov in 2005 well illustrates the experts' frustrations after years of disappointed hopes: "I will try to help WHO in any way possible, and will write again. . . . The problem, as I look back over my 25 years association with WHO, is that in spite of your efforts, and those of many others including myself, the organization still gives genetics a very low priority."[56]

The development of medical genetics seems to have received shifting and uncertain attention from the WHO, the best evidence being that it is only in 2004 that the World Health Assembly passed a resolution on "Genomics and World Health"— and later on sickle cell anemia in 2006 and birth defects in 2010. This surge of WHO interest in the 2000s was closely related to the sequencing of the human genome in the 1990s. HGP historical figures viewed the eruption of genomic technologies in the WHO program with skepticism, believing that this new technical focus and its related business stakes would undermine their clinical perspectives and conception of medical genetics as integral to primary health care worldwide. Indeed, a major paradox is that the Human Genetics Program ended up leaving its mark thanks to genomics instead of community genetics.

The WHO's limited role in the globalization of community genetics can be explained in several ways. Oral as well as written sources consistently point to the WHO's historical focus on infectious diseases. Although HGP reports highlighted the epidemiological transition in the "developing world" and the growing challenge represented by genetic diseases, in the realm of international health, genetics still "looked unimportant compared to infectious diseases, high infant mortality and lack of proper sanitation" (Williamson 2001). This view of WHO priorities was prevalent outside the organization as well. Michael Katz, senior vice president for research and global programs at the March of Dimes, states that WHO authorities "all came from a generation that thought infectious diseases were the most important"; thus, hereditary diseases "disturbed their pattern of thinking. It was like throwing some sand into a system."[57]

Another explanation is that the HGP work on community genetics coincided with a period of financial crisis at the WHO (Chorev 2012). This is reflected in documents from the late 1980s. Facing regular requests for financial support for different projects around the world, the head of the HGP usually refused "due to severe financial cutbacks." Boulyjenkov insists, "We have never been in the WHO's priorities. Therefore, we had a little amount of catalytic funds. . . . Then each year this budget was reduced, reduced, reduced and reduced."[58]

Transregional Health Encounters: Indian Ayurveda, African Markets, and the WHO's Guiding Principles

If we want to look to a place where the WHO holds sway over Asian herbal medicines and their pharmaceuticalization, we need to switch national partners to focus on the export of Ayurvedic medicines from India to Kenya. In contrast to Chinese practitioners and medicines, which have been in Africa for decades (Hsu 2002), Indian Ayurveda has only recently been introduced to and inscribed in East Africa's medical, political, and economic fields (Meier zu Biesen 2017). Here, the WHO plays a dual and ambivalent role in the growing market for complementary and alternative medicines (CAM), to which Ayurveda belongs. It is an actor that strongly influences the promotion of traditional medicine and also a powerful but "neutral" global institution that epitomizes governance of non-biomedical therapies. Although the WHO sets limits on what counts as traditional medicine through a homogenized transnational category of traditional medicine (legitimized by law, policy, and scientific research within the biomedical paradigm), Indian pharmaceutical companies use this "symbolic categorical acknowledgment" from the WHO to boost support for drugs that are otherwise marginalized by the Kenyan state (McNamara 2020). At the same time, and outside of the WHO's discourses, medical entrepreneurs transcend the biopolitical order established by WHO regulations and create new networks that play an equally important role in carving out an "African Ayurveda market."

In 1978, the WHO-UNICEF conference at Alma-Ata specifically mentioned the role of herbal medicine and traditional practitioners in primary health and recommended their incorporation into healthcare delivery systems (Akerele 1987). Thereafter, the WHO (in addition China, India, and members of the African Union) grappled with how to best exploit traditional therapies "in the service of development." On some level, this was a practical move, but it also represented a symbolic departure from colonization and/or a return to indigenous values (World Health Organization 1978; Boyo, Cao et al. 1983; World Health Organization 2002; McMillen 2004). In particular, the WHO began to support the investigation of plant products. In general, traditional medicines barely figure into global health programs and the forms of knowledge the field values. The WHO is, in this respect, an exception since it persistently advocates for integration—albeit in the forms of "professionalization," standardization, and pharmaceuticalization (Feierman 1985; Last and Chavunduka 1986). As we have seen with the case of artemisinin, the role of the WHO has therefore shifted toward facilitating the worldwide circulation of industrialized herbal preparations, thus enabling a process critical to the globalization of health but still marginal to the field of global health.

During the 1990s, traditional medicine moved from being a strategy for national self-reliance to being a tool for managing the impact of structural adjustment programs by incorporating useful elements of traditional therapies into national healthcare systems (Langwick 2011). Indeed, the WHO proposed locally produced herbal medicines as one way to meet the global strategy for Health for All by the Year 2000 objectives.

Four decades after the Alma-Ata Declaration, the WHO, through its own Traditional Medicine Unit, has invested significant energy and resources in the development of non-biomedical therapies (Bode 2013). At the same time, Chinese and Indian firms have put the production and consumption of Asian preparations on their agenda (Pordié and Gaudillière 2014b). This business strategy has less to do with traditional medicine as a solution to fiscal tightening and more to do with the growing demand for "natural" forms of healing among patients (Craig 2012). This move is also based on the oft-cited WHO statistic that up to 80 percent of the Global South relies primarily or exclusively on traditional medicines to meet their primary health care needs (Bode 2013).

When herbal products, such as Ayurvedic preparations, began to circulate globally, the WHO naturally saw an increase in its influence as a regulator and promoter of such treatments. At the same time, the number of global actors pushing the industrialization of herbal medicines increased to include the World Trade Organization (WTO), the World Intellectual Property Organization (WIPO), and the World Bank. The global expansion of the market for Asian medicines has contributed to the inscription of these products within a larger system of health governance, which has evolved in parallel to the expansion of the circulation itself (Coderey 2020). This system is an assemblage of local, national, and global actors; trade rules and guidelines; financial resources; and market interests—permeated by significant power relations, which are also sources of friction. For instance, while global pharmaceutical regulations set by the WHO and WTO are essential for accelerating the movement of herbal drugs at the state level, WHO trade and migration policies can also impact drug flows. As exemplified in Kenya, expensive licenses for Ayurvedic practitioners and imported medicines act as barriers to market entry. However, as we will show, national arrangements regulating Ayurvedic drugs not only cause friction, they also create opportunities for intermediate traders by providing new transnational drug channels circumventing the WHO's regulatory authority.

At the macro level, the WHO sets policy frameworks determining which *materia medica* should be allowed to be traded according to research protocols and legal and ethical codes. In this sense, the WHO acts as the directing and coordinating authority on international health work (Brown, Cueto et al. 2006). In order for Ayurvedic pharmaceuticals to be marketed, they must be registered in their country of origin, they have to meet the safety requirements of the recipient country, and they must demonstrate that they adequately suit the receiving country's "needs" (World Health Organization 2005). Of course, these needs are subject to different interpretations. Kenyan drug regulation authorities determine, for instance, whether Ayurvedic drugs are classified as food supplements or herbal therapeutic products; marketing authorization for the latter is more complicated. Therefore, in addition to the WHO, African authorities have a huge impact on the mobility of Ayurvedic drugs in East Africa. Pharmaceutical facility inspections conducted by African drug authorities in India illustrate one important prerequisite for drug registration.

Large and profitable Indian enterprises, such as The Himalaya Drug Company, which successfully convert the Ayurvedic herbal tradition into cutting-edge medical technology (see chapter 4, Markets, Medicines, and Health Globalization; Pordié and Gaudillière 2014) and become integrated into a growing market through their capacity to adhere to WHO's normative standards, such as "good manufacturing practices" (Bhattacharya, Reddy et al. 2014). The representatives of these enterprises acknowledge that the "WHO-filter" (i.e., licensing and inspection procedures) is an indispensable element of drug quality, as well as a way to control the broader market (Meier zu Biesen 2017). Big firms value such regulations as a means to "wipe out the competition," as the WHO's transnationally valid quality assurance requirements that regulate the transition of herbs and traders across borders cannot be easily undertaken by smaller companies that lack the financial and technological means. As a consequence, small-scale Indian entrepreneurs and firms that cannot comply with the border regimes operate more and more on the illicit side of the pharmaceutical trade. In response to the harsh conditions they face—such as arbitrary seizures, high drug taxes, and onerous administrative regimes—these smaller companies build their own networks that enable Ayurveda drug flow.

Ayurvedic entrepreneurs and medical practitioners in Nairobi are often known by word-of-mouth, especially in Westland, where the largest part of the ethnically Indian population is concentrated (Chand 2010). These Ayurvedic entrepreneurs—practitioners, private enterprises, small-scale pharmaceutical companies—bypass the official regulations governing the circulation of goods and operate in a complex system of trade stratification, of which diaspora networks are an important example. A distinctive aspect of Indian engagement in East Africa takes the form of the large diaspora, which is a constitutive influence in India's multifaceted relations with the continent today, including the formation of new trade networks under the slogan of "South-South cooperation" (Bhattacharya 2010; Duclos 2012; Chorev 2019). The diaspora communities are important as potential consumers of Ayurvedic medicines and as indispensable players in their marketing strategy. Intermediate traders—Indian merchants, commercial intermediaries, and brokers—have mobilized transnational networks offering alternative infrastructures for Ayurvedic drug flow. Their modes of trade include cross-border drug delivery and movements via physical and electronic means, constituting transnational medical spaces and drug channels through real-world practices (Zanini, Raffaetà et al. 2013; Quet, Pordié et al. 2018).

Thus, "medicines on the move" must be analyzed through the prism of global institutional power while the WHO—acting as a "boundary organization" (McNamara 2020)—remains embedded in policy developments, even though there are ways in which it is also marginal as a governing institution. Despite its relative power, the WHO and other global health actors have erased neither the central role of the state nor those of innumerable local and national actors who actualize Ayurvedic medicines in the form of South-South partnerships. Medical entrepreneurs operating between India and Africa do so sometimes in conjunction with the state and global health actors and sometimes in opposition to these actors (Coderey 2020). Moreover, the Kenyan state maintains centrality and decides how to apply WHO guidelines. It can also circumvent the WHO and determine its own norms regarding manufacturing practices, drug laws, drug prices, and border regimes. Hence, the way the state organizes health depends significantly on local sociopolitical and economic configurations, local assumptions about safety and efficacy, market desires, and globally linked entrepreneurship. In addition to legal requirements, purchasing power and cultural preferences play a key role in Ayurveda's transregional trade.

A ROAD TO AFRICA: CHINA AND GLOBAL HEALTH

In 1975, when the WHO and UNICEF issued their first major document on what would become the primary health care strategy, mainland China had just been given the organization's member seat that Taiwan had occupied until 1972. In spite of the novelty of its presence within the WHO, Chinese health policy in general—the experiences of barefoot doctors in rural communities, the integration of Chinese traditional medicines into biomedicine—became important resources in the preparation of the 1978 Alma-Ata conference. However, there was one area of Chinese medical diplomacy that barely affected the WHO agenda during these years and the following decades: the numerous projects aiming at "cooperation and solidarity" in the domain of health that the country was advancing in Africa. Yet this parallel project had many consequences for the relationship between China and the WHO. We can analyze this relationship in two different stages: the first starts in the 1960s, at the inception of Chinese development policies in Africa; the second, much more recent period, refers to the launch of China's Belt and Road Initiative, under the mandate of Xi Jinping in 2013.

China first established diplomatic relations with African countries in the late 1950s.[59] Medical cooperation between China and Africa started as early as 1963, when China sent its first medical team to Algeria (A. Li 2011). In 1966, the Chinese government formalized its first development policies in relation to Africa. Between 1965 and 1969, the total amount of Chinese aid to Africa amounted to $200 million.[60] After China's economic reforms in in 1978, China-Africa relations changed from a model of "grant aid" to that of "bilateral cooperation."

Since 1963, when the first Chinese medical team went to Africa,[61] more than 23,000 Chinese health professionals have been sent to sixty-nine countries and regions around the world, treating hundreds of millions of patients. Currently, China has more than sixty medical teams in sixty-six different countries, including fifty-one in Africa. They provide services to nearly 270 million people and train tens of thousands of local doctors. Wang Liji, deputy director of the Department of International Cooperation at the National Commission on Health and Family Planning, states, "Through this selfless assistance over the past 50 years, China has gained the confidence of African countries, which has helped to strengthen Sino-African friendship."[62]

After China's economic reforms and opening to the global market from 1978 onward, China-Africa relations changed from a model of "grant aid" to that of "bilateral cooperation" based on the growth of economic exchange. In 1999, China's annual trade with Africa reached $64.8 billion, rising from about $1 billion in 1990. In 2000, the first Forum on China-Africa Cooperation was held in Beijing, with forty-five African countries attending.[63] This meeting encouraged the establishment of more than 600 Chinese companies in Africa. In 2006, the country put forward its official "policy towards Africa," the stated aims of which were to "develop a new type of strategic partnership . . . featuring political equality and mutual trust, economic cooperation in a win-win economic spirit, and cultural exchange."[64]

For five decades, China has engaged in bilateral cooperation with Africa, based on a palette of activities including sending Chinese medical teams to provide free medical services, offering free facilities and medication, training African medical personnel, and building hospitals in various African countries. (A. Li 2011) Foreign aid is thus a critical piece of China's role in health globalization. Health aid is delivered through medical teams, hospital construction, pharmaceutical and equipment donation, health professional training programs, and public-health/health-security-program support, including malaria control (Chen, Pender et al. 2019).[65] Although Chinese medical teams are highly visible in African countries, several researchers have pointed to their lack of inclusion within the field of global health, highlighting their operational flaws and lack of alignment with other international donor programs (Chen, Pender et al. 2019).

In September and October 2013, during his visit to Central and Southeast Asian countries, President Xi Jinping proposed a major initiative that garnered much attention from the international community. In March 2015—with the authorization of the State Council—China's National Development and Reform Commission, the Ministry of Foreign Affairs, and the Ministry of Commerce jointly issued the "Vision and Action for Promoting the Construction of the Silk Road Economic Belt and the 21st Century Maritime Silk Road," which included expanding "cooperation in the field of medicine."

Traditional Chinese medicine is an important part of the exchange and cooperation between countries along the New Silk Road.[66] In December 2016, in order to actively respond to the Belt and Road Initiative,[67] the State Administration of Traditional Chinese Medicine and the National Development and Reform Commission jointly issued the "'One Belt and One Road' Development Plan for Chinese Medicine," that aims to strengthen exchange and cooperation with countries along the New Silk Road in the field of Chinese medicine. According to the planning requirements, by 2020, thirty centers for traditional Chinese medicine were envisioned to be established in cooperation with countries along the route; twenty international standards for Chinese medicine promulgated; 100 Chinese medicine products registered; and fifty Chinese medicine pharmacopoeia "demonstration bases" highlighting international cooperation and exchange built. The goal, according to the People's Republic of China, is that, by that time, "the value of Chinese medicine medical care and health care will be widely recognized by people along the route."

Under the guidance of national promoters of the route, various Chinese regional authorities have formulated corresponding support policies. For example, the Thirteenth Five-Year Plan for the Development of Traditional Chinese Medicine (TCM) in Shaanxi Province proposes to support TCM enterprises, medical institutions, and units in the province; to carry out TCM education and training within key countries in the Belt and Road, as well as in Hong Kong, Macao, and Taiwan; and to foster multi-level and multi-field cooperation, especially in terms of creating overseas TCM treatment centers and of promoting health tourism. "Guangdong Province's Implementation Plan for the Outline of the Strategic Plan for the

Development of Traditional Chinese Medicine (2016–2030)" supports TCM institutions in carrying out investment and cooperation in the field of TCM health in the countries along the Belt and Road and encourages pharmaceutical enterprises selling TCM preparations to apply for overseas trademark registration and to build internationally renowned brands.

As a result of its dramatic economic growth, China seeks a profound transformation of its presence abroad, regardless of the country of destination, from a simple "made in China" label to an overall appreciation for the "conceptual dynamics of creation/initiative in China" (Wang 2019). In this way, China is attempting to become an exporter of standards and values at the international level, moving beyond the industrial products attached to its current image as the "factory of the world." Chinese medicine is emerging as a diplomatic tool when promoting the interests of the Chinese state and pursuing international recognition of Chinese knowledge (see Wang 2019 for more details).

While in European countries, Chinese medicine is viewed as an alternative and complementary practice, a holistic medicine that relies on less "technical" forms of listening and intervention and that responds to criticisms of biomedicine; in some African countries, TCM is a tool of primary health care. In fact, the export of TCM is one strategy in the overall Chinese project of strengthening and reorganizing entire healthcare systems—systems that are considered deeply deficient and in a state of permanent crisis. In general terms, regardless of the country of destination, the new Chinese health diplomacy, in general, and the recent Belt and Road Initiative, in particular, operate without any links to or coordination with the classical players of global health, including the WHO, thus contributing to the latter's provincializing. While the WHO has drawn inspiration from China—for instance, when developing its "Health for All" policies—our analysis shows that the reverse cannot be claimed. Instead, it looks like Chinese developmental policies toward Africa, following their own trajectories, have approached the WHO as peripheral.

Conclusion

Seen from inside the organization, the WHO's adaptation to global health could be summed up as a refocusing on its deep historical roots. By mediating its own operational ambition and concentrating on normative activities—guidelines and epidemiological reporting, for instance—the WHO under Director General Gro Harlem Brundtland experienced shifts that created an organization that somehow resembled the League of Nations Health Organization (LNHO) (Cueto, Brown et al. 2019). This predecessor of the WHO had also come to prominence after a World War (WWI) by focusing on similar activities (Borowy 2009).

Yet, we argue that the recent provincialization of the WHO bears only superficial resemblance to that of the LNHO between the wars. In the 1920s, the LNHO operated in a complex web of states that allowed for the normative activities of an international political body. In the 1990s, in an environment of economic globalization, critique of the U.N. system, and proliferation of nonstate actors, the context was less amenable to international political oversight.

On the one hand, the rise of DOTS is an example of the WHO trying to renew its normative role, providing a global standard for how to run national tuberculosis programs. But if we look deeper, we see that the standard was created by others and was in direct opposition to the WHO's previous control strategy. In reality, it was the World Bank that made the WHO the face of a program that directly contradicted WHO's principles and policies. In our second archival exploration, the case of the relationship between the WHO and World Bank, we discover an approach on the side of the WHO that can be summarized as adaptive learning. In this case, the WHO used its relationship with the World Bank to increase the legitimacy and the resources available for its primary health care strategy, take into account the mounting economization of health, and update tropical diseases research. This collaboration does not only reveal unexpected roots for the World Bank health turn but also sheds light on the tensions this turn and the development agenda more broadly created in the very same organization that sidelined the WHO with regards to tuberculosis and DOTS. In our third case, that of medical genetics, we see a different set of challenges. The role of the WHO in this novel field was limited from the start, partially because of the organization's traditional focus on infectious disease control and partially because of a lack of interest of many Southern states in the implications of genetic conditions and their role in public health. In our fourth study, in Kenya we have an exemplary case of authority under erosion, where the WHO's normative activities around Ayurvedic medicines and their proliferation are increasingly evaded by a trade that is first and foremost regional, leaving the WHO's normative role a memory of past days of Anglo-European dominance. Finally, in our story about China and the WHO, we see that despite an early sympathy with the WHO's policies on primary health care, the Chinese government took a divergent path of bilateral health aid in Africa. The importance and impact of this alternative agenda expanded with China's escalating role in the world economy with initiatives enlarged to the global promotion of traditional Chinese medicine.

Ultimately, the WHO's role in global health remains both inadequate and indispensable. In a world of neoliberal governance and medico-economic interests, be they corporate, humanitarian, or any combination of the two, the WHO signals the continued need for political processes, with their elements of representation, public accountability, and strategic debates about health needs. In the case of the WHO, that such processes (whatever their limitations might be) come part and parcel with the production of rich, publicly accessible data is not a coincidence. Rather, they are one of the foundations on which such a role can be built.

Epilogue

GLOBAL HEALTH FOR ALL: COVID-19 AND BEYOND

Claudia Lang, Andrew McDowell, Claire Beaudevin,
and Jean-Paul Gaudillière

On March 13, 2020, an aircraft landed in Rome. Nine people disembarked and immediately stopped next to the jet bridge for a group photo. Behind their masks, the team of doctors in reflective burgundy-colored "China Health" jackets smiled for Associated Press cameras. In the background, under the watchful eye of customs officials, airport personnel unloaded boxes of respirators, face masks, and other supplies labeled in Mandarin. The first medical team from China had arrived to support Italian health system responses to COVID-19, a novel airborne infectious disease that would soon cause a pandemic.

Over the weeks that followed, the arrival scene appeared repeatedly on social networks and news channels. For China, the scene enacted a new form of health intervention, an expansion of its health diplomacy expanded from a focus on Africa, where China was already the leading builder of hospitals, to other countries that, like Italy, were more accustomed to providing international development aid than to receiving it. For most of Europe and North America, the episode shed a harsh light on the disorganization, shortages, and systemic failures that characterized the COVID-19 responses. Global interest in the scene and its multiple interpretations highlight this book's central questions: How do medical techniques, commodities, and ideas move across space and time? What are the effects of those movements and connections? What does health intervention reveal about the power imbalances established by providing care? How do flows of medicine and healthcare reveal the dynamics of comparability and difference at work in attending to the health of others?

The arrival of Chinese medical personnel and goods in Italy is of such popular interest because it presents the convergence and inversion of global health's assumed directionality from North (Europe and North America) to South (Africa, Asia, and South America). It reinforces what we have argued throughout this book: The easy image of North-South donor-recipient flows is far more complicated when viewed through the lenses of global health and health globalization. Like the massive production of pharmaceuticals and the experimental global health projects in the South, Chinese expert intervention and donations to Italy and other countries has required disrupting the analytics that only see health exchanges as moving from North to South. These circulations insist that we consider collaborations between people and institutions based in Africa, South America, and Asia as well as their effects on people and institutions in Europe and North America when attending to health at a global scale. Moreover, the shortages of medical supplies and staff and disjointed public health responses to the rapid spread of COVID-19 in most European countries and in the United States pose serious questions about what seems to be vanishing differences between the health systems of supposedly affluent countries and those labeled as low- or middle-income. Indeed, COVID-19's trajectory in Europe and in North America, in parallel with the rise of noncommunicable diseases in Latin America, Asia, and Africa, which concern the global health actors documented in this book, may be a decisive event in the convergence of worldwide health problems and health system deficiencies.

The COVID-19 pandemic and *Global Health for All*, though in a smaller way, challenge one of global health's central dichotomies. They defy an imagined polarity between centers of expertise in the North and sites of interventions and experimentation in the South. In fact, they trouble not only the dichotomy itself but the very meaning of its categories. In the process, they highlight the inadequacy of assumptions that medical expertise, in infectious disease management in particular and health issues in general, is solely located in Europe and North America. Moreover, they challenge the view that expert and technical knowledge as well as health-related tools, finances, and priorities always move along a North-South gradient. Our notion of multidirectional arenas of health globalization indicates what the pandemic has brought to the fore: Health with a global aspiration is less than ever a matter of intervening in the health of others. Rather, targets and sites of experimentation and intervention have diversified; expertise, pandemic knowledge, and pharmaceutical and nonpharmaceutical tools increasingly circulate along alternative East-North, East-South or even South-South pathways.

What is at stake here is more than the blurring of an already nebulous North-South boundary by the existence of a global infectious disease without a technical solution. It is a story about who—scientists, economists, markets, states, global philanthropic organizations, technology producers, the World Health Organization (WHO),—can and should intervene in the health of others and how. It also troubles assumptions about who those others might be. New international hierarchies and rapidly increasing inequalities within countries have emerged to reorganize relations of health intervention and prioritization. Consider the relationships between new global players, like China, and those who have benefited less from globalization, like most countries in sub-Saharan Africa. Consider how COVID-19 has disproportionately killed the elderly, the socially and racially marginalized, and those with other health conditions. Our attention to measurement, triage, standardization, and hospital infrastructures in *Global Health for All* suggests that these themes were emerging well before COVID-19. Their ubiquity, however, is a powerful testimony of the emerging new hierarchies between entire regions of the world health landscape as well as within countries and communities.

Attending to the ways in which COVID-19 challenges and reinforces imaginaries of health at a global scale helps situate the most recent wave of health globalization in what has become a shared human experience of precarious and connected health. Nonetheless, forms of inequality within and across states and regions have become somberly clear. COVID-19 is a stark reminder for scholars of health at any scale that we need to develop ways to consider health inequalities beyond the geopolitically imagined North and South paradigm and engage health's entanglement with inequalities associated with race, class, age, gender, and comorbidity at multiple, often overlapping, scales.

Chinese medical aid to Europe and the (relatively) successful development and implementation of pandemic control measures such as the "test, trace, isolate" strategy in China, South Korea, and Taiwan—like many features of the global trajectory of the COVID-19 pandemic—confirm the bifocal lenses of global health and health globalization that *Global Health for All* proposes. Chinese pandemic aid to the Italian healthcare system is an intervention that foregrounds Asian countries as models for pandemic control, although China neither participates in institutions in the global health field nor follows its rules. However, it is clearly part of larger processes of health globalization. Throughout this book, we have shown the key relevance of the dynamic interconnections between the *field* of global health and the less formalized and more variegated *arenas* of health globalization. The institutions and the forms of knowledge and instruments mobilized in programs and by self-defined practitioners of global health are inseparable from broader circulations of health personnel, patients, drugs, or other technologies. However, in spite of all their interactions and connections, the actors involved in both realms of globalization, the targets they select, and the way they intervene are not the same. The difference between field and arenas helps to elucidate health universalism's profound discrepancies. It reveals a separation between global health's practices of knowing and intervening with their strong reliance on biomedicine and techno-packs, on the one hand, and the renewed forms of social medicine and knowledge put in place to stop a global plague, on the other.

Beyond the dialectics of field and arenas, the COVID-19 pandemic's double discourse of systemic transformation and aspirational return to normalcy reinforces several of this book's central themes. It sheds critical light on the ways the pandemic challenges global health and raises anew the question of continuity and change we started with. For example, the COVID-19 pandemic and its management undoubtedly reinforce our argument about the indispensable but inadequate role of the WHO in global health. The U.N. organization can rely on a certain degree of continuity and on the legacy of its long-term interests in epidemiological data gathering, social determinants of health, and the organization of public health institutions. However, this very same WHO has been the central, and perhaps only, global health institution in a guiding role since the beginning of the COVID-19 crisis. Here too, the WHO's power has remained largely a soft power of advising but not directly intervening in pandemic responses, even as COVID-19 responders complain about its inaction and insist on its reform.

Indeed, actors and institutions that populate the field of global health have largely remained invisible. For example, the Institute for Health Metrics and Evaluation, the key provider of data in global health, remains largely in the background. Comparison continues nonetheless. Institutes that produce national data are at work, and alternative metrics—such as Ro, the COVID-19 reproduction rate—used as proxies for infections and social behavior have become a new currency of global comparability. Similarly, other actors that are part of health globalization arenas but not of the global health field—such as nation-states, manufacturers of protective equipment, digital health developers, or even traditional medicine manufacturers—dominate the landscape of COVID-19 strategy and response. When key global health players like the Gates Foundation and the World Bank did come onstage, they promoted initiatives focusing on biomedical innovation—for example, promoting vaccination as the only serious and definite preventive response and identifying (again and this time incorrectly) Africa as the primary region at risk.

With global health's favorite tools, pharmaceuticals and vaccines, unavailable during the first phases of the pandemic, response strategies such as lockdowns, social distancing, and "test, trace, isolate" are reminiscent of earlier health regimes like social medicine and sanitation campaigns. Mass action combined with highly technical second-line interventions, such as assisted respiration and molecular diagnostics, reveals what we might call "sociopacks." Sociopacks add social action to global health's conglomerations of technology and techniques that we have called "technopacks." Emerging modular pandemic socio-techno-packs change healthcare systems and ideas about risk and security, as we have argued in this book. And perhaps more importantly, they affect everyday conduct and ethics, even as they spark political controversies. From another perspective, masks, protective equipment, PCR tests, and vaccines for COVID-19 reinforce what we have called the central importance of markets (including black markets) in the arenas of health globalization. They do so even as debates about the local or global production and market-oriented circulation of these goods reveal and reinforce structural inequalities on global, national, and local scales.

Much like global health responses to tuberculosis, HIV, and malaria, when COVID-19 containment or prevention strategies fail, disease interventions center on the hospital. In a stunning example, the Mumbai tuberculosis (TB) clinic, in this book's introduction, continued to provide TB care and COVID-19 referrals even though mandates to stay-at-home silenced the busy road on which it sits. This is simultaneously surprising and predictable: Hospitals have often been neglected in global health but have remained the main sites of medical care during the pandemic. Vertical programs in the global fights against infectious disorders have largely ignored hospitals despite relying on them. Hospitals are, at the very least, critical loci of care, research, and training the world over. As we have shown here, they are a central node where global health and health globalization overlap.

Like the persistence of hospitals, COVID-19 responses lay the transformed endurance of the state bare. It is one of our central arguments that the state has remained crucial in global health even if its role as provider and organizer of health-care has been transformed. Neoliberal reason and its practitioners have often rendered the state an implementer of health programs designed elsewhere rather than a space for debate about them. Yet, when faced with a novel challenge, it becomes evident that the state continues to be the primary organizer of healthcare and population management while at the same time trying to implement strategies conceived of in the realms of global health.

Finally, state-organized pandemic responses leave little space for global health interventions. They have challenged the epistemic power of neoliberal rationality and economization and, in doing so, question the legitimacy of global health's role as a central knowledge clearinghouse for evaluating interventions and apportioning collective resources. The institutional response to the pandemic utilizes little of global health's vocabulary of efficiency, cost-effectiveness, and operability. It is, however, replete with the experimentation, tinkering, and bricolage that we revealed in processes of localization, on the one hand, and in needs-based medical triage (what we call political triage), on the other. COVID-19 has not only led to a massive public debate about who should be protected and at what cost, it has starkly revealed the centrality of *clinical* triage on a global scale, as countries attempt to respond to the virus with limited resources. Pandemic responses like rationing, identifying "essential workers," and lockdown practices are a macabre confirmation that cost-based triage is central to health at a global scale.

What does all of this mean for global health, anthropology, sociology, and history? To us, change accompanies continuity, and an important part of the historian's work is to accommodate this dialectic through periodization. The genealogy of global health we propose here insists on its break with the 1960s and 1970s international public health initiatives as well as with the Primary Health Care Strategy's original form of social medicine for the South. These forms have lingered in health globalization, but the neoliberal reforms of the 1980s and 1990s limited their power to organize interventions. Neoliberal reforms paved the way for the strong endorsement of biomedicine, the priority given to vertical programs and the decisive role of economic triage. They set the stage for what we call the field of global health.

Our book does not offer an alternative grand narrative of health universalism. Instead, it argues for a change in the granularity of the analysis and timeline used to understand health at a global scale by looking at heterogeneous temporalities as well as various combinations of change and continuity. We show, for instance, that depending on the perspective, the history of the WHO blurs the three-phase story of global health interventions, which traditionally moves from institution building in the period after World War II to the primary health care moment in the 1960s and 1970s to neoliberal reforms in the 1990s and 2000s. Of course, a diversity of temporalities does not imply an avoidance of chronology. Attention to multiple timelines, places, and ways of knowing confirms the idea that certain critical moments ground the deployment of global health's universal aspirations as well as its limitations. Periodization thus helps understand why, after global health's 1990s emergence alongside the creation of a new focus on chronic disorders, the field and its leading actors did not establish large programs targeting these afflictions. It might even explain why movements like global mental health, which surfaced later, remain at its periphery, operating instead within the arenas of health globalization.

The COVID-19 pandemic will certainly appear as another critical moment for ways of knowing and intervening on the health of others. It will have far-reaching and diverse consequences for many of the institutions and logics we have presented here. It is already moving across scales, jostling the circulations and knowledge systems that are central to imagining who the others are and what might be at stake in attending to their health. Moreover, COVID-19 has indeed revealed deep entanglements of health with political economies and social inequalities and also, importantly, with ecologies. It remains to be seen if a larger debate about anthropogenic causes of the COVID-19 pandemic and the human, more-than-human, and ecological effects of strategies to contain it will reframe imaginaries of health on a global scale to include its entanglement with more-than-human and planetary ecologies. In resonance with the complex trajectories of the pandemic, not only does *Global Health for All* reflect on global health's meaning and limits, but it also highlights the necessity of a reconceived international and decidedly more social and ecological approach to health. This new framework is now more essential than ever.

Leipzig, New Orleans, Grenoble, and Paris, December 2020

Acknowledgments

We are deeply indebted to interlocutors and archivists the world over. Without their guidance, spirit of openness, and willingness to help, our task to sketch health at a global scale would have been impossible. Similarly, we thank Cindy Hemery, Jean-Guy Gay, Ursula Read, Camille Gasnier, Anabel Rodriguez, Bego Alic, Tara Dankel, Celine Eschenbrenner, Kimberly Guinta, and two anonymous reviewers who were essential to the research and writing of this book. The European Research Council's generous advanced grant funding made the GLOBHEALTH project (From international to global: knowledge, disease, and the postwar government of health) possible. Cermes3 (Paris), the Institut National de la Santé et de la Recherche Médicale (INSERM), and Oslo University made the project's everyday running a reality.

We must also express our gratitude to the colleagues who took part in manifold events and conversations with us over the years: Vincanne Adams, Marine Al Dahdah, Joseph A. Alter, Dominique Béhague, Dörte Bemme, Roberto Beneduce, Anne-Emanuelle Birn, Gunnar Bjune, Christian Bonah, Catherine Bourgain, Nils Brimnes, Alila Brossard Antonielli, Elise Burton, Carlo Caduff, Maurice Cassier, Soraya de Chadarevian, Sangeeta Chattoo, Nitsan Chorev, Sara Cooper, Thomas Cousins, Mary-Jo Del Vecchio Good, Blandine Destremau, Hansjörg Dilger, Emilio Dirilkov, Erica Dwyer, Nora Engel, Didier Fassin, Steven Feierman, Heidi Fjeld, Duana Fullwiley, Wenzel Geissler, Rene Gerrets, Sahra Gibbon, Byron Good, Tine Hanrieder, Ian Harper, Emily Harrison, Cori Hayden, Matthew M. Heaton, Nicolas Henckes, Sarah Hodges, Nancy Rose Hunt, Craig Jeffery, Kriti Kapila, Janina Kehr, Hanna Kienzler, Laurence Kirmayer, Stephan Kloos, Erin Koch, Wen-Hua Kuo, Lakshmi Kutty, Anne Kveim Lie, Guillaume Lachenal, Laurence Louër, Ilana Löwy, David Macfadyen, Harilal Madhavan, Manjari Mahajan, Lenore Manderson, Dominik Mattes, James H. Mills, Elia Mmbaga, Kåre Moen, Kirubel Mussie, Vinh-Kim Nguyen, Mark Nichter, Kris Peterson, Sarah Pinto, Ruth Prince, Mathieu Quet, Mohan Rao, Ursula Rao, Hans L. Rieder, Abril Saldaña-Tejeda, Emilia

Sanabria, Katharina Schramm, Judith Schühle, Andrea Solnes Miltenburg, Anubha Sood, Katerini Storeng, Alice Street, Johanne Sundby, Kaushik Sunder Rajan, Steve Sturdy, Noelle Sullivan, Merete Taksdal, Josiane Tantchou, Marlee Tichenor, Helen Tilley, Anitha Tingira, Catherine Trundle, Megan Vaughan, Bharat Venkat, Ayo Wahlberg, Catherine Waldby, Alexis Walker, Andrea S. Winkler, Harry Yi-Jui Wu, Mei Zhuan, and many others. We are grateful to Amron Gravett and Tara Dankel for their invaluable help in finalizing this book.

Notes

CHAPTER 1 — LOCALIZATION IN THE GLOBAL

1. Interview with Anver Kuliev, Chicago, December 2018.

2. Accounting for the high prevalence of hemoglobinopathies in the (sub)tropics, scientists argue that blood disorders emerged in areas where malaria was endemic, meaning that carrying a single copy of the mutated gene protects against malaria.

3. Interview with Bernadette Modell, London, November 2016.

4. Interview with Bernadette Modell, London, November 2016.

5. This is a humoristic reference to the French company that bears this name and runs holiday resorts in various countries.

6. "From 1977, cases were sent to London and Athens, but also to Jerusalem," in order to get prenatal diagnosis (Angastiniotis and Hadjiminas 1981, 369–370).

7. "Factors Limiting the Effective Delivery of Fetal Diagnosis for Thalassaemia," M. A. Angastiniotis, Archbishop Makarios Thalassaemia Centre, Nicosia, Cyprus, presented at the WHO/SERONO Meeting on Perspectives in Fetal Diagnosis of Hereditary Diseases, Geneva, May 2–4, 1984, G3-181-129, World Health Organization Records and Archives.

8. Cyprus's size by landmass is similar to Sardinia, also known as a successful example of thalassemia care and prevention.

9. M. Angastiniotis, "Prevention of Thalassaemia in Cyprus," circa 1983–1984, G3-181-129, WHO archives.

10. "Factors Limiting," WHO archives.

11. Interview with Bernadette Modell, November 2016.

12. Interview with Anver Kuliev, December 2018.

13. For instance, the blood bank was deemed "one of the best examples of community involvement in our health system" (Angastiniotis, Kyriakidou et al. 1986, 295).

14. Memorandum from Anver Kuliev (Hereditary Diseases Programme) to the Director of the Department of Noncommunicable Diseases, March 13, 1984, G3-181-129, WHO archives.

15. Memorandum from Victor Bulyzhenkov to EMRO Regional Director, April 2, 1990, for the "Re-designation of the Archbishop Makarios Thalassaemia Centre, Nicosia, Cyprus, as a WHO collaborating Centre," G3-286-2 Jac 5, WHO archives.

16. Interview with Anver Kuliev, December 2018.

17. K. Styblo and WHO Tuberculosis Program, "The National Tuberculosis/Leprosy Programme in Tanzania," WHO/TB/88.153, WHO archives, https://apps.who.int/iris/handle/10665/61230.

18. Interview with physician, Geneva, Switzerland, May 2018.

19. Interview with project administrator, Mumbai, India, August 2016.

20. Interview with M. P., Mumbai, India, August 2017.

21. Interview L. S., Patna, India, January 2014.

22. For instance, in 1983, a study sponsored and published by the Pan American Health Organization (PAHO) proposed a metric that was supposed to measure community participation by assigning a score to "agents of community participation" (e.g., health promoters and health committees) and "participatory activities" in a given community (Agudelo 1983).

23. Interestingly enough, at the very same time that the WHO reiterated the "spirit" of community participation (as proposed in Alma-Ata) and was promoting the concept of "community action in health," the WHO/Canadian Department of Health and Welfare gave birth to the Ottawa Charter on health promotion in 1986. See International Conference on Health Promotion (1986, Ottawa, Canada) and World Health Organization. Division of Health Education and Health Promotion, "Health Promotion: Ottawa Charter—Promotion santé, Charte d' Ottawa," unpublished paper, 1995, WHO/HPR/ HEP/95.1, WHO archives, https://apps.who.int/iris/handle/10665/59557. On the link between the primary health care strategy and the Ottawa Charter, see Cueto, Brown et al. (2019, 199).

24. See, in particular, the background document for the technical discussions (World Health Assembly, 40, *Economic Support for National Health for All Strategies: Background Document*, May 1987, Geneva, WHO A40/Technical Discussions/2, WHO archives, https:// apps.who.int/iris/handle/10665/164144). This technical discussion had been prepared with the support of the World Bank, which endorsed four policy measures: user charges in government health facilities, insurance of other risks, use of nongovernmental resources, and decentralization of government health services (J. Akin, N. Birdsal, and A. R Measham to J. North, May 27, 1987, "Back to Office Report," 30158262, World Bank Group Archives, Washington, DC). Community funding seems to have been a WHO idea.

25. For instance, as Chorev contends, at the end of the 1990s, the WHO objected to "users' fees," which were endorsed by the World Bank, using the same economic reasoning that was prevalent at the time (Chorev 2012, 172–174).

CHAPTER 2 — METRICS FOR DEVELOPMENT

1. GBD data visualizations and the GBD Compare tool are available at the Institute for Health Metrics and Evaluation (IHME) website (http://www.healthdata.org/data -visualization/gbd-compare).

2. The Washington Consensus has become the conventional way to describe neoliberal economic reforms and policies that the International Monetary Fund (IMF), the World Bank, and later the World Trade Organization (WTO) shared and implemented in the 1980s and 1990s.

3. How audit culture works in global health vertical programs in AIDS, tuberculosis, and malaria has been illustrated in Eboko (2015).

4. According to the Institute for Health Metrics and Evaluation, the GBD process examines over 350 causes of death and injury and almost 3,000 conditions resulting from disease and injury, as well as risk factors and health states.

5. De Ferranti, "Sector Financing: An Overview of the Issues," November 30, 1983, Draft Population, Health, and Nutrition Paper, Folder 19831130, and De Ferranti, "Health Resources in Developing Countries: How Should They Be Allocated?," May 14, 1985, Draft Population, Health, and Nutrition Paper, Folder 1104184, World Bank Group Archives, Washington, DC.

6. "This indicator can evaluate the impact, expressed in units of time, of specific diseases on a given society, and has the advantage of presenting a common metric of health loss for all

causes and states. . . . In this sense, AVISAs [DALYs] can be used to estimate the health needs of a population, evaluate the effectiveness of interventions, establish research priorities and care, and measure the technical efficiency of service production" (FUNSALUD 1994, 125).

7. The data in the report constitute a baseline in the sense that later calculations for the same categories of disease are compared to it. The metrics in the 1990 report can also be reiterated later, using more comprehensive data for the same "baseline" period.

8. Interview with Dan Chisolm, WHO health economist, by A. Lovell, May 3, 2019.

9. Interview with Dan Chisolm, May 3, 2019.

10. The IHME compiles data from audits of financial records and budget and program-level information for all major global health assistance (Charlson, Dieleman et al. 2017).

11. Interview with Dan Chisolm, May 3, 2019. Chisholm authored the above-cited WHO report.

12. See http://www.healthdata.org/disease-burden-india.

13. See http://www.healthdata.org/disease-burden-india.

14. See Roychowdhury (2019), citing Vinod Paul, a member of NITI Aayog.

15. Interview with P. Jeemon by C. Lang, Thiruvananthapuram, India, January 2018.

16. Interview with Gopalakrishnan Gururaj and Matthew Varghese, two of the authors of the National Mental Health Survey, by C. Lang, Bengaluru, India, February 2018.

17. Interview with Gopalakrishnan Gururaj by C. Lang, Bengaluru, February 2018.

18. Interview with Gopalakrishnan Gururaj, February 2018.

19. Jocalyn Clark (Lancet), comments delivered at the workshop on "Measuring Global Health: An International Workshop on the Political, Social and Ethical Aspects of Metrics and Quantification in Global Health," King's College, London, January 27, 2017.

20. However, the World Mental Health authors noted an absence of mental health statistics and systematic data at the WHO while they were preparing their report in the early 1990s (interview with Robert Desjarlais by A. Lovell, C. Lang, and U. Read, June 22, 2017).

21. Interview with Robert Desjarlais by A. Lovell, C. Lang and U. Read, June 22, 2017.

22. An unintended effect of field research is that the researcher's questions can provoke changes in an area up until then ignored. In this case, the current mental health leadership expresses interest in statistics.

23. Joy Lawn was, for ten years, the director of the Global Evidence and Policy for Saving Newborn Lives program (funded by the Gates Foundation) of Save the Children.

24. Interview with Bernadette Modell, geneticist, by Jean-Paul Gaudillière and Claire Beaudevin, November 24, 2016.

25. Interview with Bernadette Modell, November 24, 2016.

26. Interview with Bernadette Modell, November 24, 2016.

27. The database is a research output of UCL (University College London). A list of core resources and associated work is available at http://www.mgdb.info/.

28. Interview with Bernadette Modell, November 24, 2016.

29. Interview with Bernadette Modell, November 24, 2016.

30. Interview with Dan Chisolm, May 3, 2019.

CHAPTER 3 — TRIAGE BEYOND THE CLINIC

1. For one of the best analyses of the PHC context (i.e., its links to the rise of the Third World as well as its relations with the 1970s U.N. agenda for a "new international economic order"), see *The World Health Organization between North and South*, especially chapter 3 (Chorev 2012).

2. What follows is a prelude to a proper thematic analysis of the Alma-Ata preparatory debates, especially in WHO regional offices, beginning with the Southeast Asia regional

office (SEARO), for which there is a wealth of material in the WHO archives. All quotes are from the final report of the conference (International Conference on Primary Health Care, World Health Organization et al. 1978).

3. A. Yazbeck, J. P. Tan, and V. L. Tanzi, "Public Spending in Health in the 1980s: The Impact of Adjustment Lending Programs," August 1995, Internal report, Folder 39272, World Bank Group Archives, Washington, DC.

4. D. De Ferranti, "Health Resources in Developing Countries: How Should They Be Allocated?," February 1985, Draft memo, Folder 1104184, World Bank Group Archives.

5. World Bank Archives De Ferranti, "Health Resources in Developing Countries: How Should They Be Allocated?," May 14, 1985, Draft Population, Health, and Nutrition Paper, Folder 1104184, World Bank Group Archives, quote p. 14.

6. Interview of an Ahmedabad-based health economist, conducted by A. McDowell and J.-P. Gaudillière, New Delhi, India, January 2017.

7. Nils Brimnes's detailed study of India's postcolonial TB intervention supports the argument that the early program was to act in the interim to treat those who suffered from TB in the present (Brimnes 2016).

8. Though caused by a single species of bacteria, TB's bodily manifestations can be varied. Most often TB afflicts the lungs, but it can also afflict lymph nodes, the intestine and stomach, bones, the uterus, and the brain.

9. WHO mission report submitted to SIDA office, New Delhi, January 23, 1992. Rijksarkivet-Täby, Arninge, Sweden. SIDA Indien Bistankontoret 1.24 Ind 22.7 Rapporter Tuberculosisbekampning 1979–1993 F22: 3.

10. World Bank Aide-Memoire, "India: Proposed Tuberculosis Control Project, Preappraisal Mission," February 28, 1995, M. D. Clark, Annex B, p. 10, File 30283576, World Bank Group Archives.

11. Personal interview, Delhi, India, August 2016.

12. Personal interview, Mumbai, India, September 2016.

13. Qaboos bin Said Al Said died on January 10, 2020. His successor is one of his cousins, Haitham bin Tariq Al Said.

14. At the time, besides some military facilities, there were only two missionary hospitals, the small British Consulate hospital, and the hospital of the national oil company—for a total of about 250 beds in the country.

15. Oman's first Minister of Health, personal interview, C. Beaudevin, Muscat, Oman, November 30, 2008.

16. Oman's first Minister of Health, personal interview, C. Beaudevin, Muscat, Oman, November 30, 2008.

17. Interview with B. Modell conducted by J.-P. Gaudillière and C. Beaudevin, London, November 2016.

18. Task shifting is defined by the WHO as situations where "specific tasks are moved, where appropriate, from highly qualified health workers to health workers with shorter training and fewer qualifications in order to make more efficient use of the available human resources for health" (World Health Organization, PEPFAR et al. 2008).

19. These high-risk groups include (a) patients on palliative care, (b) caregivers for all diseases, (c) persons with a history of deliberate self-harm, (d) recent life events such as job loss, (e) substance abuse, and (f) spouses of those with substance abuse.

20. Interview conducted by C. Lang, Thiruvananthapuram, India, January 2018.

21. All interviews were conducted in the Thiruvananthapuram district, between 2016 and 2019.

22. Interview conducted by C. Lang, Thiruvananthapuram, January 2018

23. Village councils are a South Asian form of local self-governance or participatory local democracy that gained new political power in Kerala with the People's Campaign for Decentralized Planning, launched in 1996, which emphasized participatory, community-based sustainable development (Isaac and Franke 2002). Under the new system, policymakers brought primary health centers and subcenters under the responsibility of the *panchayats*.

CHAPTER 4 — MARKETS, MEDICINES, AND HEALTH GLOBALIZATION

1. See World Bank Memo to Indian Ministry of Health and Family Welfare, Department of Economic Affairs. 25 February, 1998. WHO Archive T/ 16/181/M2/119, TSA (B).

2. WHO prequalification aims to ensure that medicines meet global quality, safety, and efficacy standards. The prequalification process consists of a scientifically sound assessment including drug testing, performance evaluation, and site visits to drug manufacturers. It also aims to ensure the similarity of a generic to the reference medicine by requiring that manufacturing plants comply with the Current Good Manufacturing Practices and that the generic is bioequivalent to the original medicine.

3. There is no shortage of criticism leveled at WHO policy. The WHO's response to this criticism is swift but measured. International aid organizations have been demanding that the WHO validate generic drugs demonstrating suitability as an alternative to Coartem. Several public–private partnerships are acting on this demand for local alternatives.

4. Prequalifying a medicine is very costly for the firm and requires investments that local firms cannot afford.

5. Artesunate-amodiaquine is also cheaper than artemether-lumefantrine.

6. Himalaya Ayurveda specialists realize that the need for a preparation like Menosan is therefore not due to the recognition of a previously invisible, unrecognized disorder but the emergence of a new problem, whose roots are in the changing structure of families and in processes of individualization and urbanization. In other words, menopause is a disease of modernity.

7. Two international surveys, conducted by Political and Economic Risk Consultancy in 2011 and Transparency International in 2013, identify Cambodia as one of the most corrupt countries in the world (cited in Bourdier, Man et al. 2014, 8).

CHAPTER 5 — TECH FOR ALL

1. Development scholars and economists coined this term for Kerala's development experience, which is characterized by low rates of birth and infant mortality and high life expectancy and literacy among men and women, in spite of relatively low levels of economic development. The Kerala model is often celebrated as an alternative to market-driven development.

2. The packages of care for depression in low- and middle-income countries include regular screening, psychoeducation, generic antidepressants, and practical skills for managing stress.

3. The *mhGAP Intervention Guide* is a technical tool developed by WHO to assist in the implementation and scaling up of services for mental, neurological, and substance use disorders in low- and middle-income countries. The program includes technopackages of assessment/detection and pharmacological and psychosocial interventions for prioritized conditions. For depression, it includes psychosocial interventions such as psychoeducation, social support, and reduction of stress, and promotes functioning in daily life and pharmacological treatments such as amitriptyline and fluoxetine.

4. Interview with pilot clinic physician, Delhi, July 2016; interview with pilot project laboratory technologist, July 2016.

5. Communication between SIDA offices in New Delhi and Stockholm. Rijksarkivet-Täby, Arninge, Sweden. SIDA Indien Bistankontoret 1.24/1 Ind 22.7 Tuberculosisbekampning 1994 F22: 8.

6. Interview, with pilot project director, New Delhi, August 2016.

7. Letter from Arata Kochi to Karel Styblo. WHO Archive, T9.Ind., 1994.

8. Internal memo sent between SIDA New Delhi and SIDA Stockholm. Rijksarkivet-Täby, Arninge, Sweden. SIDA Indien Bistankontoret 1.24 Ind 22.7 Rapporter Tuberculosisbekampning 1979–1993 F22: 3.

9. SNPs are locations in the DNA sequence where individuals differ at a single DNA base. SNPs that are close together on the same chromosome tend to be inherited in blocks. A pattern of SNPs on a block is a haplotype. Because they are inherited together in a block, identifying only a few SNPs (called tag SNPs) can be enough to determine the haplotype they form. This greatly reduces the information that needs to be read in sequencing projects, from the 10 million SNPs existing in a genome to roughly 500,000 tag SNPs. These techniques of selection—of tag SNPs, often on the basis of frequency—and deduction determined which tag SNPs would be designated as the ones marking a haplotype, what future researchers would look for, and what they would ignore when determining the haplotype of the population they studied.

10. For example, the ABC-A1 gene variant R230C has been associated with obesity and diabetes in Mexican mestizos and described as a variant exclusive to Amerindian and "descent populations" (Acuña-Alonzo et al. 2010; Villarreal-Molina et al. 2008). Such a description shows the use of a genetic marker to distinguish and simultaneously connect population groups. The Indigenous component is taken to be the living representation of the ancestral Amerindian population. It appears to contribute the disease-prone gene variant to the mestizo profile but is also what makes the mestizo genome singular.

11. A summary of the study's findings was published in *PNAS: Proceedings of the National Academy of Sciences of the United States of America* (Silva-Zolezzi, Hidalgo-Miranda et al. 2009).

CHAPTER 6 — PERSISTENT HOSPITALS

1. See chapter 3, "Triage beyond the Clinic," for more information about primary health care in Oman.

2. This situation is of course not unique to Oman, however. Cuts in the resources allocated to health (related to financial crises and structural adjustments) have major impacts on healthcare systems and individual health decision making worldwide, the most recent European examples being Greece and Spain (Pfeiffer and Chapman 2010; Brand, Rosenkotter et al. 2013; Karanikolos, Mladovsky et al. 2013; Kehr 2014).

3. WhatsApp does not store messages on servers, though (except when delivery fails), which makes this messenger service a somehow safer solution than email for circulating medical information.

4. Among these databases are RefSeq or ClinVar. The latter, according to the National Center for Biotechnology Information, is introduced as "a freely accessible, public archive of reports of the relationships among human variations and phenotypes, with [accessible] supporting evidence" (https://www.ncbi.nlm.nih.gov/clinvar/intro/).

5. Interview with Kibong'oto hospital director, February 2018.

6. LHL International is a branch of the Norwegian Heart and Lung Association while KNCV (Koninklijke Nederlandse Centrale Vereniging tot bestrijding der Tuberculose) is a Royal Dutch NGO.

7. In opposition to natural ventilation, a mechanical system refers to technical systems that improve circulation and air quality in buildings.

8. Interview with Kibong'oto hospital director, February 2018.

9. Interview with Kibong'oto hospital nurse, thirty-five year old, head of quality improvement unit, February 2018.

10. Interview with nurse M, twenty-six year old, February 2017.

11. Interview with Nurse R, fifty-six years old and working in Kibong'oto since 1981, February 2018.

12. Interview, medical attendant, fifty-five years old, February 2018.

13. Interview Nurse M., twenty-six years old, February 2017.

14. Interview with a neighbor who worked in the Kibong'oto hospital for forty years (from 1958 until 1998), February 2017.

15. Global mental health also ignores other forms of Indigenous mental healthcare, such as traditional medicine or ritual healing (Sax and Lang 2020).

16. Interview with the psychiatrist, Bengaluru, India, February 2018.

17. "Designation and Activities of the WHO Collaborating Center for Research and Training in Mental Health—The National Institute of Mental Health and Neurosciences—Bangalore India," 1986, folder M4/286/4(U), WHO archives.

18. Many of these projects are assembled in the Mental Health Innovation Network, "a community of mental health innovators—researchers, practitioners, policy-makers, service user advocates, and donors from around the world—sharing innovative resources and ideas to promote mental health and improve the lives of people with mental, neurological and substance use disorders," as its website states (https://www.mhinnovation.net/about).

19. National Institute of Mental Health and Neurosciences, "NIMHANS Centre Well Being," web page, last updated June 28, 2018, http://www.nimhans.ac.in/nimhans-centre-well-being.

CHAPTER 7 — PROVINCIALIZING THE WHO

1. See, most recently, Cueto, Brown et al. (2019, 239–279), where the authors analyzed the 1990s, a decade in which the WHO was in a deep crisis with regards to political influence and finance. N. Chorev (2012) authored a comprehensive analysis of the WHO from the 1970s to the 1990s, which also views the period as one of crisis. For the Rockefeller Foundation, see Farley (2004).

2. The WHO is modernizing its Geneva headquarters campus. The journey to WHO's new headquarters campus will take eight years, from 2017 to 2024; see "An Overview of the WHO Building Renovation Strategy," 2016 brochure, https://www.who.int/about/structure/modernizing-who-headquarters.pdf.

3. The perspective of India during this period is well described by Brimnes (2016).

4. Additional details about the MRC trials are collected in Fox, Ellard et al. (1999); McMillen (2015, chap. 8 and 9).

5. East African Tuberculosis Trials," memorandum, December 2, 1962, Kew, Richmond/UK, FD 12/552, 13, The National Archives.

6. Letter from Mahler to Rouillon, April 21, 1983, T9/348/2, No. 3, WHO archives.

7. Interview with Arata Kochi, former director of the WHO's tuberculosis programs, November 2017.

8. J. Lee, "WHO/IBRD [International Bank for Reconstruction and Development]," February 19, 1975, Draft memo, File 30134432, World Bank Group Archives, Washington, DC (hereafter WB archives).

9. S. Boskey, "Visit to WHO," March 19, 1975, memo, File 30134432, WB archives.

10. Boskey, "Visit to WHO," 4.

11. Boskey, "Visit to WHO," 5.

12. "Collaboration with IBRD in Family Planning," letter from K. Kanagaratnam (WB), January 14, 1981, P13-372-5, Jacket 3, WHO archives.

13. Cable WPRO to Geneva, April 13, 1978, P-3-372-5, Jacket 2 (1975–79), WHO archives.

14. Lee Howard, "Major Issues Affecting the Mobilization of Resources for Health for All by the Year 2000," 1981, Folder B 12/87/4 (80), J1, WHO archives

15. "Report on the Consultation on the Health 2000 Resources Group Geneva," December 10–11, 1979, HRG/CON/79.7, Folder B 12/87/4, J1, WHO archives.

16. "Report of the First Meeting of the Health 2000 Resources Group," May 1–2, 1980, Folder B 12/87/4 (80), J 1, WHO archives.

17. "Report of the First Meeting of the Health 2000 Resources Group." In 1979, for the first time, the regular budget was less than half of the total amount expended.

18. "Report of the First Meeting of the Health 2000 Resources Group."

19. "Report on the Consultation on the Health 2000 Resources Group Geneva."

20. "Report on the Consultation on the Health 2000 Resources Group Geneva."

21. "Report on the Consultation on the Health 2000 Resources Group Geneva."

22. The group also included representatives of the Christian Medical Commission, the USSR, and Malawi in representation of "developing countries," along with WHO secretariat members.

23. Cited in "J. Kilgour to Members of the HRG Steering Committee," February 5, 1981, B 12/87/4 (81), J1, WHO archives.

24. "Guidelines for Analysis of Country Resource Utilization for Primary Health Care," 1981, B 12/87/4 (80), J1, WHO archives.

25. "H. Mahler to Regional Directors," April 23, 1981, B 12/445/2 SRL, WHO archives.

26. "Health Resources Group for Primary Health Care. Report on the Second Meeting of the Steering Committee, Geneva," July 2–3, 1981, B 12/87/4(81), J1, WHO archives.

27. "J. Evans to J. Kilgour," February 2, 1982, B12/87/4(81), J2 (cf), WHO archives.

28. "J. Mashler to J. Kilgour," July 20, 1982, B 12/87/4, WHO archives.

29. "Health Resources Group for Primary Health Care (HRG) Progress Report as at 31 October 1983 HRG/Prog. Rep/83.2," B 12/87/4 (83), WHO archives.

30. "Health Resources Group for PHC—Second Meeting of the Steering Committee, Geneva," July 2–3, 1981, summary records, B 12/87/4(81), J1, WHO archives.

31. Mr. Warford, WB representative, "Draft: Health Resources Group for Primary Health Care—Report on the Third Meeting of the Committee of the HRG, Geneva," December 12–13, 1983, B 12/87/4(83), WHO archives, p. 12.

32. Mr. Warford, "Draft: Health Resources Group for Primary Health Care."

33. "Health Resources Group for Primary Health Care. Progress Report as at 30 June 1984," B12/87/4 (84), WHO archives.

34. "H. Mahler to Regional Directors," May 31, 1985, B 12/87/4 (85), WHO archives. Despite the termination of the HRG, until the end of the 1980s, WHO headquarters continued to be solicited for assistance with CRUs in member countries.

35. World Health Organization Executive Board, "Planning of the Finances of Health for All: Economic Strategies to Support the Strategy for Health for All: Report by the Director-General," November 4, 1985, Provisional agenda item 11.2, EB77/INF.DOC./1, WHO archives.

36. "Proposal for Task Group Meeting on HMG Programme," Memorandum from Kuliev to Director-General, May 15, 1981, G3-87-5, WHO archives.

37. Interview with A. Kuliev conducted by L. Ruault, Chicago, December 2018.

38. Interview with R. Williamson, Paris, January 2019.

39. The temporary advisers invited to the Task Group Meeting on WHO HGP were W. Schull (United States), N. Bochkov (USSR), J. Edwards (United Kingdom), F. Epstein

(Switzerland), A. Boyo (Nigeria), and I. C Verma (India). The "difficulty" of reforming the HGP by focusing on hemoglobinopathies notably stemmed from the commitment of these older experts to the study of the impact of radiation on human genetics. For instance, J. V. Neel (professor of human genetics, Michigan), member of the Expert Advisory Panel on Human Genetics since 1957, commented in a 1983 draft report of the November 1982 meetings in Geneva: "The statement there, about the 'urgent need' for a definitive statement on the impact of radiation by an expert group of *human* geneticists, is about the sharpest statement that appears in the entire document. I agree with it wholeheartedly." Letter sent by James V. Neel to Anver Kuliev, March 24, 1983. WHO archives, G3-87-6.

40. Interview with B. Modell, London, November 2016.

41. "Report of a WHO Advisory Group, Community Approaches to the Control of Hereditary Diseases, Geneva," October 3–5, 1985, HDP/WG/85.10, WHO archives.

42. Interview with A. Kuliev, Chicago, December 2018.

43. Or, conversely, the articulation of "prevention and care," as it was sometimes called, starting in the late 1990s, under the influence of the pediatrician Arnold Christianson, who had long been caring for children with Down syndrome. The prevailing order of words ("prevention" coming before "care") somehow reflects the emphasis put on prospective strategies among WHO experts.

44. Interview with A. Kuliev, Chicago, December 2018.

45. "Report of a WHO Advisory Group, Community Approaches to the Control of Hereditary Diseases, Geneva," October 3–5, 1985; see also Modell, Kuliev et al. (1991).

46. Interview with R. Williamson, Paris, January 2019.

47. From the minutes of a meeting held in Cagliari, Sardinia, September 6, 1981, in association with the International Congress on Recent Advances in Thalassaemia, to discuss the desirability of a WHO program for the control of hemoglobinopathies, p.3, Robert Williamson's personal archives.

48. "Report of a WHO Advisory Group, Community Approaches to the Control of Hereditary Diseases," Geneva, October 3–5, 1985.

49. These various reports from the WHO archives included, for example, *Guidelines on the Prevention and Control of Congenital Hypothyroidism* (1990, WHO/HDP/CON.HYPO/GL/90.4) and *on PKU* (1990, WHO/HDP/PKU/GL/90.4); *Guidelines for the Development of National Programmes for Monitoring Birth Defects* (1993, WHO/HDP/ICBDMS/GL/93.4) and *for the Control of Haemoglobin Disorders* (1994, WHO/HDP/HB/GL/94.1); *Guidelines on Ethical Issues in Medical Genetics and the Provision of Genetics Services* (1995, WHO/HDP/GL/ETH/95.1); *Guidelines for the Diagnosis and Management of Cystic Fibrosis* (1996, WHO/HGN/ICF(M)A/GL/96.2). Such reports multiply from 1994 to 1997.

50. See Boyo, Cao et al. (1983); "Report of a WHO Advisory Group, Community Approaches to the Control of Hereditary Diseases, Geneva," October 3–5, 1985.

51. "Letter from Bulyzhenkov to Nemat Hashem (Professor of Paediatrics and Genetics, Cairo)," January 11, 1994, G3-370-1, WHO archives.

52. The first mention of this concept in EMRO annual reports dates back to 1993.

53. See, in particular, Alwan and Modell (1997).

54. A January 1999 meeting in The Hague paid tribute to the involvement of the Pan American Health Organization (PAHO) and EMRO over the previous ten or fifteen years (see World Health Organization 1999).

55. The standard formulation that opens these report is, "This document is not a formal publication of the World Health Organization. . . . The views expressed in documents by named authors are solely the responsibility of those authors..

56. Email sent by Robert Williamson to Victor Boulyjenkov, April 2005, Williamson's personal archives.

57. Interview with M. Katz, New York, December 2018.

58. Interview with V. Boulyjenkov, Geneva, April 2019.

59. On the establishment of diplomatic relations with other African countries, see the table from the Ministry of Foreign Affairs of the People's Republic of China, October 18, 2004, http://www.fmprc.gov.cn/ce/ceza/eng/zghfz/zfgx/t165322.htm.

60. African countries for this assistance include Tanzania, Zambia, Guinea, and Somalia. See consultations of the Chinese archives, the Central People's Government of the People's Republic of China, 2010–2012, http://www.gov.cn/zwgk/2010-12/23/content_1771638.htm.

61. See A. Li (2000).

62. "Aux petits soins pour l'Afrique," July 7, 2015, *La Chine au présent*, http://french.peopledaily.com.cn/n/2015/0707/c96852-8916700.html.

63. The forum takes place every three years. The last one was held in 2018 in Beijing.

64. English translation of this policy is available at https://www.fmprc.gov.cn/zflt/eng/zgdfzzc/t481748.htm..

65. See Men and Barton (2011, 47), especially the table on China supported anti-malaria centers in Africa.

66. State Administration of Traditional Chinese Medicine, "'One Belt, One Road'" Development Plan for Traditional Chinese Medicine (2016–2020)," May 16, 2017, http://bgs.satcm.gov.cn/gongzuodongtai/2018-03-24/1330.html.

67. Initially known as the One Belt, One Road Initiative.

References

Acuña-Alonzo, V., T. Flores-Dorantes., J. K. Kruit, T. Villarreal-Molina, O. Arellano-Campos, T. Hünemeier, A. Moreno-Estrada, M. G. Ortiz-López, H. Villamil-Ramírez, P. León-Mimila, M. Villalobos-Comparan, L. Jacobo-Albavera, S. Ramírez-Jiménez, M. Sikora, L. H. Zhang, T. D. Pape, A. Granados-Silvestre Mde, I. Montufar-Robles, A. M. Tito-Alvarez, C, Zurita-Salinas, J. Bustos-Arriaga, L. Cedillo-Barrón, C. Gómez-Trejo, R. Barquera-Lozano, J. P. Vieira-Filho, J. Granados, S. Romero-Hidalgo, A. Huertas-Vázquez, A. González-Martín, A. Gorostiza, S. L. Bonatto, M. Rodríguez-Cruz, L. Wang, T. Tusié-Luna, C. A. Aguilar-Salinas, R. Lisker, R. S. Moises, M. Menjivar, F. M. Salzano, W. C. Knowler, M. C. Bortolini, M. R. Hayden, L. J. Baier, and S. Canizales-Quinteros. 2010. "A Functional ABCA1 Gene Variant is Associated with Low HDL-Cholesterol Levels and Shows Evidence of Positive Selection in Native Americans." *Human Molecular Genetics* 19 (14): 2877–2885.

Adams, V. 2016a. "Metrics of the Global Sovereign: Numbers and Stories in Global Health." In *Metrics: What Counts in Global Health*, edited by Vincanne Adams, 19–57. Durham, NC: Duke University Press.

———, ed. 2016b. *Metrics: What Counts in Global Health*. Durham, NC: Duke University Press.

Adams, V, and J. Biehl. 2016. "The Work of Evidence in Critical Global Health." *Medicine Anthropology Theory* 3 (2): 123–126. doi:10.17157/mat.3.2.432.

Agarwal, S. P., and L. S. Chauhan. 2005. *Tuberculosis Control in India*. New Delhi: Directorate General of Health Services, Ministry of Health and Family Welfare.

Agudelo, C. A. 1983. "Community Participation in Health Activities: Some Concepts and Appraisal Criteria." *Bulletin of the Pan American Health Organization* 17 (4): 375–386.

Akerele, O. 1987. "The Best of Both Worlds: Bringing Traditional Medicine Up to Date." *Social Science and Medicine* 24:177–181.

Akin, J. 1987. *Financing Health Services in Developing Countries: An Agenda for Reform*. Washington, DC: World Bank.

Akrich, M. 1992. "The De-scription of Technical Objects." In *Shaping Technology/Building Society: Studies in Sociotechnical Change*, edited by Wiebe E. Bijker and John Law, 205–224. Cambridge, MA: MIT Press.

Al-Araimi, M. S. 2016. *Genetic Counselling Training Course*. Muscat, Oman: National Genetic Centre.

Al Dahdah, M. 2017. "Health at Her Fingertips: Development, Gender and Empowering Technologies." *Gender, Technology and Development* 21 (1–2): 135–151.

Al-Riyami, A. 2000. *National Genetic Blood Disorders Survey.* Muscat, Oman: Ministry of Health.

Alwan, A., and B. Modell B. 1997. *Community Control of Genetic and Congenital Disorders.* EMRO Technical Publications Series. Alexandria: World Health Organization, Eastern Mediterranean Regional Office.

Amin, A. 2014. "Lively Infrastructure." *Theory, Culture, and Society* 31 (7–8): 137–161.

Amrith, S. 2004. "In Search of a 'Magic Bullet' for Tuberculosis: South India and Beyond, 1955–1965." *Social History of Medicine* 17 (1): 113–130.

Amrith, S. S. 2006. *Decolonizing International Health: India and Southeast Asia, 1930–65.* Cambridge Imperial and Post-Colonial Studies Series. Basingstoke, UK: Palgrave Macmillan.

Andersen, S., and D. Banerji. 1963. "A Sociological Inquiry into an Urban Tuberculosis Control Programme in India." *Bulletin of the World Health Organization* 29 (5): 685–700.

Andersen, S., and G. Dahlstrom. 1983. *Review of SIDA/GoI Cooperation: Tuberculosis.* Copenhagen: Swedish International Development Agency.

Aneesh, A. 2015. *Neutral Accent: How Language, Labor, and Life Became Global.* Durham, NC: Duke University Press.

Angastiniotis, M. A., and M. G. Hadjiminas. 1981. "Prevention of Thalassaemia in Cyprus." *The Lancet* 14:369–371.

Angastiniotis, M. A., S. Kyriakidou, and M. G. Hadjiminas. 1986. "How Thalassaemia Was Controlled in Cyprus." *World Health Forum* 7:291–297.

Angastiniotis, M. A., B. Modell, P. Englezos, and V. Boulyjenkov. 1995. "Prevention and Control of Haemoglobinopathies." *Bulletin of the World Health Organization* 73 (3): 375–386.

Appadurai, A. 1996. *Modernity at Large: Cultural Dimensions of Globalization.* Minneapolis: University of Minnesota Press.

———. 2006. "The Thing Itself." *Public Culture* 18 (1): 15–21.

Arnesen, T., and E. Nord. 1999. "The Value of DALY Life: Problems with Ethics and Validity of Disability Adjusted Life Years." *British Medical Journal* 319 (7222): 1423–1425.

Arora, V., and R. Sarin. 2000. "Revised National Tuberculosis Control Programme: Indian Perspective." *Indian Journal of Chest Diseases and Allied Sciences* 42:21–26.

Attewell, G. 2007. *Refiguring Unani Tibb: Plural Healing in Late Colonial India.* Hyderabad, India: Orient Longman.

Ayimpam, S. 2014. *Economie de la débrouille à Kinshasa: Informalité, commerce et réseaux sociaux.* Paris: Karthala.

Banerjee, A. 2012. "BMC Rethinks Khar TB Clinic Upgrade Proposal." *Indian Express,* February 1.

Banerjee, A. V., E. Duflo, and R. Glennerster. 2008. "Putting Band-Aid on a Corpse: Incentives for Nurses in the Indian Public Health Care System." *Journal of the European Economic Association* 6 (2): 487–500.

Banerjee, M. 2009. *Power, Knowledge, Medicine. Ayurvedic Pharmaceuticals at Home and in the World.* Hyderabad, India: Orient Blackswan.

Banerji, D. 1967. "Behaviour of Tuberculosis Patients towards a Treatment Organisation Offering Limited Supervision." *India Journal of Tuberculosis* 14 (3): 156–172.

———. 1971. "Tuberculosis as a Problem of Social Planning in India." *NIHAE Bulletin* 4 (1): 9–25.

Baqué, M-H, and C. Biewer. 2013. *L'empowerment, une pratique émancipatrice?* Paris: La Découverte.

Bate, R. 2008. *Local Pharmaceutical Production in Developing Countries: How Economic Pro-tectionism Undermines Access to Quality Medicines*. London: Campaign for Fighting Diseases.

Baxter, A. J., G. Patton, K. M. Scott, L. Degenhardt, and H. A. Whiteford. 2013. "Global Epidemiology of Mental Disorders: What Are We Missing?" *PLoS One* 8 (6): e65514.

Baxter, A. J., K. M. Scott, A. J. Ferrari, R. E. Norman, T. Vos, and H. A. Whiteford. 2014. "Challeng-ing the Myth of an "Epidemic" of Common Mental Disorders: Trends in the Global Prevalence of Anxiety and Depression between 1990 and 2010." *Depression and Anxiety* 31 (6): 506–516.

Beaudevin, C. 2010. "Faqr al-dam, l'indigence du sang, comme héritage: représentation et enjeux sociaux des hémoglobinopathies héréditaires au sultanat d'Oman." PhD the-sis, Anthropology, Aix-Marseille University.

———. 2013. "Of Red Cells, Translocality and Origins: Inherited Blood Disorders in Oman." In *Regionalizing Oman: Political, Economic and Social Dynamics*, edited by Stef-fen Wippel, 91–105. Dordrecht: Springer Science.

———. 2015. "Cousin Marriages and Inherited Blood Disorders in the Sultanate of Oman." In *Cousin Marriage: Between Tradition, Globalisation and Genetic Risk*, edited by Alison Shaw and Aviad E. Raz, 65–87. London: Berghahn.

Becker, G. 1995. *Human Capital and Poverty Alleviation*. Vol. 52, *Human Resources Devel-opment and Operations Policy Working Papers*. Washington, DC: World Bank.

Behrends, A., S.-J. Park, and R. Rottenburg. 2014. "Travelling Models: Introducing an Analytical Concept to Globalisation Studies." In *Travelling Models in African Conflict Management: Translating Technologies of Social Ordering*, edited by Andrea Behrends, Sung-Joon Park, and Richard Rottenburg, 1–40. Leiden: Brill.

Bhattacharya, S. B. 2010. "Engaging Africa: India's Interest in the African Continent, Past and Present." In *The Rise of China and India in Africa: Challenges, Opportunities and Critical Interventions*, edited by F. Cheru and C. Obi, 63–76. London: Zed Books.

Bhattacharya, S. B., K.R.C Reddy, and A. K. Mishra. 2014. "Export Strategy for Ayurvedic Products from India." *International Journal of Ayurvedic Medicine* 5 (1): 125–128.

Bhore Committee. 1946. *Report of the Health Survey and Development Committee*. Delhi: Manager Publications.

Bieh, K. L., R. Weigel, and H. Smith. 2017. "Hospitalized Care for MDR-TB in Port Har-court, Nigeria: A Qualitative Study." *BMC Infectious Diseases* 17 (1): 50.

Biehl, J. 2007. "Pharmaceuticalization: AIDS Treatment and Global Health Politics." *Anthropological Quarterly* 80 (4): 1083–1126.

Biehl, J., and A. Petryna, eds. 2013. *When People Come First: Critical Studies in Global Health*. Princeton, NJ: Princeton University Press.

Birn, A.-E. 2006. *Marriage of Convenience: Rockefeller International Health and Revolu-tionary Mexico*. Rochester, NY: Boydell & Brewer.

———. 2009. "The Stages of International (Global) Health: Histories of Success or Suc-cesses of History?" *Global Public Health* 4 (1): 50–68.

Birn, A.-E., Y. Pillay, and T. H. Holtz. 2009. *Textbook of International Health: Global Health in a Dynamic World*. New York: Oxford University Press.

Blencowe, H., S. Moorthie, M. W. Darlison, S. Gibbons, B. Modell, and Congenital Disorders Expert Group. 2018. "Methods to Estimate Access to Care and the Effect of Interventions on the Outcomes of Congenital Disorders." *Journal of Community Genetics* 9 (4): 363–376.

Boateng, K. P. 2009. "A Study to Determine the Factors Affecting the Compliance of Local Pharmaceutical Manufacturers to International Best Practices in the Pharmaceutical Industry: A Case Study of Danadams Pharmaceutical Industry Limited," MBA thesis, Strategic and Project Management, Paris Graduate School of Management.

Bobadilla, J. L., P. Cowley, P. Musgrove, and H. Saxenian. 1994. "Design, Content and Financing of an Essential National Package of Health Services." *Bulletin of the World Health Organization* 72 (4): 653–662.

Boccagni, P. 2012. "Rethinking Transnational Studies: Transnational Ties and the Transnationalism of Everyday Life." *European Journal of Social Theory* 15 (1): 117–132.

Bode, M. 2008. *Taking Traditional Knowledge to the Market*. Hyderabad, India: Orient Longman.

———. 2013. "Evidence Based Traditional Medicine: For Whom and to What End?" *eJournal of Indian Medicine* 6:1–20.

Bonneuil, C., P.-B. Joly, and C. Marris. 2008. "Disentrenching Experiment: The Construction of GM-Crop Field Trials as a Social Problem." *Technology and Human Values* 33 (2): 201–229.

Borowy, I. 2009. *Coming to Terms with World Health: The League of Nations Health Organisation 1921–1946*. Frankfurt am Main: Lang.

Bourdier, F., B. Man, and P. Res. 2014. "La circulation non contrôlée des médicaments en Asie du Sud-Est et au Cambodge." *L'Espace Politique* 24.

Bourdieu, P. 1976. "Le champ scientifique." *Actes de la Recherche en Sciences Sociales* 2 (2–3): 88–104.

———. 1984. *Homo Academicus*. Paris: Editions de Minuit.

Bowker, G., and S. L. Star. 1999. *Sorting Things Out: Classification and Its Consequences*. Cambridge, MA: MIT Press.

Boyer, R. 1990. *The Regulation School*. New York: Columbia University Press.

Boyo, A., A. Cao, V. Der Kaloustian, J. Hercules, A. Kuliev, D. Loukopoulos, B. Modell, A. Motulsky, S. Pantelakis, A. Piel, J. Rosa, P. Wasi, D. Weatherall, and R. Williamson. 1983. "Community Control of Hereditary Anaemias: Memorandum from a WHO Meeting." *Bulletin of the World Health Organization* 61 (1): 63–80.

Brand, H., N. Rosenkotter, T. Clemens, and K. Michelsen. 2013. "Austerity Policies in Europe—Bad for Health." *British Medical Journal* 346 (June 13): f3716–f3716.

Brimnes, N. 2008. "BCG Vaccination and WHO's Global Strategy for Tuberculosis Control 1948–1983." *Social Science and Medicine* 67 (5): 863–873.

———. 2016. *Languished Hopes: Tuberculosis, The State and International Health in Twentieth Century India*. New Delhi: Orient Black Swan.

Brives, C., F. Le Marcis, and E. Sanabria. 2016. "What's in a Context? Tenses and Tensions in Evidence-Based Medicine." *Medical Anthropology* 35 (5): 369–376.

Brodwin, P. 2013. *Everyday Ethics: Voices from the Front Line of Community Psychiatry*. Berkeley: University of California Press.

———. 2015. "Technologies of the Self and Ethnographic Praxis." *Medical Anthropology* 36 (1): 77–82.

Brown, P. J. 2017. "Anthropologists in MalariaWorld." *Medical Anthropology* 36 (5): 479–484.

Brown, T. M., M. Cueto, and E. Fee. 2006. "The World Health Organization and the Transition from 'International" to 'Global' Public Health." *American Journal of Public Health* 96 (1): 62–72.

Brown, W. 2015. *Undoing the Demos: Neoliberalism's Stealth Revolution*. New York: Zone Books.

Bullard, A. 2007. "Imperial Networks and Postcolonial Independence: The Transition from Colonial to Transcultural Psychiatry." In *Psychiatry and Empire*, edited by Sloan Mahone and Megan Vaughan. London: Palgrave Macmillan.

Bureau-Point, E., M. To, and C. Baxerres. 2016. "Automédication ou Prescription? Les relations entre les vendeurs et les acheteurs de médicaments au Cambodge." In *Actes du Colloques "L'automédication en question."* Nantes, France: Université de Nantes.

Caduff, C. 2015. *The Pandemic Perhaps: Dramatic Events in a Public Culture of Danger.* Oakland: University of California Press.

Caminero, L. J. 2003. *A Tuberculosis Guide for Specialist Physician.* Paris: International Union Against TB and Lung Disease.

Carpenter, D. 2010. *Reputation and Power: Organizational Image and Pharmaceutical Regulation at the FDA.* Princeton, NJ: Princeton University Press.

Casper, M. J., and A. E. Clarke. 1998. "Making the Pap Smear into the 'Right Tool' for the Job: Cervical Cancer Screening in the USA, circa 1940–95." *Social Studies of Science* 28 (2): 255–290.

Cassier, M., and Correa, M. 2003. "Patents, Innovation and Public Health: Brazilian Public-Sector Laboratories' Experience in Copying AIDS Drugs." In *Economics of AIDS and Access to HIV/AIDS Care in Developing Countries: Issues and Challenges,* 89–107. Paris: ANRS.

———. 2009. "Eloge de la copie: le reverse engineering des antirétroviraux contre le VIH/Sida dans les laboratoires pharmaceutiques brésiliens." *Sciences Sociales et Santé* 27 (3): 77–103.

Caton, S. 2005. *Yemen Chronicle: An Anthropology of War and Mediation.* New York: Macmillan.

Chabrol, F. 2018. "Viral Hepatitis and a Hospital Infrastructure in Ruins in Cameroon." *Medical Anthropology* 37 (8): 645–658.

Chadarevian, S. de. 2015. "Human Population Studies and the World Health Organization." *Dynamics* 35 (2): 359–388.

Chakrabarty, D. 2008. *Provincializing Europe: Postcolonial Thought and Historical Difference.* New ed. Princeton, NJ: Princeton University Press.

Chand, M. 2010. "Comparing India with China in Africa." *Africa Quarterly* 50 (2): 14–21.

Chandler, C.I.R., and U. Beisel. 2017. "The Anthropology of Malaria: Locating the Social." *Medical Anthropology* 36 (5): 411–421.

Charlson, F. J., J. Dieleman, L. Singh, and H. A. Whiteford. 2017. "Donor Financing of Global Mental Health, 1995–2015: An Assessment of Trends, Channels, and Alignment with the Disease Burden." *PloS One* 12 (1): e01693841.

Chattoo, S. 2018. "Inherited Blood Disorders, Genetic Risk and Global Public Health: Framing 'Birth Defects' as Preventable in India." *Anthropology and Medicine* 25 (1): 30–49.

Chaudhuri, S. 2015. "Can Foreign Firms Promote Local Production of Pharmaceuticals in Africa?" In *Making Medicines in Africa,* edited by M. Mackintosh, G. Banda, P. Tibandebage, and W. Wamae. London: Palgrave Macmillan.

Chauveau, S. 1999. *L'invention pharmaceutique. La pharmacie française entre l'Etat et la société au XXè siècle.* Paris: Les Empecheurs de Penser en Rond.

Chavali, A. 2011. "World Health Partners." Center for Health Market Innovations and Indian School of Business, https://globalhealthsciences.ucsf.edu/sites/globalhealthsciences.ucsf.edu/files/pub/worldhealthpartners.pdf.

Chen, A. 2016. "A New Health Care Project Won Awards. But Did It Really Work?" *NPR: Goats and Soda,* October 22. https://www.npr.org/sections/goatsandsoda/2016/10/22/497672625/a-new-health-care-project-won-awards-but-did-it-really-work.

Chen, A., K. H. Jacobsen, A. A. Deshmuk, and S. B. Cantor. 2015. "The Evolution of the Disability-Adjusted Life Year (DALY)." *Socio-economic Planning Sciences* 49:10–15.

Chen, S., M. Pender, N. Jin, M. Merson, S. Tang, and S. Gloyd. 2019. "Chinese Medical Teams in Africa: A Flagship Program Facing Formidable Challenges." *Journal of Global Health* 9 (1): 0103011.

Chisholm, D., K. Sweeny, P. Sheehan, B. Rasmussen, F. Smit, P. Cuijpers, and S. Saxena. 2016. "Scaling-up Treatment of Depression And Anxiety: A Global Return on Investment Analysis." *The Lancet Psychiatry* 3 (5): 415–424.

Chorev, N. 2007. *Remaking U.S. Trade Policy: From Protectionism to Globalization*. Ithaca, NY: Cornell University Press.

———. 2012. *The World Health Organization between North and South*. Ithaca, NY: Cornell University Press.

———. 2015. "Narrowing the Gaps in Global Disputes: The Case of Counterfeits in Kenya." *Studies in Comparative International Development* 50 (2): 157–186.

———. 2016. "Good Drugs, Good Intentions, and the (Bumpy) Road to Development." *World Development Perspectives* 1 (C): 4–5.

———. 2019. *Give and Take: Development Foreign Aid and the Pharmaceutical Industry in East Africa*. Princeton, NJ: Princeton University Press.

Choy, T. 2011. *Ecologies of Comparison: An Ethnography of Endangerment in Hong Kong*. Durham, NC: Duke University Press.

Christianson, A., C. P. Howson, and B. Modell. 2006. *March of Dimes Global Report on Birth Defects: The Hidden Toll of Dying and Disabled Children*. New York: March of Dimes Birth Defects Foundation.

Clarke, A. E., and M. J. Casper. 1996. "From Simple Technology to Complex Arena: Classification of Pap Smears, 1917–90." *Medical Anthropology Quarterly* 10 (4): 601–623.

Clifford, J. 1997. *Routes: Travel and Translation in the Late Twentieth Century*. Cambridge, MA: Harvard University Press.

Coderey, C. 2020. "Introduction: Governance and Circulation of Asian Medicines." In *Circulation and Governance of Asian Medicine*, edited by Céline Coderey and Laurent Pordié, 1–23. London: Routledge.

Cohen, A., S. Chatterjee, and H. Minas. 2016. "Time for a Global Commission On Mental Health Institutions." *World Psychiatry* 15 (2): 116–117.

Cohen, A., and H. Minas. 2017. "Global Mental Health and Psychiatric Institutions in the 21st Century." *Epidemiology and Psychiatric Sciences* 26 (1): 4–9.

College of Medicine and Health Sciences. 2016. *College of Medicine and Health Science: Sultan Qaboos University Hospital—Annual Report 2015*. Muscat, Oman: Sultan Qaboos University.

Collier, S. J. 2011. *Post-Soviet Social: Neoliberalism, Social Modernity, Biopolitics*. Princeton NJ: Princeton University Press.

Collier, S. J., A. Lakoff, and P. Rabinow. 2004. "Biosecurity: Towards an Anthropology of the Contemporary." *Anthropology Today* 20 (5): 307.

Comaroff, J. 2007. "Beyond Bare Life: AIDS, (Bio)Politics, and the Neoliberal Order." *Public Culture* 19 (1): 197–219.

Condrau, F. 2007. "The Patient's View Meets the Clinical Gaze." *Social History of Medicine* 20: 525–540.

Connelly, M. 2008. *Fatal Misconception: The Struggle to Control World Population*. Cambridge, MA: Harvard University Press.

Conti, J. A, and M. O'Neil. 2007. "Studying Power: Qualitative Methods and the Global Elite." *Qualitative Research* 7 (1): 63–82.

Cooke, B., and U. Kothari. 2001. "The Case for Participation as Tyranny." In *Participation: The New Tyranny?*, edited by Bill Cooke and Uma Kothari, 1–17. New York: Zed Books.

Cooper, F. 2005. *Colonialism in Question: Theory, Knowledge, History*. San Francisco: University of California Press.

Cowan, R. S. 2008. *Heredity and Hope. The Case for Genetic Screening*. Cambridge, MA: Harvard University Press.

Craig, S. 2012. *Healing Elements: Efficacy and the Social Ecologies of Tibetan Medicine*. Berkeley: University of California Press.

Crane, J. 2013. *Scrambling for Africa: AIDS, Expertise, and the Rise of American Global Health Science*. Ithaca, NY: Cornell University Press.

Crooks, V., L. Turner, J. Snyder, R. Johnston, and P. Kingsbury. 2011. "Promoting Medical Tourism to India: Messages, Images, and the Marketing of International Patient Travel." *Social Science and Medicine* 72:726–732.

Cueto, M. 2004. "The Origins of Primary Health Care and Selective Primary Health Care." *American Journal of Public Health* 94 (11): 1864–1874.

———. 2007. *Cold War, Deadly Fevers: Malaria Eradication in Mexico, 1955–1975*. Washington, DC: Woodrow Wilson Center Press.

———. 2013. "A Return to the Magic Bullet? Malaria and Global Health in the Twenty-First Century." In *When People Come First: Critical Studies in Global Health*, edited by J. Biehl and A. Petryna, 10–30. Princeton, NJ: Princeton University Press.

Cueto, M., T. M. Brown, and E. Fee. 2019. *The World Health Organisation: A History*. Cambridge: Cambridge University Press.

Das, V. 1996. *Critical Events: An Anthropological Perspective on Contemporary India*. London: Oxford University Press.

Das, V., and D. Poole, eds. 2004. *Anthropology in the Margins of the State: Comparative Ethnographies*. Santa Fe, NM: School of American Research Press.

Davis, B., J. Ladner, K. Sams, E. Tekinturhan, D. de Korte, and J. Saba. 2013. "Artemisinin-Based Combination Therapy Availability and Use in the Private Sector of Five AMFm Phase 1 Countries." *Malaria Journal* 12:135–144.

Davis, E. A. 2018. "Global Side Effects: Counter-Clinics in Mental Health Care." *Medical Anthropology* 37 (1): 1–16.

de Laet, M., and A. Mol. 2000. "The Zimbabwe Bush Pump: Mechanics of a Fluid Technology." *Social Studies of Science* 30 (2): 225–263.

Desjarlais, R., L. Eisenberg, B. Good, and A. Kleinman. 1995. *World Mental Health: Problems and Priorities in Low-Income Countries*. New York: Oxford University Press.

Desrosières, A. 2002. *The Politics of Large Numbers: A History of Statistical Reasoning*. Cambridge, MA: Harvard University Press.

Director General of the World Health Organization and Executive Director of the United Nations Children's Fund. 1978. *Primary Health Care: A Joint Report*. Geneva: World Health Organization.

Dirlikov, E. 2015. "BRICS Health and Tuberculosis Control Collaborations during an Era of Global Health." *Medicine Anthropology Theory* 2 (1): 136.

Ditiu, L., and B. Kumar. 2012. "Tuberculosis Care: Why the Words We Use Matter." *International Journal of Tuberculosis and Lung Disease* 16 (6): 711.

Duclos, V. 2012. "Building Capacities: The Resurgence of Indo-African Techno Economic Cooperation." *India Review* 11 (4): 209–225.

Dumit, J. 2012. *Drugs for Life: How Pharmaceutical Companies Define Our Health*. Durham, NC: Duke University Press.

Dumoulin Kervran, D., M. Kleiche-Dray, and M. Quet. 2018. "Going South: How STS Could Think Science in and with the South?" *Tapuya: Latin American Science, Technology and Society* 1 (1): 280–305.

Eboko, F. 2015. *Repenser l'action politique en Afrique. Du sida à l'analyse de la globalisation des politiques publiques*. Vol. 45. Paris: Karthala.

Eboko, F., F. Bourdier, and C. Broqua. 2011. "Introduction." In *Les Suds face au sida: Quand la société civile se mobilise*, edited by F. Eboko, F. Bourdier, and C. Broqua. Marseille: IRD Editions.

Ecks, S. 2016. "Commentary: Ethnographic Critiques of Global Mental Health." *Transcultural Psychiatry* 53 (6): 804–808.

Elamon, J., R. W. Franke, and B. Ekbal B. 2000. "Decentralization of Health Services: The Kerala People's Campaign." *International Journal of Health Services* 34 (4): 681–708.

Engel, N. 2015. *Tuberculosis in India: A Case of Innovation and Control.* London: Orient Blackswan.

Epstein, H. 2007. *The Invisible Cure: Africa, the West, and the Fight against AIDS.* London: Penguin Books.

Erikson, S. 2019. "Global Health Futures? Reckoning with a Pandemic Bond." *Medicine Anthropology Theory* 6 (3): 77–108.

Ernst, W. 2007. "Madness and Colonial Spaces—British India, c. 1800–1947." In *Madness, Architecture and the Built Environment: Psychiatric Spaces in Historical Context,* edited by James Moran, Leslie Topp, and Johnathan Andrews. London: Routledge.

Escobar, A. 1995. *Encountering Development: The Making and Unmaking of the Third World.* Princeton Studies in Culture/Power/History. Princeton, NJ: Princeton University Press.

———. 2001. "Culture Sits in Places: Reflections on Globalism and Sublatern Strategies of Localization." *Political Geography* 20 (2): 139–174.

Evans, J., V. Crooks, and P. Kingsbury. 2009. "Theoretical Injections: On the Therapeutic Aesthetics of Medical Spaces." *Social Science and Medicine* 69 (5): 716–721.

Farley, J. 2004. *To Cast Out Disease: A History of the International Health Division of the Rockefeller Foundation (1913–1951).* London: Oxford University Press.

Farmer, P. 2005. *Pathologies of Power: Health, Human Rights, and the New War on the Poor.* Berkeley: University of California Press.

Fassin, D. 2007. *When Bodies Remember: Experiences and Politics of AIDS in South Africa.* Berkeley: University of California Press.

———. 2011. *Humanitarian Reason: A Moral History of the Present.* Berkeley: University of California Press.

———. 2012. "That Obscure Object of Global Health." In *Medical Anthropology at the Intersections: Histories, Activisms, and Futures,* edited by M. C. Inhorn and E. A. Wentzell, 95–115. Durham, NC: Duke University Press.

Feierman, S. 1985. "Struggles for Control: The Social Roots of Health and Healing in Modern Africa." *African Studies Review* 28 (2–3): 73–147.

———. 2019. "Writing History: Flow and Blockage in the Circulation of Knowledge: Keynote for the Regional Assembly of the African Humanities Program, Dar es Salaam, 30 January 2019." *Journal of Contemporary African Studies* 37 (1): 3–13.

Ferguson, J. 1990. *The Anti-Politics Machine: Development," Depoliticization, and Bureaucratic Power in Lesotho.* Cambridge: Cambridge University Press.

———. 2006. *Global Shadows: Africa in the Neoliberal World Order.* Durham, NC: Duke University Press.

Fernández, A., J. Haro, M. Martinez-Alonso, K. Demyttenaere, T. Brugha, J. Autonell, G. De Girolamo, S. Bernert, J. Lepine, and J. Alonso. 2007. "Treatment Adequacy for Anxiety and Depressive Disorders in Six European Countries." *British Journal of Psychiatry* 190 (2): 172–173.

Fitzgerald, D., N. Rose, and I. Singh. 2016. "Living Well in the Neuropolis." *Sociological Review* 64 (1): 221–237.

Foucault, M. 1973. *The Birth of the Clinic: An Archaeology of Medical Perception.* London: Routledge.

———. 1984. *The History of Sexuality, Vol. 3: The Care of the Self.* London: Penguin Books.

Foucault, M., M. Senellart, and Collège de France. 2008. *The Birth of Biopolitics: Lectures at the Collège de France, 1978–79.* New York: Palgrave Macmillan.

Fox, W., G. A. Ellard, and D. A. Mitchison. 1999. "Studies on the Treatment of Tuberculo-sis Undertaken by the British Medical Research Council Tuberculosis Units, 1946–1986, with Relevant Subsequent Publications." *International Journal of Tuberculosis and Lung Disease* 3 (10): S231–S279.

Frenk, J., J. L. Bobadilla, J. Sepulveda, and M. L. Cervantes. 1989. "Health Transition in Middle-Income Countries: New Challenges for Health Care." *Health Policy and Planning* 4 (1): 29–39.

Frenk, J., R. Lozano, and M. Á. González-Block. 1994. *Economía y Salud: Propuestas para el avance del sistema de salud en México, informe final*. Mexico City: Fundación Mexicana para la Salud.

Friedman, J. 1990. "Being in the World: Globalization and Localization." *Theory, Culture, and Society* 7 (2–3): 311–328.

Funk, M., B. Saraceno, N. Drew, and E. Faydi. 2008. "Integrating Mental Health into Pri-mary Healthcare." *Mental Health Family Medicine* 5 (1): 5–8.

FUNSALUD. 1994. *Economía y Salud: Propuestas para el avance del sistema de salud en Mexico, informe final*. Mexico City: Fundación Mexicana para la Salud.

García-Deister, V. 2014. "Laboratory Life of the Mexican Mestizo." In *Race Mixture, Nation, and Science in Latin America*, edited by Peter Wade, Carlos López-Beltrán, Eduardo Restrepo and Ricardo Ventura-Santos, 161–182. Durham, NC: Duke University Press.

Gaudillière, J.-P. 2008. "How Pharmaceuticals Became Patentable: The Production and Appropriation of Drugs in the Twentieth Century." *History & Technology* 24 (2): 99–106.

———. 2014a. "De la santé publique internationale à la santé globale: l'OMS, la Banque Mondiale et le gouvernement des thérapies chimiques." In *Le gouvernement des sciences à l'échelle globale*, edited by D. Pestre, 65–96. Paris: La Découverte.

———. 2014b. "An Indian Path to Biocapital? The Traditional Knowledge Digital Library (TKDL), Drug Patents and the Reformulation Regime of Contemporary Ayurveda." *East Asian Science Technology and Society* 8 (4): 391–415.

———. 2016. "Un nouvel ordre sanitaire international? Performance, néolibéralisme et outils du gouvernement médico-économique." *Ecologie et politique* 52 (1): 107–124.

Gaudillière, J.-P., and C. Gasnier. 2020. "From Washington DC to Washington State: The Global Burden of Disease Data Basis and the Political Economy of Global Health." In *Data Journeys in the Sciences*, edited by S. Tempini and N. Leonelli, 321–339. Berlin: Springer.

Gaudillière, J.-P., and V. Hess, eds. 2013. *Ways of Regulating Drugs in the 19th and 20th Cen-turies*. London: Palgrave Macmillan.

Gaudillière, J.-P., and U. Thoms, ed. 2015. *The Development of Scientific Marketing in the Twentieth Century*. New York: Pickering & Chatto.

Geissler, P. W. 2013a. "Public Secrets in Public Health: Knowing Not to Know While Mak-ing Scientific Knowledge." *American Ethnologist* 40 (1): 13–34.

———. 2013b. "Stuck in Ruins, or Up and Coming? The Shifting Geography of Urban Health Work in Kisumu, Kenya." *Africa* 83 (4): 539–560.

Gerrets, R. 2012. "Governing Malaria: How and Old Scourge Troubles Percepts in Social Theory." In *Rethinking Biomedicine and Governance in Africa*, edited by P. Wenzel Geissler, R. Rottenburg, and J. Zenker, 23–42. Bielefeld, Germany: Transcript Verlag.

Go, J., and M. Krause. 2016. *Fielding Transnationalism*. London: Wiley Blackwell.

Goffman, E. 1961. *Asylums*. New York: Anchor Books.

Goud, M. T., S. M. Al-Harassi, S. A. Al-Khalili, K. K. Al-Salmani, S. M. Al-Busaidy, and A. Rajab. 2005. "Incidence of Chromosome Abnormalities in the Sultanate of Oman." *Saudi Medical Journal* 26 (12): 1951–1957.

Gradmann, C. 2019. "Treatment on Trial: Tanzania's National Tuberculosis Program, the International Union Against Tuberculosis and Lung Disease, and the Road to DOTS, 1977–1991." *Journal of the History of Medicine and Allied Sciences* 74 (3): 316–343.

Greene, J. 2007. *Prescribing by Numbers: Drugs and the Definition of Disease*. Baltimore: Johns Hopkins University Press.

———. 2011. "Making Medicines Essential: The Emergent Centrality of Pharmaceuticals in Global Health." *BioSocieties* 6 (1): 10–33.

Greenwood, D. 2008. *Antimicrobial Drugs: Chronicle of a Twentieth Century Triumph*. Oxford: Oxford University Press.

Guinzburg, C., J. Tedeschi, and A. C. Tedeschi. 1993. "Microhistory: Two or Three Things That I Know about It." *Critical Inquiry* 20 (1): 10–35.

Gujit, I., and M. K. Shah. 1998. "Waking Up to Power, Conflict and Process." In *The Myth of Community: Gender Issues in Participatory Development*, edited by I. Gujit and M. K. Shah, 1–23. London: Intermediate Technology Publications.

Gupta, A., and J. Ferguson. 1992. "Beyond "Culture": Space, Identity and the Politics of Difference." *Cultural Anthropology* 7 (1): 6–23.

Gurav, R. 2011. "Khar TB Clinic to Be Upgraded to Hospital?" *Mid-day*, May 10. https://www.mid-day.com/articles/khar-tb-clinic-to-be-upgraded-to-hospital/121372.

Gururaj, G., M. Varghese, V. Benegal, G. Rao, K. Pathak, L. Singh, R. Mehta, D. Ram, T. Shibukumar, A. Kokane, R. Lenin Singh, B. Chavan, P. Sharma, C. Ramasubramanian, P. Dalal, S. Saha, S. Deuri, A. Giri, A. Kavishvar, V. Sinha, J. Thavody, R. Chatterji, B. Akoijam, S. Das, A. Kashyap, V. Ragavan, S. Singh, R. Misra, and NMHS Collaborators Group. 2016. *National Mental Health Survey of India, 2015–16: Prevalence, Patterns and Outcomes*. Bengaluru: National Institute of Mental Health and Neurosciences.

Gusterson, H. 1997. "Studying Up Revisited." *PoLAR* 20 (1): 114–119.

Halliburton, M. 1998. "Suicide: A Paradox of Development in Kerala." *Economic and Political Weekly* 33 (36/37): 2341–2345.

Haraway, D. J. 1997. *Modest Witness@Second_Millenium.FemaleMan©_Meets_On coMouse™: Feminism and Technoscience*. New York: Routledge.

Hardon, A., and R. Pool. 2016. "Anthropologists in Global Health Experiments." *Medical Anthropology* 35 (5): 447–451.

Hardon, A., and E. Sanabria. 2017. "Fluid Drugs: Revisiting the Anthropology of Pharmaceuticals." *Annual Review of Anthropology* 46:117–132.

Harper, I. 2014. *Development and Public Health in the Himalaya: Reflections on Healing in Contemporary Nepal*. London: Routledge.

Harper, I., and M. Parker. 2014. "The Politics and Anti-Politics of Infectious Disease Control." *Medical Anthropology* 33 (3): 198–205.

Harper, J., and M. Gyansa-Lutterodt. 2007. *The Viability of Pharmaceutical Manufacturing in Ghana to Address Priority Endemic Diseases in the West Africa Sub-Region*. Accra: Ghana Publishing.

Hayden, C. 2003. *When Nature Goes Public: The Making and Unmaking of Bioprospecting in Mexico*. Princeton, NJ: Princeton University Press.

———. 2007. "A Generic Solution? Pharmaceuticals and the Politics of the Similar in Mexico." *Current Anthropology* 48 (4): 475–495.

Hsu, E. 2002. ""The Medicine from China Has Rapid Effects": Chinese Medicine Patients in Tanzania." *Anthropology and Medicine* 9 (3): 291–313.

Hutchby, I. 2001. "Technologies, Texts and Affordances." *Sociology* 35 (2): 441–456.

Huvila, I. 2011. "The Politics of Boundary Objects: Hegemonic Interventions and the Making of a Document." *Journal of the American Society for Information Science and Technology* 62 (12): 2528–2539.

Inda, J. X., and R. Rosaldo, eds. 2002. *The Anthropology of Globalization: A Reader.* Oxford: Blackwell.

Indu, P. S., T. V. Anilkumar, R. Pisharody, P.S.S. Russell, D. Rajub, P. S. Sarma, S. Remadevi, K.R.L.I. Amma, A. Sheelamonic, and C. Andrade. 2017. "Prevalence of Depression and Past Suicide Attempt in Primary Care." *Asian Journal of Psychiatry* 27:48–52.

Ingold, T. C. 1997. "Eight Themes in the Anthropology of Technology." *Social Analysis: The International Journal of Social and Cultural Practice* 41 (1): 106–138.

Institute of Communications, Operations Research, and Community Involvement. 1988. *In-Depth Study on National Tuberculosis Program of India.* Bangalore: Institute of Communications, Operations Research, and Community Involvement.

International Conference on Primary Health Care, World Health Organization, and United Nations Children's Fund. 1978. *Primary Health Care: Report of the International Conference on Primary Health Care, Alma-Ata, USSR, September 6–12, 1978.* Geneva: World Health Organization.

International HapMap Consortium. 2005. "A Haplotype Map of the Human Genome." *Nature* 437 (7063): 1299–1320.

Isaac, M. 1986. *A Decade of Rural Mental Health Centre Sakalawara: 1976–86.* Bangalore: National Institute of Mental Health and Neurosciences. https://communitypsychiatry nimhans.files.wordpress.com/2012/10/sakalwara-nimhans.pdf.

Isaac, T. M. T. and R. W. Franke. 2002. *Local Democracy and Development: The Kerala People's Campaign for Decentralized Planning.* Lanham, MD: Rowman and Littlefield.

Jackson, M. D. 1989. *Paths Toward a Clearing: Radical Empiricism and Ethnographic Inquiry.* Bloomington: Indiana University Press.

Jacquemot, P. 2012. "Les systèmes de santé en Afrique et l'inégalité face aux soins." *Afrique contemporaine* 243 (3): 95–97.

Jagota, P. 2000. *Annals of the National Tuberculosis Institute, Bangalore.* Bangalore: The Institute.

Jain, S., and S. Jadhav. 2009. "Pills That Swallow Policy: Clinical Ethnography of a Community Mental Health Program in Northern India." *Transcultural Psychiatry* 46 (1): 60–85.

Jain, S., and P. Murthy. 2006. "Madmen and Specialists: The Clientele and the Staff of the Lunatic Asylum, Bangalore." *International Review of Psychiatry* 18 (4): 345–354.

Jamison, D. T., W. H. Mosley, A. R. Measham, and J. L. Bobadilla, eds. 1993. *Disease Control Priorities in Developing Countries.* New York: Oxford University Press.

Janes, C. 2002. "Buddhism, Science, and Market: The Globalisation of Tibetan Medicine." *Anthropology and Medicine* 9 (3): 267–289.

Janes, C., and K. Corbett. 2009. "Anthropology and Global Health." *Annual Review of Anthropology* 38:167–183.

Jerven, M. 2013. *Poor Numbers: How We Are Misled by African Development Statistics and What to Do about It.* Ithaca, NY: Cornell University Press.

Jiménez-Sánchez, G. 2003. "Developing a Platform for Genomic Medicine in Mexico." *Science* 300 (5617): 295–296.

Kachur, S. P., C. Black, S. Abdulla, and C Goodman. 2006. "Putting the Genie Back in the Bottle? Availability and Presentation of Oral Artemisinin Compounds at Retail Pharmacies in Urban Dar-es-Salaam." *Malaria Journal* 5 (1): 25.

Kahssay, H. M., and P. Oakley. 1999. *Community Involvement in Health Development: A Review of the Concept and Practice.* Geneva: World Health Organization.

Kamat, V. R. 2013. *Silent Violence: Global Health, Malaria, and Child Survival in Tanzania.* Tucson: University of Arizona Press.

Kapur, D., P. Lewis, and R. Webb. 1997. *The World Bank: Its First Half a Century.* Washington, DC: The Brookings Institution.

Karanikolos, M., P. Mladovsky, J. Cylus, S. Thomson, S. Basu, D. Stuckler, and M. McKee. 2013. "Financial Crisis, Austerity, and Health in Europe." *The Lancet* 381 (9874): 1323–1331.

Kehr, J. 2014. "Against Sick States: Ebola Protests in Austerity Spain." *Somatosphere*, October 22. http://somatosphere.net/2014/10/against-sick-states.html.

Kehr, J., and F. Chabrol. 2018. "L'hôpital." *Anthropologie & Santé* 16. http://journals .openedition.org/anthropologiesante/2997.

Kent, P. W. 1976. "Tanzania Tuberculosis Survey." *Bulletin of the International Union Against Tuberculosis and Lung Diseases* 51 (1): 303–309.

Keshavjee, S. 2014. *Blind Spot: How Neoliberalism Infiltrated Global Health.* California Series in Public Anthropology. Oakland: University of California Press.

Khatib, R. A., M. Selemani, G. A. Mrisho, I. M. Masanja, M. Amuri, M. H. Njozi, D. Kajungu, I. Kuepfer, S. M. Abdulla, and D. de Savigny. 2013. "Access to Artemisinin-based Antimalarial Treatment and Its Related Factors in Rural Tanzania." *Malaria Journal* 12 (155): 1–8.

Kim, J. Y. 2000. *Dying for Growth: Global Inequality and the Health of the Poor.* Monroe, ME: Common Courage Press.

Kleinman, A., and J. Kleinman. 1996. "The Appeal of Experience; The Dismay of Images: Cultural Appropriations of Suffering in Our Times." In *Social Suffering*, edited by Arthur Kleinman, Veena Das, and Margaret Lock, 1–24. Berkeley: University of California Press.

Koch, E. 2011. "Local Microbiologies of Tuberculosis: Insights from the Republic of Georgia." *Medical Anthropology* 30 (1): 81–101.

———. 2013. *Free Market Tuberculosis: Managing Epidemics in Post-Soviet Georgia.* Nashville, TN: Vanderbilt University Press.

Kochi, A. 1990–1991. "Ten-Year Collaboration of the IUATLD with National Tuberculosis Programmes in Developing Countries: WHO Standpoint." *Bulletin of the International Union Against Tuberculosis and Lung Diseases* 66 (supp.): 43–44.

Kohrt, B. A., L. Asher, A. Bhardwaj, M. Fazel, M.J.D. Jordans, B. B. Mutamba, A. Nadkarni, G. A. Pedersen, D. R. Singla, and V. Patel. 2018. "The Role of Communities in Mental Health Care in Low- and Middle-Income Countries: A Meta-Review of Components and Competencies." *International Journal of Environmental Research and Public Health* 15 (6): 1279.

Kuliev, A. M. 1986. "Thalassaemia Can Be Prevented." *World Health Forum* 7 (3): 286–290.

Kwankam, S. Y. 2004. "What e-Health Can Offer." *Bulletin of the World Health Organization* 82 (10): 1105–1107.

Lachenal, G., C. Lefève, and V.-K. Nguyen, eds. 2014. *La médecine du tri: Histoire, éthique, anthropologie.* Paris: Presses Universitaires de France.

Lakoff, A. 2010a. *Disaster and the Politics of Intervention.* New York: Columbia University Press.

———. 2010b. "Two Regimes of Global Health." *Humanity: An International Journal of Human Rights, Humanitarianism, and Development* 1 (1): 59–79.

———. 2017. *Unprepared: Global Health in a Time of Emergency.* Oakland: University of California Press.

Lakoff, A., and S. J. Collier. 2008. *Biosecurity Interventions: Global Health and Security in Question.* New York: Columbia University Press.

Landecker, H. 2013. "When the Control Becomes the Experiment." Sentinel Devices, *LIMN* 3.

Lang, C. 2018. *Depression in Kerala: Ayurveda and Mental Health Care in 21st Century India.* Routledge Studies in Health and Medical Anthropology. New York: Routledge.

———. 2019. "Inspecting Mental Health: Depression, Surveillance and Care in Kerala, South India." *Culture, Medicine and Psychiatry* 43:596–612.

Langford, J. 2002. *Fluent Bodies: Ayurvedic Remedies for Postcolonial Imbalance.* Durham, NC: Duke University Press.

Langwick, S. A. 2011. *Bodies, Politics, and African Healing: The Matter of Maladies in Tanzania.* Indianapolis: Indiana University Press.

Lantenois, C., and B. Coriat. 2014. "La 'préqualification' OMS: origines, déploiement et impacts sur la disponibilité des antirétroviraux dans les pays du Sud." *Sciences sociales et santé* 32 (1): 71–99.

Last, M., and G. L. Chavunduka. 1986. *The Professionalisation of African Medicine.* Manchester: Manchester University Press.

Latour, B., P. Mauguin, and G. Teil. 1992. "A Note on Socio-Technical Graphs." *Social Studies of Science* 22 (1): 33–57.

Latour, B., and S. Woolgar. 1979. *Laboratory Life: The Construction of Scientific Facts.* Beverly Hills, CA: Sage Publications.

Laxminarayan, R., J. Chow, and S. A. Sahid-Salles. 2010. "Intervention Cost-Effectiveness: Overview of Main Messages." In *Disease Control Priorities in Developing Countries.* 2nd ed., edited by Dean T. Jamison, Joel G. Breman, Anthony R. Measham, George Alleyne, Mariam Claeson, David B. Evans, Prabhat Jha, Anne Mills, and Philip Musgrove, 35–86. New York: Oxford University Press and the World Bank.

Leal, P. A. 2010. "Participation: The Ascendancy of a Buzzword in the Neo-Liberal Era." In *Deconstructing Development Discourse: Buzzwords and Fuzzwords*, edited by A. Cornwall and D. Eade, 539–548. Warwickshire, UK: Practical Action.

Levin, C., and D. Chisholm. 2013. "Cost-Effectiveness and Affordability of Interventions, Policies and Platforms." In *Mental, Neurological, and Substance Use Disorders*, edited by Vikram Patel, Dan Chisholm, Tarun Dua, Ramanan Laxminarayan, and Maria Elena Medina-Mora, 219–236. Washington, DC: World Bank Group.

Li, A. 2000. *A History of Chinese Overseas in Africa.* Beijing: Overseas Chinese Publishing House.

———. 2011. *Chinese Medical Cooperation in Africa: With Special Emphasis on the Medical Teams and Anti-Malaria Campaign.* Uppsala, Sweden: Nordiska Afrikainstitutet.

Li, T. M. 2011. "Rendering Society Technical: Government Through Community and the Ethnographic Turn at the World Bank in Indonesia." In *Adventures in Aidland: The Anthropology of Professionals In International Development*, edited by David Mosse, 57–80. New York: Berghahn.

Lindee, S. 2014. "Scaling Up: Human Genetics as a Cold War Network." *Studies in History and Philosophy of Biological and Biomedical Science* 47:185–190.

Lisker, R., A. Loria, S. Ibarra, and L. Sánchez-Medal. 1965. "Estudio sobre las características genéticas hematológicas en la Costa Chica de Oaxaca y Guerrero." *Salud Pública de México* 7 (1): 45–50.

Lisker, R., G. Zárate, and A. Loria. 1966. "Studies on Several Genetic Hematologic Traits of Mexicans IX: Abnormal Hemoglobins and Erythrocytic Glucose-6-Phosphate Dehydrogenase Deficiency in Several Indian tribes." *Blood* 27 (6): 824–830.

Livingston, J. 2012. *Improvising Medicine: An African Oncology Ward in an Emerging Cancer Epidemic.* Durham, NC: Duke University Press.

Lo, T. Q.-K. 2011. "Telemedicine Provision Centers and Reproductive Age Women in Rural Uttar Pradesh, India." PhD dissertation, Public Health, University of California at Berkeley. https://escholarship.org/uc/item/33w37940.

Lock, M., and V.-K. Nguyen. 2018. *An Anthropology of Biomedicine.* 2nd ed. New York: Wiley-Blackwell.

Loveday, M., K. Wallengren, J. Brust, J. Roberts, A. Voce, B. Margot, J. Ngozo, I. Master, G. Cassell, and N. Padayatchi. 2015. "Community-Based Care vs. Centralised Hospitalisation for MDR-TB Patients, KwaZulu-Natal, South Africa." *International Journal of Tuberculosis and Lung Disease* 19 (2): 163–171.

Lovell, A. M. Forthcoming. "Bringing Psychiatric Epidemiology to Senegal's 'Living Laboratory': Knowledge-Production and Erasure in the Margins of Science." In *Reimagining Psychiatric Epidemiology in a Global Frame: Towards a Social and Conceptual History*, edited by Anne M. Lovell and Gerald Oppenheimer. Rochester, NY: University of Rochester Press.

Lovell, A. M., U. Read, and C. Lang. 2019 "Genealogies and New Anthropologies of Global Mental Health." *Culture, Medicine, and Psychiatry* 43 (4): 519–547.

Lovell, A. M., and F. Susser E. 2014. "What Might Be a History of Psychiatric Epidemiology? Towards a Social History and Conceptual Account." *International Journal of Epidemiology* 43:i1–i5.

Löwy, I. 2001. *Virus, moustiques et modernité: La fièvre jaune au Brésil, entre science et politique*. Paris: Editions des archives contemporaines.

Ma, L. 2013. "Indian Ambassador Discusses Trade Ties." *Phnom Penh Post*, July 19, 2013.

Mackintosh, M., G. Banda, P. Tibandebage, and W. Wamae, eds. 2015. *Making Medicines in Africa*. London: Palgrave McMillan.

Maes, K. 2015. "Task-Shifting in Global Health: Mental Health Implications for Community Health Workers and Volunteers." In *Global Mental Health. Anthropological Perspectives*, edited by Brandon A. Kohrt and Emely Mendenhall, 291–308. Walnut Creek, CA: Left Coast Press.

Mahajan, M. 2018. "Philanthropy and the Nation-State in Global Health: The Gates Foundation in India." *Global Public Health* 13 (10): 1357–1368.

———. 2019. "The IHME in the Shifting Landscape of Global Health Metrics." *Global Policy* 10:110–120.

March, D., and G. M. Oppenheimer. 2014. "Social Disorder and Diagnostic Order: The U.S. Mental Hygiene Movement, the Midtown Manhattan Study and the Development of Psychiatric Epidemiology in the 20th Century." *International Journal of Epidemiology* 43:129–142.

Marcheco-Teruel, B. 2009. "Cuba's National Medical Genetics Program." *Medicc Review* 11 (1): 11–13.

Marcus, G. 1995. "Ethnography in/of the World System: The Emergence of Multi-Sited Ethnography." *Annual Review of Anthropology* 24:95–117.

Markovits, C., J. Pouchepadass, and S. Subrahmanyam. 2003. "Introduction: Circulation and Society under Colonial Rule." In *Society and Circulation: Mobile People and Itinerant Cultures in South Asia, 1750–1950*, edited by Claude Markovits, Jacques Pouchepadass, and Sanjay Subrahmanyam. New Delhi: Permanent Black.

Marks, H. M. 1997. *The Progress of Experiment: Science and Therapeutic Reform in the United States, 1900–1990*. New York: Cambridge University Press.

Martin, J. L. 2003. "What Is Field Theory?" *American Journal of Sociology* 109 (1): 1–49.

Maude, R. J., C. J. Woodrow, and L. J. White. 2010. "Artemisinin Antimalarials: Preserving the 'Magic Bullet.'" *Drug Development Research* 71 (1): 12–19.

McGoey, L. 2015. *No Such Thing as a Free Gift: The Gates Foundation and the Price of Philanthropy*. London: Verso.

McKay, R. 2018. *Medicine in the Meantime: The Work of Care in Mozambique*. Durham, NC: Duke University Press.

McMillen, C. W. 2015. *Discovering Tuberculosis: A Global History, 1900 to Present*. New Haven, CT: Yale University Press.

McMillen, H. 2004. "The Adapting Healer: Pioneering through Shifting Epidemiological and Sociocultural Landscapes." *Social Science and Medicine* 59 (5): 889–902.

McNamara, K. 2020. "WHOse Guidelines Matter? The Politics Of Regulating Traditional Medicine in Bangladesh." In *Circulation and Governance of Asian Medicine*, edited by Céline Codery and Laurent Pordié, 24–47. London: Routledge.

McQueston, K. 2014. "The Known Unknown: Estimating the Global Burden of Disease." *Center for Global Development*, June 19. https://www.cgdev.org/blog/known-unknown -estimating-global-burden-disease.

Meier zu Biesen, C. 2013. *Globale Epidemien—Lokale Antworten: Eine Ethnographie der Heilpflanze Artemisia annua in Tansania*. Frankfurt: Campus Verlag.

———. 2017. "From Coastal to Global: The Transnational Flow of Ayurveda and Its Relevance for Indo-African Linkages." *Global Public Health* 13 (3): 339–354.

———. 2019. "Globalized Planta Medica and Processes Of Drug Validation: The Artemisinin Enterprise." In *Circulation and Governance of Asian Medicine*, edited by C. Coderey and L. Pordié. London: Routledge.

Men, J., and B. Barton. 2011. *China and the European Union in Africa: Partners or Competitors?* Farnham, U.K.: Ashgate.

Méndez-Rosado, L. A., O. Quiñones, O. Molina Gamboa, N. González, M. del Sol, L. Maceiras, and Y. Bravo. 2014. "Antenatal Cytogenetic Testing in Havana, Cuba." *Medicc Review* 16 (3–4): 27–34.

Mercer, A. 2014. *Infections, Chronic Disease, and the Epidemiological Transition*. Rochester, NY: University of Rochester Press.

Merry, S. E. 2011. "Measuring the World: Indicators, Human Rights, and Global Governance." *Current Anthropology* 52 (S3): 583–593.

Mills, J. 2001. "The History of Modern Psychiatry in India, 1858–1947." *History of Psychiatry* 12 (48): 431–458.

Ministry of Health, Oman. 2017. *Annual Health Report 2016*. Muscat, Oman: Department of Health Information and Statistics, Directorate General of Planning.

———. 2020. *Annual Health Report 2019*. Muscat, Oman: Department of Health Information and Statistics, Directorate General of Planning.Modell, B., R. J. Berry, C. A. Boyle, A. Christianson, M. Darlison, H. Dolk, C. P. Howson, P. Mastroiacovo, P. Mossey, and J. Rankin. 2012. "Global Regional and National Causes of Child Mortality." *The Lancet* 380 (9853): 1556, author reply 1556–1557.

Modell, B., and A. Kuliev. 1998. "The History of Community Genetics: The Contribution of the Haemoglobin Disorders." *Community Genetics* 1:3–11.

Modell, B., A. N. Kuliev, and M. Wagner. 1991. *Community Genetic Services in Europe: Report on a Survey*. Vol. 38, WHO Regional Publications European Series. Copenhagen: World Health Organization. Regional Office for Europe.

Mohanan, M., K. Babiarz, J. Goldhaber-Fiebert, G. Miller, and M. Vera-Hernandez. 2016. "Effect of a Large-Scale Social Franchising and Telemedicine Program on Childhood Diarrhea and Pneumonia Outcomes in India." *Health Affairs* 35 (10): 1800–1809.

Mohanan, M., S. Giardili, V. Das, T. Rabin, S. Raj, J. Schwartz, A. Seth, J. Goldhaber-Fiebert, G. Miller, and M. Vera-Hernandez. 2017. "Evaluation of a Social Franchising and Telemedicine Programme and the Care Provided for Childhood Diarrhoea and Pneumonia, Bihar, India." *Bulletin of the World Health Organization* 95 (5): 313–388.

Moorthie, S., H. Blencowe, M. W. Darlison, S. Gibbons, J. E. Lawn, P. Mastroiacovo, J. K. Morris, B. Modell, and Congenital Disorders Expert Group. 2018. "Chromosomal Disorders: Estimating Baseline Birth Prevalence and Pregnancy Outcomes Worldwide." *Journal of Community Genetics* 9 (4): 377–386.

Moorthie, S., H. Blencowe, M. W. Darlison, J. E. Lawn, P. Mastroiacovo, J. K. Morris, and B. Modell. 2018. "An Overview of Concepts and Approaches Used in Estimating the Burden of Congenital Disorders Globally." *Journal of Community Genetics* 9 (4): 347–362.

Morgan, L. 1993. *Community Participation in Health: The Politics of Primary Care in Costa Rica*. Cambridge: Cambridge University Press.

———. 2001. "Community Participation in Health: Perpetual Allure, Persistent Challenge." *Health Policy and Planning* 16 (3): 221–230.

Morgan, M. 2012. *The World in the Model: How Economists Work and Think*. New York: Cambridge University Press.

Mudaliar Committee. 1962. *Report on the Health Survey and Planning Committee*. New Delhi: Government of India, Ministry of Health.

Muller, A. 1982. *The Health of Nations: A North–South Investigation*. London: Faber & Faber.

Muller, J. Z. 2018. *The Tyranny of Metrics*. Princeton, NJ: Princeton University Press.

Münster, D. 2012. "Farmers' Suicides and the State in India: Conceptual and Ethnographic Notes from Wayanad, Kerala." Special issue, *Contributions to Indian Sociology* 46 (1 + 2): 181–208.

Murphy, M. 2017. *The Economization of Life*. Durham, NC: Duke University Press.

Murray, C.J.L. 1994. "Quantifying the Burden of Disease: The Technical Basis for Disability-Adjusted Life Years." *Bulletin of the World Health Organization* 72 (3): 429–445.

Murray, C.J.L., E. Dejonghe, H. J. Chum, D. S. Nyangulu, A. Salomao, and K. Styblo. 1991. "Cost Effectiveness of Chemotherapy for Pulmonary Tuberculosis in Three Sub-Saharan African Countries." *The Lancet* 338 (8778): 1305–1308.

Murray, C.J.L., M. Ezzati, A. D. Flaxman, S. Lim, R. Lozano, C. Michaud, M. Naghavi, J. A. Salomon, K. Shibuya, T. Vos, and A. D. Lopez. 2012. "GBD 2010: Design, Definitions, and Metrics." *The Lancet* 380 (9859): 2063–2066.

Murray, C.J.L., A. D. Lopez, World Health Organization, World Bank, and Harvard School of Public Health, eds. 1996. *The Global Burden of Disease: A Comprehensive Assessment of Mortality and Disability from Diseases, Injuries, and Risk Factors in 1990 and Projected to 2020*. Cambridge, MA: Harvard University Press.

Murray, C.J.L., K. Styblo, and A. Rouillon. 1990. "Tuberculosis in Developing Countries: Burden, Intervention and Cost." *Bulletin of the International Union Against Tuberculosis and Lung Diseases* 65 (1): 6–24.

Murthy, P., M. Isaac, and H. Dabholkar. 2017. "Mental Hospitals in India in the 21st Century: Transformation and Relevance." *Epidemiology and Psychiatric Sciences* 26 (1): 10–15.

Nader, L. 1972. "Up the Anthropologist: Perspectives Gained from Studying Up." In *Reinventing Anthropology*, edited by Dell Hymes, 284–311. New York: Pantheon Books.

Nagpaul, D. R. 1967. "District Tuberculosis Control Programme in Concept and Outline." *India Journal of Tuberculosis* 14 (4): 186–198.

———. 1975. "A Tuberculosis Programme for Big Cities." *Indian Journal of Tuberculosis* 22 (3): 96–103.

Nagpaul, D. R., N. Naganathan, and M. Prakash. 1979. "Some Aspects of Sputum Examination in Tuberculosis Case-Finding." *Indian Journal of Tuberculosis* 26 (1): 11–16.

Narain, R., S. S. Nair, K. Naganna, P. Chandrasekhar, G. Ramanatha Rao, and P. Lal. 1968. "Problems of Defining a "Case" of Pulmonary Tuberculosis in Prevalence Surveys." *Bulletin of the World Health Organization* 39 (5): 701–729.

National Tuberculosis and Leprosy Control Unit. 1987. *Manual of the National Tuberculosis/Leprosy Programme in Tanzania for the District Tuberculosis/Leprosy Coordinators*. 2nd ed. Dar-es-Salaam: Ministry of Health.

Nguyen, V.-K. 2009. "Government-by-Exception: Enrolment and Experimentality in Mass HIV Treatment Programmes in Africa." *Social Theory and Health* 7 (3): 196–217.

———. 2010. *The Republic of Therapy: Triage and Sovereignty in West Africa's Time of AIDS*. Durham, NC: Duke University Press.

Nichter, M., and N. Vuckovic. 1994. "Agenda for an Anthropology of Pharmaceutical Practice." *Social Science and Medicine* 39 (11): 1509–1525.

Nichter, M. M., ed. 1996. *Anthropology and International Health: Asian Case Studies*. London: Routledge.

Novartis. 2010. "Coartem in Africa. Gaining Momentum on the Ground." Accessed July 1, 2020, https://www.novartis.com/our-company/corporate-responsibility.

Oakley, P. 1989. *Community Involvement in Health Development: An Examination of the Critical Issues*. Geneva: World Health Organization.

Ogden, J., G. Walt, and L. Lush. 2003. "The Politics of 'Branding' in Policy Transfer: The Case of DOTS for Tuberculosis Control." *Social Science and Medicine* 57 (1): 179–188.

Oman News Agency. 2015. "Steps Taken to Cut Govt Expenses: H E Balushi." *Muscat Daily*, December 29, 2015. https://www.menafn.com/qn_news_story_s.aspx?storyid=1094506380&title=Oman-Steps-taken-to-cut-govt-expenses-H-E-Balushi&src=RSS.

———. 2016. "28% Fall in Oman's Exports." *Muscat Daily*, June 11. Accessed July 11, 2016. http://www.muscatdaily.com/Archive/Oman/28-fall-in-Oman-s-exports-4uvk.

Ong, A., and S. J. Collier. 2005. "Global Assemblages, Anthropological Problems." In *Global Assemblages. Technology, Politics and Ethics as Anthropological Problems*, edited by A. Ong and S. J. Collier. Malden, MA: Blackwell.

Packard, R. M. 2016. *A History of Global Health: Interventions into the Lives of Other Peoples*. Baltimore: Johns Hopkins University Press.

Parker, M., and T. Allen. 2014. "De-politicizing Parasites: Reflections on Attempts to Control the Control of Neglected Tropical Diseases." *Medical Anthropology* 33 (3): 223–239.

Patel, V., S. Saxena, C. Lund, G. Thornicroft, F. Baingana, P. Bolton, D. Chisholm, P. Y. Collins, J. L. Cooper, J. Eaton, H. Herrman, M. M. Herzallah, Y. Huang, M.J.D. Jordans, A. Kleinman, M. E. Medina-Mora, E. Morgan, U. Niaz, O. Omigbodun, M. Prince, A. Rahman, B. Saraceno, B. K. Sarkar, M. De Silva, I. Singh, D. J. Stein, C. Sunkel, and J. UnUtzer. 2018. "The Lancet Commission on Global Mental Health and Sustainable Development." *The Lancet* 392 (10157): 1553–1598.

Patel, V., G. Simon, N. Chowdhary, S. Kaaya, and R. Araya. 2009. "Packages of Care for Depression in Low- and Middle-Income Countries." *PLoS Medicine* 6 (10): e1000159 –e1000159.

Patel, V., and G. Thornicroft. 2009. "Packages of Care for Mental, Neurological and Substance Use Disorders in Low- and Middle-Income Countries." *PLoS Medicine* 6 (10): e100160.

Perkins, M. 2000. "New Diagnostic Tools for Tuberculosis." *International Journal of Tuberculosis and Lung Disease* 4 (12): S182–184.

Pestre, D. 2003. *Science, argent et politique. Un essai d'interprétation, Sciences en questions*. Paris: Editions Quae.

Peterson, K. 2014. *Speculative Markets: Drug Circuits and Derivative Life in Nigeria*. Durham, NC: Duke University Press.

Petryna, A. 2009. *When Experiments Travel: Clinical Trials and the Global Search for Human Subjects*. Princeton, NJ: Princeton University Press.

Petryna, A., and A. Kleinman. 2006. "The Pharmaceutical Nexus." In *Global Pharmaceuticals: Ethics, Markets, and Practices*, edited by A. Petryna, A. Kleinman, and A. Lakoff. Durham, NC: Duke University Press.

Petryna, A., A. Kleinman, and A. Lakoff, eds. 2006. *Global Pharmaceuticals: Ethics, Markets, and Practices.* Durham, NC: Duke University Press.

Pfeiffer, J. 2013. "The Struggle for a Public Sector: PEPFAR in Mozambique." In *When People Come First: Critical Studies in Global Health,* edited by Joao Biehl and Adriana Petryna, 166–181. Princeton, NJ: Princeton University Press.

Pfeiffer, J., and R. Chapman. 2010. "Anthropological Perspectives on Structural Adjustment and Public Health." *Annual Review of Anthropology* 39:149–165.

Pinto, S. 2014. *Daughters of Parvati: Women and Madness in Contemporary India.* Philadelphia: University of Pennsylvania Press.

Pordié, L. 2008. "Tibetan Medicine Today. Neo-Traditionalism as an Analytical Lens and a Political Tool." In *Tibetan Medicine in the Contemporary World: Global Politics of Medical Knowledge and Practice,* edited by Laurent Pordié. London: Routledge.

———. 2011. "Se démarquer dans l'industrie du bien-être. Transnationalisme, innovation et indianité." *Anthropologie et Santé* 3.

———. 2015. "Hangover Free! The Social and Material Trajectories of PartSmart." *Anthropology and Medicine* 22 (1): 34–48.

Pordié, L., and J.-P. Gaudillière. 2014a. "Introduction: Industrial Ayurveda." *Asian Medicine* 9 (1–2): 1–11.

———. 2014b. "The Reformulation Regime in Drug Discovery: Revisiting Poly-Herbals and Property Rights in the Ayurvedic Industry." *East Asian Science Technology and Society* 8:57–79.

Porter, T. M. 1996. *Trust in Numbers: The Pursuit of Objectivity in Science and Public Life.* Princeton, NJ: Princeton University Press.

Pourraz, J. 2019. "Réguler et produire les médicaments contre le paludisme au Bénin et au Ghana: une affaire d'Etat? Politiques pharmaceutiques, normes de qualité et marchés de médicaments," PhD thesis, Sociology, EHESS, Paris.

Power, M. 1997. *The Audit Society: Rituals of Verification.* Oxford: Oxford University Press.

Quet, M. 2017. "Values in Motion: Anti-Counterfeiting Measures and the Securitization of Pharmaceutical Flows." *Journal of Cultural Economy* 10 (2): 150–162.

Quet, M., L. Pordié, A. Bochaton, S. Chantavanich, N. Kiatying-Angsulee, M. Lamy, and P. Vungsiriphisal. 2018. "Regulation Multiple: Pharmaceutical Trajectories and Modes of Control in the ASEAN." *Science Technology and Society* 23 (3): 485–503.

Quirke, V. 2008. *Collaboration in the Pharmaceutical Industry: Changing Relationships in Britain and France, 1935–1965.* London: Routledge.

Radhika, P., P. Murthy, and S. Jain. 2015. *Mindscape and Landscape: An Illustrated History of NIMHANS.* Bangalore: National Institute of Mental Health and Neuroscience.

Radhika, P., P. Murthy, A. Sarin, and S. Jain. 2015. "Psychological Symptoms and Medical Responses in Nineteenth-Century India." *History of Psychiatry* 26 (1): 88–97.

Rajab, A., Q. Al Salmi, J. Jaffer, A. J. Mohammed, and M. A. Patton. 2014. "Congenital and Genetic Disorders in the Sultanate of Oman: First Attempt to Assess Healthcare Needs." *Journal of Community Genetics* 5 (3): 283–289.

Rajab, A., and M. A. Patton. 1997. "Major Factors Determining the Frequencies of Hemoglobinopathies in Oman." *American Journal of Medical Genetics* 71 (2): 240–242.

———. 1999. "Development and Use of a National Haemoglobinopathy Register in Oman." *Community Genetics* 2 (1): 47–48.

Rao, M. 2004. *From Population Control to Reproductive Health: Malthusian Arithmetic.* New Delhi: Sage.

Raviglione, M., D. Snider, and A. Kochi. 1995. "Global Epidemiology of Tuberculosis." *Journal of the American Medical Association* 273 (3): 220–226.

Ravindran, S. 2011. "Public-Private Partnerships in Maternal Health Services." *Economic and Political Weekly* 46 (48): 43–52.

Redfield, P. 2008. "Vital Mobility and the Humanitarian Kit." In *Biosecurity Interventions: Global Health and Security in Question*, edited by Andrew Lakoff and Stephen J. Collier, 147–171. New York: Columbia University Press.

———. 2013. *Life in Crisis: The Ethical Journey of Doctors Without Borders*. Berkeley: University of California Press.

Rees, T. 2010. "Being Neurologically Human Today: Life and Science and Adult Cerebral Plasticity (an Ethical Analysis)." *American Ethnologist* 37 (1): 150–166.

———. 2014. "Humanity/Plan; or, On the "Stateless" Today (Also Being an Anthropology of Global Health)." *Cultural Anthropology* 29 (3): 457–478.

Reid-Henry, S. 2010. *The Cuban Cure: Reason and Resistance in Global Science*. Chicago: University of Chicago Press.

Reubi, D. 2018. "Epidemiological Accountability: Philanthropists, Global Health and the Audit of Saving Lives." *Economy and Society* 47 (1): 83–110.

Reuters. 2016. "Oman to Cut Budget Deficit 27 Pct This Year, Minister Says," January 1, 2016. http://www.reuters.com/article/oman-budget-idUSL8N14L0G920160101.

Revel, J., ed. 1996. *Jeux d'échelle. La micro-analyse à l'expérience*. Paris: Seuil, Gallimard, EHESS.

Rheinberger, H.-J. 1997. *Toward a History of Epistemic Things: Synthesizing Proteins in the Test Tube*. Stanford, CA: Stanford University Press.

Rifkin, S. B. 1990. *Community Participation in Maternal and Child Health/Family Planning Programmes: An Analysis Based on Case Study Materials*. Geneva: World Health Organization.

Rifkin, S. B., F. Muller, and W. Bichmann. 1988. "Primary Health Care: On Measuring Participation." *Social Science and Medicine* 26 (9): 931–940.

Roberts, E., and N. Scheper-Hughes. 2011. "Medical Migrations." *Body and Society* 17 (2–3): 1–30.

Robins, S. 2004. "'Long Live Zackie, Long Live': AIDS Activism, Science and Citizenship after Apartheid." *Journal of Southern African Studies* 30 (3):651–672.

Robinson, W. 1998. "Beyond Nation-State Paradigms: Globalization, Sociology, and the Challenge of Transnational Studies." *Sociological Forum* 13 (4): 561–595.

Rosenberg, T. 2019. "Busting the Myth That Depression Doesn't Affect People in Poor Countries." *The Guardian*, April 30, 2019.

Rottenburg, R., S. E. Merry, S.-J. Park, and J. Mugler, eds. 2015. *The World of Indicators: The Making of Governmental Knowledge through Quantification*. Cambridge: Cambridge University Press.

Rouillon, A. 1991. "The Mutual Assistance Programme of the IUATLD: Development, Contribution and Significance." *Bulletin of the International Union Against Tuberculosis and Lung Diseases* 66 (4): 159–172.

Roychowdhury, V. 2019. "Making Data Drive Health Coverage." *Express Healthcare*, January 15. https://www.expresshealthcare.in/blogs/editors-blog/making-data-drive-health-coverage/406789

Ruault, L. C. Beaudevin, and J.-P. Gaudillière. 2020. "The genes of others. WHO, the invention and globalization of community genetics (1960s–2010s)." Cermes3 seminar series. Paris: January 30.

Rudan, I., and K. Y. Chan. 2015. "Global Health Metrics Needs Collaboration and Competition." *The Lancet* 385 (9963): 92–94.

Ruger, J. P. 2005. "The Changing Role of the World Bank in Global Health." *American Journal of Public Health* 95 (1): 60–70.

Sahlins, M. 1981. *Historical Metaphors and Mythical Realities: Structure in the Early History of the Sandwich Islands Kingdom.* Ann Arbor: University of Michigan Press.

Sarin, A., and S. Jain. 2013. "The 300 Ramayanas and the District Mental Health Programme." *Economic and Political Weekly* 43 (25): 77–81.

Sarin, R., and L.B.S. Dey. 1995. "Indian National Tuberculosis Programme: Revised Strategy." *Indian Journal of Tuberculosis* 42 (1): 95–100.

Sax, W., and C. Lang. 2020. *The Movement for Global Mental Health: Critical Views from South and Southeast Asia.* Amsterdam: Amsterdam University Press.

Sayers, J. 2001. "The World Health Report 2001: Mental Health—New Understanding, New Hope." *Bulletin of the World Health Organization* 79 (11): 1085.

Schnippel, K., S. Rosen, K. Shearer, N. Martinson, L. Long, I. Sanne, and E. Variava. 2013. "Costs of Inpatient Treatment for Multi-Drug-Resistant Tuberculosis in South Africa." *Tropical Medicine & International Health* 18 (1): 109–116.

Schutz, C., G. Meintjes, F. Almajid, R. J. Wilkinson, and A. Pozniak. 2010. "Clinical Management of Tuberculosis and HIV-1 Co-Infection." *European Respiratory Journal* 36 (6): 1460–1481.

Second East African/British Medical Research Council Kenya Tuberculosis Survey. 1978. "Tuberculosis in Kenya: A Second National Sampling Survey of Drug Resistance and Other Factors, and a Comparison with the Prevalence Data from the First National Sampling Survey—An East African and British Medical Research Council Co-operative Investigation." *Tubercle* 59 (3): 155–177.

Secretaría de Salud. 2001. *Programa Nacional de Salud 2001–2006: La democratización de la salud en México: hacia un sistema universal de salud.* Mexico City: Secretaría de Salud.

Sen, A. 1998. "The Concept of Development." In *Handbook of Development Economics,* edited by H. Chenery and T. N. Srinivasan. Amsterdam: Elsevier Science Publishers, 10–26.

Shapin, S., and S. Schaffer. 1985. *Leviathan and the Air-Pump: Hobbes, Boyle, and the Experimental Life.* Princeton, NJ.: Princeton University Press.

Sharan, P., A. Mahapatra, D. Das, and A. Sarin. Forthcoming. "Evolution of Community Epidemiological Studies in India: A Subaltern Critique." In *Reimagining Psychiatric Epidemiology in a Global Frame: Towards a Social and Conceptual History,* edited by Anne M. Lovell and Gerald Oppenheimer, Rochester, NY: University of Rochester Press.

Sharma, A. 2008. *Logics of Empowerment: Development, Gender and Governance in Neoliberal India.* Minneapolis: Minnesota University Press.

Shen, X. S., Q. Su, Z. P. Qiu, J. Y. Xu, Y. X. Xie, H. F. Liu, and Y. Liu. 2010. "Effects of artemisinin derivative on the growth metabolism of Tetrahymena thermophila BF5 based on expression of thermokinetics." *Biological Trace Elements Research* 136 (1):117–125.

Shore, C., and S. Wright. 2000. "Coercive Accountability. The Rise of Audit Culture in Higher Education." In *Audit Cultures: Anthropological Studies in Accountability, Ethics, and the Academy,* edited by Marilyn Strathern, 57–89. Oxford: Routledge.

SIGMA Type 2 Diabetes Consortium. 2014. "Sequence Variants in SLC16A11 Are a Common Risk Factor for Type 2 Diabetes in Mexico." *Nature* 506 (7486): 97–101.

Silva-Zolezzi, I., A. Hidalgo-Miranda, J. Estrada-Gil, J. C. Fernández-López, L. Uribe-Figueroa, A. Contreras, E. Balam-Ortiz, L. del Bosque-Plata, D. Velázquez-Fernández, C. Lara, R. Goya, E. Hernández-Lemus, C. Dávila, E. Barrientos, S. March, and G. Jiménez-Sánchez. 2009. "Analysis of Genomic Diversity in Mexican Mestizo Populations to Develop Genomic Medicine in Mexico." *PNAS* 106 (21): 8611–8616.

Smith, J. N. 2015. *Epic Measures: One Doctor, Seven Billion Patients.* New York City: Harper Wave.

Staples, A.L.S. 2006. *The Birth of Development: How the World Bank, Food and Agriculture Organization, and World Health Organization Changed the World, 1945–1965*. Kent, OH: Kent State University Press.

Stoler, A. L. 2009. *Along the Archival Grain: Epistemic Anxieties and Colonial Common Sense*. Princeton, NJ: Princeton University Press.

Strathern, M. 2000. "Introduction: New Accountabilities." In *Audit Cultures: Anthropological Studies in Accountability, Ethics, and the Academy*, edited by Marilyn Strathern, 1–18. Oxford: Routledge.

Street, A. 2012. "Affective Infrastructure Hospital Landscapes of Hope and Failure." *Space and Culture* 15 (1): 44–56.

———. 2014. *Biomedicine in an Unstable Place: Infrastructure and Personhood in a Papua New Guinean Hospital*. Experimental Futures. Durham, NC: Duke University Press.

Sudre, P., G. Ten Dam, and A. Kochi. 1992. "Tuberculosis: A Global Overview of the Situation Today." *Bulletin of the World Health Organization* 70 (2): 149.

Sullivan, N. 2011. "Mediating Abundance and Scarcity: Implementing an HIV/AIDS-Targeted Project within a Government Hospital in Tanzania." *Medical Anthropology* 30 (2): 202–221.

———. 2017. "Multiple Accountabilities: Development Cooperation, Transparency, and the Politics of Unknowing in Tanzania's Health Sector." *Critical Public Health* 27 (2): 193–204.

Sunder Rajan, K. 2006. *Biocapital: The Constitution of Postgenomic Life*. Durham, NC: Duke University Press.

———. 2017. *Pharmocracy: Value, Politics and Knowledge in Global Biomedicine*. Durham, NC: Duke University Press.

Swai, O. B., E. A. Edwards, R. Thiong'o, J. H. Darbyshire, R. Stephens, D. A. Mitchison, M. Kinyanjui, W. Fox, and M. Caplin. 1989. "Tuberculosis in Kenya 1984: A Third National Survey and a Comparison with Earlier Surveys in 1964 and 1974—A Kenyan/British Medical Research Council Co-operative Investigation." *Tubercle* 70 (1): 5–20.

Tarimo, E., E. G. Webster, and World Health Organization. 1994. *Primary Health Care Concepts and Challenges in a Changing World: Alma-Ata Revisited*. Geneva: World Health Organization.

Taylor, M., and I. Harper. 2014. "The Politics and Anti-Politics of the Global Fund Experiment: Understanding Partnership and Bureaucratic Expansion in Uganda." *Medical Anthropology* 33 (3): 206–222.

Taylor-Alexander, S., and E. Schwartz-Marín. 2013. "Bioprophecy and the Politics of the Present: Notes on the Establishment of Mexico's National Genomics Institute (INMEGEN)." *New Genetics and Society* 32 (4): 333–349.

Theron, G., L. Zijenah, D. Chanda, P Clowes, A. Rachow, M. Lesosky, W. Bara, S. Mungofa, M. Pai, M. Hoelscher, D. Dowdy, A. Pym, P. Mwaba, P. Mason, J. Peter, K. Dheda and the TB-NEAT team. 2014. "Feasibility, Accuracy, and Clinical Effect of Point-of-Care Xpert MTB/RIF Testing for Tuberculosis in Primary-Care Settings in Africa: A Multicentre Randomised, Controlled Trial." *The Lancet* 383 (9915): 424–435.

Thornicroft, G., T. Deb, and C. Henderson. 2016. "Community Mental Health Care Worldwide: Current Status and Further Developments." *World Psychiatry* 15 (3): 276–286.

Thornicroft, G., and M. Tansella. 2004. "Components of a Modern Mental Health Service: A Pragmatic Balance of Community and Hospital Care: Overview of Systematic Evidence." *British Journal of Psychiatry* 185:283–290.

Tibandebage, P., S. Wangwe, M. Mackintosh, and P.G.M. Mujinja. 2016. "Pharmaceutical Manufacturing Decline in Tanzania: How Possible Is a Turnaround to Growth?" In *The*

Political Economy of Industrializing for Local Health, edited by M. Mackintosh, G. Banda, P. Tibandebage, and W. Wamae, 45–64. London: Palgrave.

Tichenor, M. 2016. "The Power of Data: Global Malaria Governance and the Senegalese Data Retention Strike." In *Metrics: What Counts in Global Health*, edited by Vincanne Adams, 105–124. Durham, NC: Duke University Press.

Tobell, D. 2011. *Pills, Power and Policy: The Struggle for Drug Reform in Cold War America and Its Consequences*. Berkeley: University of California Press.

Towghi, F., and K. Vora. 2014. "Bodies, Markets, and the Experimental in South Asia." *Ethnos* 79 (1): 1–18.

Tsing, A. 2005. *Friction: An Ethnography of Global Connection*. Princeton, NJ: Princeton University Press.

Udwadia, Z. F., R. A. Amale, K. K. Ajbani, and C. Rodrigues. 2012. "Totally Drug-Resistant Tuberculosis in India." *Clinical Infectious Disease* 54 (4): 579–581.

Valeri, M. 2007. *Le Sultanat d'Oman: Une Révolution en trompe-l'oeil*. Paris: Karthala.

———. 2018. *Oman: Politics and Society in the Qaboos State*. 2nd ed. London: Hurst/ Columbia University Press.

van der Geest, S. 2011. "The Urgency of Pharmaceutical Anthropology: A Multilevel Perspective." *CURARE* 34 (1/2): 9–15.

van der Geest, S., S. Reynolds Whyte, and A. Hardon. 1996. "The Anthropology of Pharmaceuticals: A Biographical Approach." *Annual Review of Anthropology* 25 (1): 153–178.

van Ginneken, N., S. Jain, V. Patel, and V. Berridge. 2014. "The Development of Mental Health Services within Primary Care in India: Learning from Oral History." *International Journal of Mental Health Systems* 8:30.

Varma, S. 2016. "Disappearing the Asylum: Modernizing Psychiatry and Generating Manpower in India." *Transcultural Psychiatry* 53 (6): 783–803.

Villarreal-Molina, M. T., M. T. Flores-Dorantes, O. Arellano-Campos, M. Villalobos-Comparan, M. Rodríguez-Cruz, A. Miliar-García, A. Huertas-Vazquez, M. Menjivar, S. Romero-Hidalgo, N. H. Wacher, M. T. Tusie-Luna, M. Cruz, C. A. Aguilar-Salinas, and S. Canizales-Quinteros. 2008. "Metabolic Study Group. Association of the ATP-binding Cassette Transporter A1 R230C Variant with Early-onset Type 2 Diabetes in a Mexican Population." *Diabetes* 57 (2): 509–513.

von Mises, L. 1944. *Bureaucracy*. New Haven, CT: Yale University Press.

Wade, P. 2017. *Degrees of Mixture, Degrees of Freedom: Genomics, Multiculturalism, and Race in Latin America*. Durham, NC: Duke University Press.

Walsh, J. A., and K. S. Warren. 1979. "Selective Primary Health Care: An Interim Strategy for Disease Control in Developing Countries." *New England Journal of Medicine* 301:967–974.

Wang, P. S., O. Demler, and R. C. Kessler. 2002. "Adequacy of Treatment for Serious Mental Illness in the United States." *American Journal of Public Health* 92 (1): 92–98.

Wang, S. 2019. "Les nouvelles circulations de la médecine chinoise: après l'Afrique, l'Europe." *Mouvements* 98:133–141.

Watkins, E. 2007. *The Estrogen Elixir: A History of Hormone Replacement Therapy in America*. Baltimore: Johns Hopkins University Press.

Watson, J. L., ed. 2006. *Golden Arches East: McDonald's in East Asia*. Stanford, CA: Stanford University Press.

Weisz, G., A. Cambrosio, and J.-P. Cointet. 2017. "Mapping Global Health: A Network Analysis of a Heterogenous Publication Domain." *Biosocieties* 12 (4): 520–542.

Weisz, G. T., and N. Tousignant. 2019. "International Health Research and the Emergence of Global Health in the Late Twentieth Century" *Bulletin of the History of Medicine* 93 (3): 365–400.

Wendland, C. L. 2012. "Moral Maps and Medical Imaginaries: Clinical Tourism at Malawi's College of Medicine." *American Anthropologist* 114 (1): 108–122.

Wharton Business School. 2014. "World Health Partners: Leveraging Entrepreneurship for Health Care Delivery." *Knowledge@Wharton*, January 24. https://knowledge.wharton.upenn.edu/article/world-health-partners-leveraging-entrepreneurship-health-care-delivery/.

White, J. M., B. S. Christie, D. Nam, S. Daar, and D. S. Higgs. 1993. "Frequency and Clinical Significance of Erythrocyte Genetic Abnormalities in Omanis." *Journal of Medical Genetics* 30:396–400.

Whitfield, L., and E. Jones. 2007. "Ghana: The Political Dimensions of Aid Dependance." Centre for International Studies, Global Economic Governance Program (GEG) Working Paper No. 2007/32, University of Oxford.

Whyte, S. R., S. van der Geest, and A. Hardon. 2002. *Social Lives of Medicines*. Cambridge: Cambridge University Press.

Williamson, B. 2001. "Our Human Genome—How Can It Serve Us Well?" *Bulletin of the World Health Organization* 79 (11): 1005.

World Bank. 1993. *World Development Report: Investing in Health*. New York: Oxford University Press.

World Health Organization. 1964. *WHO Expert Committee on Tuberculosis, Eighth Report*. Technical Report Series 290. Geneva: World Health Organization.

———. 1971. "Admission of New Members: Sultanate of Oman." World Health Assembly WHA24.21, May 13. http://www.who.int/iris/handle/10665/91865.

———. 1975. *Organization of Mental Health Services in Developing Countries*. Technical Report Series. Geneva: World Health Organization.

———. 1977. *The Selection of Essential Drugs*. Technical Report Series. Geneva: World Health Organization.

———. 1978a. *Primary Health Care: Report of the International Conference on Primary Health Care, Alma Ata, USSR, 6–12 September 1978*. Geneva: World Health Organization.

———. 1978b. *The Promotion and Development of Traditional Medicine: A Report of a WHO Meeting*. Geneva: World Health Organization.

———. 1980. *Executive Board, Sixty-Fifth Session, Geneva, 9–25 January 1980: Summary Records*. Geneva: World Health Organization. https://apps.who.int/iris/handle/10665/154448.

———. 1991. *Community Involvement in Health Development: Challenging Health Services. Report of a WHO Study Group*. Technical Report Series 809. Geneva: World Health Organization. https://apps.who.int/iris/handle/10665/40624.

———. 1999. *Services for the Prevention and Management of Genetic Disorders and Birth Defects in Developing Countries*. Geneva: World Health Organization. https://apps.who.int/iris/handle/10665/66501.

———. 2000. "Annex Table 10 Health System Performance in All Member States, WHO Indexes, Estimates for 1997." In *World Health Report 2000*. Geneva: World Health Organization. https://www.who.int/whr/2000/en/annex10_en.pdf?ua=1.

———. 2001. "Antimalarial Drug Combination Therapy: Report of a WHO Technical Consultation." WHO/Global Partnership to Roll Back Malaria. https://apps.who.int/iris/handle/10665/66952.

———. 2002. *Traditional Medicine Growing Needs and Potential: WHO Policy Perspectives on Medicines*. Geneva: World Health Organization.

———. 2005a. *Control of Genetic Diseases: Report of the Secretariat*. Geneva: World Health Organization, Executive Board. https://apps.who.int/iris/bitstream/handle/10665/20404/B116_3-en.pdf.

———. 2005b. *Global Atlas of Traditional, Complementary and Alternative Medicine.* Geneva: World Health Organization, Centre for Health Development.

———. 2006. *Medical Genetic Services in Developing Countries: The Ethical, Legal and Social Implications of Genetic Testing and Screening.* Geneva: World Health Organization. http://www.who.int/genomics/publications/GTS-MedicalGeneticServices-octo6.pdf.

———. 2008a. "Primary Health Care in Action—Country Examples: Oman." In *World Health Report 2008.* Accessed March 27, 2018. https://www.who.int/whr/2008/media _centre/oman.pdf.

———. 2008b. *The World Health Report 2008: Primary Health Care (Now More than Ever).* Geneva: World Health Organization.

———. 2010a. *Good Procurement Practices for Artemisinin-based Antimalarial Medicines.* Geneva: World Health Organization.

———. 2010b. *mhGAP Intervention Guide for Mental, Neurological and Substance Use Disorders in Non-Specialized Health Settings.* Geneva: World Health Organization. https:// apps.who.int/iris/handle/10665/259161.

———. 2011. *Automated Real-Time Nucleic Acid Amplification Technology for Rapid and Simultaneous Detection of Tuberculosis and Rifampicin Resistance: Xpert MTB/RIF System: Policy Statement.* Geneva: World Health Organization.

———. 2013. *Investing in Mental Health: Evidence for Action.* Geneva: World Health Organization.

———. 2014. *Companion Handbook to the WHO Guidelines for the Programmatic Management of Drug-Resistant Tuberculosis: Models for Delivering MDR-TB Treatment and Care.* Geneva: World Health Organization.

———. 2018a. *The Transformative Role of Hospitals in the Future of Primary Health Care.* Technical Series on Primary Healthcare. Geneva: World Health Organization. https:// apps.who.int/iris/handle/10665/326296.

———. 2018b. *World Malaria Report 2018.* Geneva: World Health Organization. https:// apps.who.int/iris/handle/10665/275867.

———. 2019. *mhGAP Community Toolkit: Mental Health Gap Action Program.* Geneva: World Health Organization. https://apps.who.int/iris/handle/10665/328742.

World Health Organization, and World Family Doctors Caring for People. 2008. *Integrating Mental Health into Primary Health Care: A Global Perspective.* Geneva: World Health Organization. https://apps.who.int/iris/handle/10665/43935.

World Health Organization Global Tuberculosis Programme. 1994. "TB: A Global Emergency, WHO Report on the TB Epidemic." WHO/TB/94.177. https://apps.who.int/iris/handle /10665/58749.

World Health Organization, PEPFAR, and UNAIDS. 2008. *Task Shifting: Rational Redistribution of Tasks among Health Workforce Teams: Global Recommendations and Guidelines.* Geneva: World Health Organization. https://apps.who.int/iris/handle/10665 /43821.

World Health Partners. n.d. "WHP Bihar Program: Engaging Private Providers to Improve Management of Infectious Disease on a Large Scale." https://www.globalgiving.org/pfil /10277/projdoc.pdf.

Wylie, S. A. 2018. *Fractivism: Corporate Bodies and Chemical Bonds.* Durham, NC: Duke University Press.

Yamey, G. 2002. "Have the Latest Reforms Reversed WHO's Decline?" *British Medical Journal* 325 (7372): 1102–1112.

Yazbeck, A. S. 2002. "An Idiot's Guide to Prioritization in the Health Sector," World Bank Health, Nutrition, and Population (HNP) Discussion Paper. https://documents.worldbank

.org/en/publication/documents-reports/documentdetail/850011468013195446/an-idiots
-guide-to-prioritization-in-the-health-sector.

Yu, H., and S. Zhong. 2002. "Artemisia Species in Traditional Chinese Medicine and the
Discovery of Artemisinin." In *Artemisia: Medicinal and Aromatic Plants—Industrial
Profiles*, edited by C. W. Wright, 119–126. London: Taylor and Francis.

Zanini, G., R. Raffaetà, K. Krause, and G. Alex. 2013. "Transnational Medical Spaces:
Opportunities and Restrictions." *MMG Working Paper* (13–16): 1–35.

Notes on Contributors

SAMEEA AHMED HASSIM is a political scientist affiliated with the Center for Research on Medicine, Science, Health, Mental Health, and Society (Cermes3), Paris.

CLAIRE BEAUDEVIN is a medical anthropologist and researcher at the National Center for Scientific Research (CNRS) assigned to Cermes3 in Paris. Her work focuses on medical genetics and genomics as they entangle with global health and universal health care in Oman, with cancer in France, and with primary health care at the WHO.

FANNY CHABROL is a sociologist of medicine and health policies in sub-Saharan Africa at the French National Research Institute for Sustainable Development, Paris.

OLIVIA FIORILLI is a historian of medicine affiliated with Cermes3, Paris.

JEAN-PAUL GAUDILLIÈRE is a senior researcher at the National Institute of Health and Medical Research (INSERM), assigned to Cermes3 Paris. A historian of science, his research explores the twentieth-century life sciences and medicine, including pharmaceutical innovation and health globalization. He coordinated the European Research Council project "From International to Global: Knowledge, Diseases, and the Postwar Government of Health."

MANDY GEISE is an anthropologist and holds a PhD from the École des Hautes Études en Sciences Sociales, Paris.

CHRISTOPH GRADMANN is a historian of medicine in Europe and Africa, specializing in the history of infectious disease. He is professor of the history of medicine at the department for community medicine and global health at the University of Oslo.

CLAUDIA LANG is an associate professor (Heisenberg) of anthropology at the University of Leipzig and affiliate researcher at the Max Planck Institute for Social

Anthropology, Halle, Germany. Her research focuses on transformation processes in mental health in South Asia. She is the author of three books, including *Depression in Kerala: Ayurveda and Mental Health Care in 21st Century India.*

ANNE M. LOVELL, a medical anthropologist, works on the anthropology of disaster and on mental health in West Africa. She is senior research scientist emeritus at INSERM, assigned to Cermes3 (Paris).

ANDREW MCDOWELL is an assistant professor of anthropology at Tulane University in New Orleans, Louisiana. A cultural and medical anthropologist, his research focuses on lived experiences of tuberculosis in South Asia.

CAROLINE MEIER ZU BIESEN is a sociologist and medical anthropologist working on the Indian Ocean region and a postdoctoral fellow at the University of Leipzig's Lab Global Health.

LAURENT PORDIÉ is an anthropologist and research scientist at the National Center for Scientific Research (CNRS) assigned to Cermes3, Paris.

JESSICA POURRAZ is a sociologist and a postdoctoral research fellow with IFRIS (Institute for Research and Innovation in Society) in the research unit CEPED (IRD-Paris Descartes), Paris. Her research interests focus on issues related to science, biomedicine, the environment, and health in the Global South.

LUCILE RUAULT is a feminist socio-historian of reproductive sciences and genetics and research scientist at the National Center for Scientific Research (CNRS) at Cermes3, Paris.

VEGARD TRAAVIK STURE is a graduate student at École des Hautes Études en Sciences Sociales, Paris.

SIMENG WANG is a sociologist working on subjects at the intersection of Chinese migration in France and health/mental health and a research scientist at the National Center for Scientific Research (CNRS) assigned to Cermes3, Paris.

Index

accountability, 22, 55, 56, 58–59, 66, 171, 195. *See also* audit culture

ACTs (Artemisinin Combination Therapy), 107–113, 119

Affordable Medicines Facility-malaria (AMF-m) program (Ghana), 112–113

Africa-China relations, 192–194

African Ayurveda market, 188–191. *See also* Ayurveda

AIIMH (All India Institute of Mental Health), 164–165. *See also* NIMHANS (National Institute of Mental Health and Neuroscience)

Akrich, Madeleine, 138

Algeria, 192

All India Institute of Mental Health (AIIMH), 164–165. *See also* NIMHANS (National Institute of Mental Health and Neuroscience)

Alma-Ata conference. *See* International Conference on Primary Health Care (1978)

Alma-Ata Declaration (1978), 46–47, 82, 148, 150, 189

Alwan, Ala, 187

AMF-m (Affordable Medicines Facility-malaria) program (Ghana), 112–113

Angastiniotis, Michael, 33–34

antibiotics: introduction to, 158; resistance to, 127; use in Cambodia, 119; use in India, 103, 104; use with TB, 132, 160, 173

Antimension Combination Therapy (ACTs), 107–113, 119

antiretroviral treatments (ARVs), 79, 104

apps for mental health care, 168

arenas, 12–15, 145–146, 169, 197–199. *See also* circulations

artemether, 109, 209n5

artemisinin, 107–113, 119, 183

artesunate-amodiaquine, 209n5

ARVs (antiretroviral treatments), 79, 104

ASEAN, 120, 122

Ashwasam program, 98–101, 128–130

Asian medicines, 1, 2, 25, 123. *See also* Ayurveda; traditional Chinese medicine (TCM)

Association of Southeast Asian Nations (ASEAN), 120, 122

audit culture, 58–59, 62, 81, 206n3, 207n10. *See also* accountability

AVISAs. *See* DALYs (disability-adjusted life years)

Ayurveda: African Ayurveda market, 188–191; industrialization of, 113–118; Kerala Ayurveda, 53; standardization of, 19, 183; in wellness tourism, 51, 52. *See also* Asian medicines

Bacillus Calmette-Guérin (BCG) vaccination, 134, 173–174

Bamako Declaration (1987), 86–87

Bamako Initiative, 20

Bangladesh, 63

BCG (Bacillus Calmette-Guérin) vaccination, 134, 173–174

Becker, Gary, 86

bedaquiline, 157

Belt and Road Initiative (China), 192, 193, 194, 214n67

benflumentol, 109

Bihar, India, 44. *See also* India

Bill and Melinda Gates Foundation. *See* Gates Foundation

biocapitalist economies, 106

biological commensurability, 19. *See also* commensurability

Printed in the United States
by Baker & Taylor Publisher Services